Mind, Body, and Medicine

Mind,
Body,
and Medicine
An Integrative Text

Raphael N. Melmed

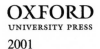
OXFORD
UNIVERSITY PRESS
2001

OXFORD
UNIVERSITY PRESS

Oxford   New York
Athens   Auckland   Bangkok   Bogotá   Buenos Aires   Calcutta
Cape Town   Chennai   Dar es Salaam   Delhi   Florence   Hong Kong   Istanbul
Karachi   Kuala Lumpur   Madrid   Melbourne   Mexico City   Mumbai
Nairobi   Paris   São Paulo   Shanghai   Singapore   Taipei   Tokyo   Toronto   Warsaw

and associated companies in
Berlin   Ibadan

Copyright © 2001 by Oxford University Press.

Published by Oxford University Press, Inc.,
198 Madison Avenue, New York, New York, 10016
http://www.oup-usa.org

Oxford is a registered trademark of Oxford University Press.

Library of Congress Cataloging-in-Publication Data
Melmed, Raphael N.
Mind, body, and medicine : an integrative text /
Ralphael N. Melmed.
p. ; cm.   Includes bibliographical references and index.
ISBN 0-19-513164-9 (cloth)
1. Medicine, Psychosomatic. 2. Mind and body.
I. Title.
[DNLM: 1. Psychophysiologic Disorders. 2.
Mental Disorders. 3. Stress, Psychological—physiopathology.
4. Stress, Psychological—therapy.
WM 90 M527m 2001]   RC49 .M444 2001   616.08—dc21   00-053023

9 8 7 6 5 4 3 2 1

Printed in the United States of America
on acid-free paper

To
Yair,
Michaela,
and Gidon,
in love
and admiration

Preface

This book deals with the psychosomatic aspects of medical practice from the vantage point of the practicing physician. This aspect of practice in the fields of internal medicine, the medical subspecialties, and primary care is widely problematic and requires serious attention in order to improve the quality of medical care in Western societies. To the best of my knowledge, there is no other book written specifically from this perspective; rather, other texts dealing with similar issues are mostly written by psychiatrists, psychologists, or sociologists for the physician.

The text integrates information in a selective way from the disciplines of internal medicine, psychiatry, social medicine, epidemiology, neuroscience, biology, and psychology. It is not intended to be exhaustive. No attempt is made to deal systematically with all conditions or states considered to be psychosomatic. The conditions and processes presented are chosen either because they are commonly encountered or because they help to illustrate important principles with general application. Certain topics, such as eating and sexual disorders, are not covered because it is my belief that they require specialized management beyond the expertise of most general physicians. In other areas, such as pain, no attempt is made to list all the known chronic or recurrent syndromes because it seems that the most important clinical principles have nearly universal application. Besides providing a theoretical basis for understanding psychosomatic states, this book, in the main, touches on aspects of patient management that are often unrecognized or largely ignored by medical practitioners. In my experience, the approach works well across a broad range of clinical problems. The therapeutic principles presented should be broadly applicable in practice.

With the role of behavioral sciences in medical education under ongoing review in many centers, I have attempted to include an important part of what I think should be taught in this field. The content is presented in a way that I hope will make the subject intelligible and relevant to anyone interested in learning more about the recognition and principles of management of psychosomatic problems in clinical practice. I have tried to present the essential elements of what we now commonly call stress management.

The content of the chapters grew out of the order that I had to create for myself from many varied and often confusing descriptions available. The process of writing for me has been an exciting one of fascination and discovery. I hope that, at least partially, the book succeeds in conveying the excitement of this understanding to the reader.

Jerusalem, Israel   R.N.M.

vii

Acknowledgments

At the beginning of my work in this field, during the phase in which I was struggling to lift myself off the floor by tugging on my own shoelaces, support from David and Catherine Shainberg and the Shainberg Family Foundation and from Shoshana and Martin Gerstel proved valuable in helping me to establish my program. Charles R. Kleeman, Professor of Medicine Emeritus at the University of California, Los Angeles, and the late Norman Cousins, by awarding me a fellowship in psychoneuroimmunology in 1987–1988 to work in the Clinical Immunology Laboratory of John Fahey at UCLA, granted me an exceptional opportunity to develop an in-depth understanding of this important field. The Feldman Family Stanford Fellowships for senior academic staff of Israeli medical schools exposed me to a valuable four-month experience in the psychophysiology laboratory of Walton T. Roth, Professor of Psychiatry and Behavioral Sciences at Stanford University. The encouragement and unstinting professional input of Patrick Wall (London); Tom Roth (Stanford); Michael Weissberg (Denver); and of Eliezer Edelstein, Lea Baider, Justin Silver, Bernard Lerer, Rami Aronson, Dina Roth, Hillel Davis, and Yisrael Steiner (all of Jerusalem) is gratefully acknowledged—though I remain solely responsible for the ideas expressed in this book. Many others offered valuable counsel or friendship. Notable among these was Daniel Kropf.

The freedom to work in an essentially new, undefined clinical field is not, I believe, something that could have happened in many comparable medical institutions of the academic world that I am familiar with. I have, therefore, a sense of gratitude to Professor Yechezkiel Stein, former head of the Department of Medicine B at the Hadassah University Hospital, who gave me the freedom and the space to choose my own path and in whose department I developed my clinical and research program in behavioral medicine, as well as to Professor Shmuel Penchas, formerly director-general of the same hospital, who by granting me a unit of behavioral medicine in internal medicine, made it clear that the institute supported my efforts.

As with all new endeavors, there is but a small nucleus of outstanding people who with courage and determination work to define the field and help establish the standards, often against very substantial practical and political difficulties. I would like to pay a special tribute to the work of Jon Kabot-Zinn of the Medical Sciences Center, University of Massachusetts, Worcester, and Herbert Benson of the New England Deaconess Hospital, Harvard Medical School, in Boston, colleagues who have made unique and historical contributions to the field of mind–body medicine and who have inspired me in various ways in my own work.

The moral support and unwavering encouragement of a number of relatives helped sustain me on what has been a long and often lonely journey. Principal among these are my brother and sister-in-law Herzl and Hazel Melmed and sister and brother-in-law Judi and Hal Bregman.

Finally, a special word of appreciation to Shirley Smith for her assistance as scientific editor, to Nili Agassi and Eilah Brand-Adel for their assistance with diagrams and illustrations, and most of all to Jeffrey W. House of Oxford University Press for his patience, persistence, and superb editorial input.

Contents

Mind, Body, and Medicine

Chapter
1

INTRODUCTION

The picture of the typical patient–doctor dynamic that has emerged from numerous studies over the last half century may be summarized as follows:

- About 70% to 90% of all bouts of illness are managed outside the established health care system (through self-care or alternative therapies such as homeopathy, chiropractic, folk medicine, or spiritual consultation).
- Of those who arrive at a primary health care clinic, over 50% have problems that cannot be classified as a formal disease entity. An estimated 25% to 75% of patients in primary care settings have psychosocial rather than biomedical reasons for their visits (Roberts and Norton, 1952; Stoeckle et al., 1964; Cummings and Vanden Bos, 1981; Kroenke and Mangelsdorff, 1989).
- Most of these patients are actually presenting a complaint different from the one they report to the doctor (Cummings and VandenBos, 1981).

Considering the enormous scientific advances over the last century, it is ironic that the established medical system in the Western world has failed to develop a style of medical practice that is sensitive to patients' feelings and needs. This failure has substantially undermined the doctor's role as a healer. Conquest of the common infective killers, as well as malnutrition, undernutrition, and many other health problems in the west has resulted in a progressive increase in life expectancy. The difficulties of old age and, for many, the psychological demands of social and economic disadvantage have brought their own burden of stress-related clinical problems. For the management of these problems, the medical profession seems poorly equipped.

It is apparent from writings in the early twentieth century that fundamental discontent of patients with the patient–physician encounter is not exclusively a latter-day phenomenon. This viewpoint was expressed by Stefan Zweig in 1931:

> Disease meant now no longer what happens to the whole man but what happens to his organs . . . And so the natural and original mission of the physician, the approach to disease as a whole changes into the smaller task of localising the ailment and identifying it and ascribing it to an already specified group of diseases . . . This unavoidable objectification and technicalization of therapy in the nineteenth century came to an extreme excess because between the physician and the patient became interpolated a third entirely mechanical thing, the apparatus. The penetrating, creative synthesising grasp of the born physician became less and less for diagnosis.

In referring to doctors in the late nineteenth century, Zweig was commenting on something that may have originated in the seventeenth century, when the English physician Thomas Sydenham began the classification and naming of diseases according to particular clinical features. This development—revolutionary in terms of its ultimate impact on medical science—began the systematic devaluation of the individually peculiar features of illness, a process that had serious consequences for medical practice. This process had the inevitable result of diminishing the value that physicians had placed on the unique meanings patients give to their experiences (Reiser, 1993).

It would seem, therefore, that alienation of the patient, which has been evolving as a trend in medical practice for 300 years, accelerated greatly during the twentieth century owing to the revolutionary advances in diagnostic methods and in the treatment of many common diseases. The growth of technology of medicine contrasted sharply with the period that Zweig refers to in the preceding extract, when the main instruments used in clinical practice were the sphygmomanometer (Hales, 1733; Poiseulle, 1828), ophthalmoscope (von Helmholz, 1851), hemoglobinometer (Gowers, 1878), and electrocardiograph (Einthoven, 1903). As the scientific basis of medicine has expanded exponentially, assuming an ever greater role in the diagnosis and treatment of disease, so the tendency Zweig calls the interposition of a "mechanical thing" between the patient and the doctor has become increasingly pronounced. The two major signs of this deepening malaise in patient–doctor interaction emerged over the course of the last century and have been expressed in part as noncompliance in drug taking as well as increasing utilization of alternative healing practices.

DISCARDING MEDICINES AND MEDICAL ADVICE

Of the patients seen by primary care physicians, regardless of their symptoms or diagnosis, more than one-third will choose not to take the medication prescribed or accept the advice given (Davis, 1966; Davis, 1968). This symptom should have alerted the medical profession to the presence of a serious problem. Most studies point to an average rate of noncompliance in the taking of medication of around 30% (Stimson, 1974), reflecting a pattern of patient behavior which has in general remained constant over many years (Legoretta et al., 1998), even when measured in relation to the treatment of serious diseases such as breast cancer (Ayres et al., 1994) or prostatic cancer (Urquhart, 1996).

With the burgeoning costs of health care, the discarding of approximately one-third of professional advice or prescribed medication must add up to an enormous waste of money when calculated in doctor-hours of consultation and quantity of medication purchased. In the commercial or industrial sector, any market product discarded *before use* by 33% of purchasers would surely be regarded as a failure by both purchaser and manufacturer. While there are probably many reasons for noncompliance by patients, the pervasiveness of the practice in the patient population points to a fundamental problem in the medical system rather than a particular problem with particular patients.

THE QUEST FOR AN ALTERNATIVE MEDICINE

The development of alternative or complementary healing practices, a trend that has also accelerated over the last three to four decades, similarly reflects patients' dissatisfaction with conventional medicine and the quest for another, more satisfactory healing system. A national household telephone survey in the United States compared trends in utilization of alternative medicine between the years 1990 and 1997 (Eisenberg et al., 1998). The use of alternative therapies increased from 34% (of 1539 adults interviewed) in 1990 to 42% (of 2055 adults interviewed) in 1997, with the biggest increase occurring in the utilization of herbal medicine, massage, megavitamins, self-help groups, folk remedies, energy healing, and homeopathy. In both surveys (i.e., in 1990 and 1997) alternative therapies were used most frequently for chronic conditions, including back problems, anxiety, depression, and headaches, although many people appear to use them for health promotion or disease prevention. Extrapolated to the U.S. population, the estimated total number of visits to alternative health practitioners, increasing from 427 million in 1990 to 629 million in 1997, would have exceeded total visits to all U.S. primary care physicians.

It is important to note that although nonscientifically based healing practices have developed into a substantial alternative health care system in scientifically

developed Western countries, patients may use them as a complement to ortho-
dox medicine rather than a replacement, much as in Asian societies such as China
and Japan (Fulder and Munro, 1985; Thomas et al., 1991; Eisenberg et al., 1993).
Such practices may have come to assume a complementary role for many, but
there is a defined subgroup of patients whose use of alternative techniques of
healing should definitely be viewed as an expression of emotional distress (Holland, 1999). In studies of patients with either breast cancer (Burstein et al., 1999)
or brain cancer (Verhoef et al., 1999), the use of alternative medical practices
appeared to be a marker of greater psychosocial distress and worse quality of
life. It would seem that while the doctor was most interested in curing the patient's disease, the patient, above all, wanted his or her illness understood and
properly managed.

DISEASE VERSUS ILLNESS

The important distinction in clinical practice between disease and illness may be
conveyed by comparing the role of the physician as perceived in the early part
of the twentieth century and today. Formerly, the physician's cures were general
in nature and of poor efficacy in a specific sense. His main influence in the therapeutic interaction was through the strength of his personality and his ability to
foster optimism and confidence in his patients and their families. The doctor focused on the patient's illness and understood little if anything of actual disease
processes. Talking about his father, who became a physician in 1905, Lewis
Thomas (1982) described medical practice then in these terms:

> During all his years in general practice he possessed only small bits of science, used
> solely for the purpose of diagnosis, and almost no science at all for therapy. What
> he did, for treating disease, was to "look after" people. This was all he, or anyone
> else, knew how to do and it had little to do with technology. Indeed, if it became
> known in the small town I grew up in that a doctor had become locally famous for
> his technical capacity to treat this or that disease, the question of medical ethics was
> automatically raised by the local establishment. Claims for being able to treat dis-
> ease were almost, not quite but almost, grounds for being charged with quackery,
> and usually the charge was warranted. In those days quackery abounded.

Thanks to scientific advances, doctors now know a great deal more about disease processes and many more have become specialists and subspecialists with
a narrow approach to medicine. Because of time pressure, communication tends
to be related to details of disease or dysfunction. A sense of unease at this trend
has helped draw attention to the important distinction between disease and illness (Eisenberg, 1977; Barondess, 1979; Jennings, 1986). The problem is by no
means merely one of semantics. Nor does it warrant being relegated, as in one
prominent medical journal, to the section on "Philosophy in Medicine" (Jennings,

1986), since it has profound practical implications for the quality of medical care. Patient management needs to be oriented toward the illness, that is, the patient's experience of disease. Thus, for example, similar degrees of organ pathology may result, in different patients, in very different accounts of pain and disorder (Beecher, 1956; Zola, 1960). Illness may occur in the absence of demonstrable disease and, as Eisenberg (1988) has pointed out, having a disease, feeling ill, and becoming a patient are not synonymous.

One of the most striking illustrations of the distinction between disease and illness is to be found in the management of chronic pain in all its forms. There is now widespread recognition of the primary role of affect in the evaluation of chronic pain, whether it be headache or migraine, facial pain including temperomandibular joint discomfort, fibromyalgia, lower back, pelvic, and abdominal pain, or phantom limb pain, to mention but a few of the chronic pain syndromes (Chapters 10 and 11). Of particular interest is the fact that studies have failed to reveal any significant psychological difference between pain patients with and without identifiable pathology, regardless of the pain's locality (Castelnuovo-Tedesco and Krout, 1970; Woodforde and Merskey, 1972; Sternbach et al., 1973; Raymer et al., 1984). These findings emphasize the key role of central neurophysiological factors in the genesis of pain in all chronic pain sufferers.

Disease and illness should not be viewed as conflicting concepts, but failure to distinguish between them could mean that the physician will overlook or underappreciate issues that may be most important in determining the natural history of a patient's condition. Physicians naturally tend to give diagnostic labels of disease categories to patients suffering from a particular constellation of symptoms. For instance, those suffering from general complaints of lassitude and easy fatigability may be diagnosed as having chronic fatigue syndrome or even postviral depression or chronic brucellosis (Chapter 15). Diagnoses have their fashion, and no doubt a substantial number of cases are overdiagnosed. In addition, however, a diagnosis may have undesirable consequences for both doctor and patient. Providing a diagnostic label may be a shortcut to bypassing the emotional aspects of the patient's problem, that is, to dealing with the patient's illness in all its aspects—leaving the patient dissatisfied and possibly even resentful. Having a diagnosis may even impair the ability to recover for those patients who feel that if they have to prove they are ill, they can't get well (Hadler, 1996).

THE QUALITY OF MEDICAL CARE: PROCESS OR OUTCOME?

As mentioned at the start of this chapter, over 60% of patients examined at primary care clinics either have no physical disorder that can be identified according to the International Classification of Diseases or are *seeking care for prob-*

lems other than those they are complaining of (Cummings and VandenBos, 1981). It is important to note that people are often unaware of the real reason for taking a particular action. When a patient consults a doctor about a particular disorder or symptom, the underlying problem is often unclear to the patient or the doctor. In this situation, the doctor who fails to explore with the patient his or her emotional condition, family and marital relationships, work situation, eating and sleeping habits, physical and sexual activities, and other relevant behaviors may lose a valuable opportunity to clarify the clinical situation. This is not only because an accurate evaluation of the clinical problem will help establish rapport and permit better directed diagnosis and treatment, but also because in today's supertechnical world, it is important to protect the patient from an unnecessarily stressful and expensive battery of tests.

While the standards of medical care are usually determined by an analysis of statistics reflecting morbidity and mortality, the *quality* of medical care seems to hinge more on the awareness of many of the topics presented in this book and on the willingness of the doctor to act on this knowledge. Clearly, medicine of the kind we are considering here will be judged more by the quality of the process than by the statistics of outcome (Ierodiakonou and Vandenbroucke, 1993), although both are undoubtedly of importance.

During the past 50 years or so, however, we have acquired a broader perspective on many of the elements influencing patients' responses to ill health, as well as a deeper understanding of the complex ways in which they communicate their problems to doctors in the clinic. Familiarity with these issues helps equip physicians with the lexicon used by patients in what may be an extremely indirect form of communication. Chapter 2 provides an account of concepts and clinical situations that, I believe, serve as a necessary background for the specifics of clinical practice in all specialties.

REFERENCES

Ayres A, Hoon PW, Franzoni JB, et al. (1994). Influence of mood and adjustment to cancer to compliance with chemotherapy among breast cancer patients. J Psychosom Res 38:393–402.

Barondess JA (1979). Disease and illness—a crucial distinction. Am J Med 66:375–376.

Beecher HK (1956). Relationship of the significance of wound to the pain experience. JAMA 161:1609–1615.

Burstein HJ, Gelber S, Guadagnoli E, et al. (1999). Use of alternative medicine by women with early-stage breast cancer. N Engl J Med 340:1733–1739.

Castelnuovo-Tedesco P, Krout BM (1970). Psychosomatic aspects of chronic pelvic pain. Int J Psychiatry Med 1:109–126.

Cummings NA, VandenBos GR (1981). The twenty years Kaiser-Permanente experience with psychotherapy and medical utilization: implications for national health policy and national health insurance. Health Policy Quarterly 1:59–75

Davis MS (1966). Variations in patients' compliance with doctor's orders: analysis of congruence between survey responses and results of empirical investigations. J Med Educ 41:1037–1048.

Davis MS (1968). Variations in patients' compliance with doctors advice: an empirical analysis of patterns of communication. Am J Public Health 58:274–288.

Eisenberg L (1977). Disease and illness: distinctions between professional and popular ideas of sickness. Cult Med Psychiatry 1:9–23.

Eisenberg L (1988). Science in medicine: too much or too little and too limited in scope? Am J Med 84:483–491.

Eisenberg DM, Davis RB, Ettner SL, et al. (1998). Trends in alternative medicine use in the United States, 1990–1997: results of a follow-up national survey. JAMA 280:1569–1575.

Eisenberg DM, Kessler RC, Foster C, et al. (1993). Unconventional medicine in the United States: prevalence, costs, and patterns of use. N Engl J Med 328:246–252.

Fulder SJ, Munro RE (1985). Complementary medicine in the United Kingdom: patients, practitioners, and consultations. Lancet 2:542–545.

Hadler NM (1996). If you have to prove you are ill, you can't get well: the object lesson of fibromyalgia. Spine 21:2397–2400.

Holland JC (1999). Use of alternative medicine: a marker for distress? N Engl J Med 340:1758–1759.

Ierodiakonou K, Vandenbroucke JP (1993). Medicine as a stochastic art. Lancet 341:542–543.

Jennings D (1986). The confusion between disease and illness in clinical medicine. Can Med Assoc J 135:865–870.

Kroenke K, Mangelsdorff AD (1989). Common symptoms in ambulatory care: incidence evaluation, therapy and outcome. Am J Med 86:262–266.

Legoretta AP, Christain-Herman J, O'Conner RD, et al. (1998). Compliance with national asthma management guidelines and speciality care: a health maintenance organization experience. Arch Intern Med 158:457–464.

Raymer D, Weininger O, Hamilton JR (1984). Psychological problems in children with abdominal pain. Lancet I:439–440.

Reiser SJ (1993). The era of the patient: using the experience of illness in shaping the missions of health care. JAMA 269:1012–1017.

Roberts BH, Norton NM (1952). Prevalence of psychiatric illness in a medical outpatient clinic. N Engl J Med 246:82–86.

Sternbach RA, Wolf SR, Murphy RW, et al. (1973). Traits of pain patients: the low back "loser." Psychosomatics 14:226–229.

Stimson GU (1974). Obeying doctors' orders: a view from the other side. Soc Sci Med 8:97–104.

Stoeckle JD, Zola JK, Davidson GE (1964). The quantity and significance of psychological distress in medical patients. J Chron Dis 17:959–970.

Thomas KJ, Carr J, Westlake L, et al. (1991). Use of non-orthodox and conventional health care in Great Britain. Br Med J 302:207–210.

Thomas L (1982). Medicine as a very old profession. In: Wyngaarden JB, Smith LH, eds. Cecil Textbook of Medicine, 17th ed. Philadelphia: WB Saunders Company, pp xli–xliii.

Urquart J (1996). Patient compliance with crucial drug regimens: implications for prostatic cancer. Eur Urol 29(Suppl 2):124–131.

Verhoef MJ, Hagen N, Pelletier G, et al. (1999). Alternative therapy use in neurological diseases: use in brain tumor patients. Neurology 52:617–622.

Woodforde JM, Merskey H (1972). Personality traits of patients with chronic pain. J Psychosom Res 16:167–172.

Zola IK (1960). Culture and symptoms: an analysis of patients presenting complaints. Am Social Rev 31:615–630.

Zweig Z (1931). Die Heilung durch den Geist (Mental Healers). Leipzig: Insel-Verlag. Quoted in: Alexander F (1950). Psychosomatic Medicine, Its Principles and Applications. New York: WW Norton.

Chapter
2

Somatization: Body Language

> A patient should complain in reasonable proportion to demonstrable pathology, report physical distress in bodily terms and emotional distress in psychological terms, and accept a doctor's opinion and advice compliantly.
>
> (Lipowski, "Somatization," 1988)

It is well-known that mental suffering may be manifested as a psychological, behavioral, or physical problem. When a physical problem represents the *principal expression* of an emotional problem, difficulties in diagnosis often arise. The close temporal association between a major stressful event, such as divorce or death of a close relative, and an exacerbation of asthma or severe migraine headaches seldom creates diagnostic difficulties. Patients themselves are often able to point to the cause-and-effect relationship between the clinical state and the stress that preceded it. But there are circumstances in which emotional stress may not be easily identified as the main mediator of a symptom complex or abnormal physical state. In these situations patients often resist the idea that their physical symptoms have an emotional basis. Their attitude may preclude effective management; for example, they may refuse to accept their doctor's recommendation that they consult a psychotherapist. This refusal by patients to contemplate an emotional cause for their symptoms may be based on a number of reasons. The range of common states that characterize this group of patients is described in this chapter.

Alexithymic subjects are so called because they are largely unaware of their emotions or moods or they have difficulty in describing them. They invariably resist the idea that their physical problem may have an emotional basis; their tendency to deny this possibility, often with great persuasiveness, may convince the doctor. Patients with persistent psychosomatic problems often show the characteristics of alexithymia and typically express their emotional discomfort through physical symptoms (Sifneos, 1973). They tend to describe the details of their pain or other symptoms endlessly and they often indicate a willingness to take action, such as accepting surgical intervention, to relieve their discomfort. As pointed out by Sifneos (1982), such patients, in the hands of unsuspecting physicians, are candidates for interventional procedures. Physicians are often impressed by a patient's detailed description of symptoms without any reference to psychological distress and may consequently be inclined to believe that some sort of invasive procedure is warranted. Extensive physical investigations and surgical procedures, while well meant, may have a crippling effect on these patients (Blumer and Heilbronn, 1982).

Sifneos (1973) predicted that alexithymic individuals, because of their inability to express their emotions verbally and their typically restricted or nonexistent fantasy life, would be unlikely to derive benefit from dynamic psychotherapy, which emphasizes verbal expression and requires a capacity for emotional interaction. Often better suited to this type of personality are supportive psychotherapy and behavioral interventions of the kind described in this book.

EXPRESSING EMOTION THROUGH PHYSICAL SYMPTOMS: SOMATIZATION

Lipowski (1988) defines *somatization* as "the tendency to communicate psychological distress in the form of physical symptoms, and to seek medical help for them." Most doctors are familiar with somatization in children, who may express anxiety or tension as stomach pain or headache (Apley and Nish, 1958). It is also common in adults and characterizes a broad range of clinical situations (Kirmayer and Robbins, 1991), including

- Patients who present with exclusively physical symptoms despite evident emotional distress.
- Patients who are convinced they have a disease or worry about their health despite an absence of objective supporting evidence.
- Patients who repeatedly seek medical help, disabled by medically unexplained somatic symptoms.

What all of these situations have in common is that the medically unexplained symptoms are related in some way to underlying social or psychological difficulties. Recognition by doctors of the true situation can help strengthen their resolve to protect such patients from excessive investigation and unnecessary medical or surgical intervention and, where necessary, help guide the patient toward appropriate psychotherapeutic or behavioral treatment. The doctor's approach in such cases will largely depend on an ability to diagnose the clinical state accurately. Problems of investigation and management arise when the doctor does not fully understand the problem. In such cases there is a tendency both to overinvestigate and to overtreat in an attempt—nearly always unsuccessful—to alleviate the patient's distress.

SOMATIZATION DISORDER: A DIAGNOSTIC DILEMMA

Determining the criteria for defining the diagnostic entity "somatization disorder" (SD) presents a major dilemma. The *Diagnostic and Statistical Manual of Mental Disorders* (DSM-IV; American Psychiatric Association, 1994) now accepts eight symptoms (i.e., any symptoms, but without demonstrable underlying pathological change) for a diagnosis of SD. The International Classification of Disease (ICD-10; World Health Organization, 1994) accepts a more realistic six or more symptoms from at least two separate groups including gastrointestinal, cardiovascular, genitourinary, and skin and pain symptoms; in addition, the symptoms should have been present for at least two years. The DSM-IV stipulates that symptoms should have begun before the age of 30 and lasted for "several" years. In the somatizing patient, anxiety and depressed mood are frequent, with patients often seeking help for depression. Antisocial behavior and occupational, interpersonal and marital difficulties are common. The disorder is seldom diagnosed in males but may be observed in 10%–20% of female first-degree relatives. Related medical conditions must be excluded as a cause of the symptoms; factitious etiologies or malingering should also be excluded.

In evaluating the prevalence of somatization among 3132 randomly selected community respondents, Escobar et al. (1987b) applied a much less stringent construct in which criteria for diagnosis were at least four symptoms for men and six symptoms for women. With these more permissive criteria, 4.4% of respondents received the diagnosis, and their reported use of health services was heavier than that of the general population. Of those respondents with a psychiatric diagnosis, usually dysthymic disorder or depression, who were also somatizers, the tendency was to use medical rather than mental health services (Escobar et al., 1987a). In addition, somatizers reported more disability than nonsomatizers. There appears to be a spectrum of severity of somatization in which various degrees of ill health, dysfunction, and disability are correlated with the number of symptoms (Katon et al., 1991). However, even if symptoms are few in number, they may be indicators of significant psychosocial distress.

ILLNESS BEHAVIOR

Mechanic (1961), who was influential in developing the notion of illness behavior as a relevant field of study, describes it as "the manner in which individuals monitor their bodies, define and interpret their symptoms, take remedial action, and utilize sources of help as well as the more formal health care system. It also is concerned with how people monitor and respond to symptoms and symptom change over the course of an illness and how this affects behavior, remedial action taken, and response to treatment."

Implicit in this definition is the premise that all forms of illness experience are shaped by cultural, social, and psychological factors in addition to biological ones. Illness behavior is fashioned by the individual's broader cultural context, social network, personality, and life experience, as well as by the response of the health care system to the patient's complaints. All of these factors influence the individual's response to symptoms (Mechanic, 1986). Kroenke and Mangelsdorf (1989) studied 567 new symptom complaints in an internal medicine practice and found that only 16% had an identifiable physical cause, implying that in the rest of the group (84%) the symptom reflected somatization and was an indication of psychosocial distress.

The concept of illness behavior is described by Pilowsky (1978) in different terms: "Anyone who has worked in the field of workers' compensation becomes aware that illness or disability can be seen as a 'property' of an organism that can be traded for money in one market place and for health care in another. It is obvious, however, that an illness always costs somebody something, whether it is cashed in for 'sick role unit' or 'money.' "

This perspective on one important aspect of illness behavior has received support from a study by Cassidy et al. (2000) showing how the elimination of compensation for pain and suffering following whiplash injury (through so-called no-fault insurance, which covers only the expense of medical care and financial losses directly attributable to the injury) results in a decreased incidence of disability and improved prognosis. Similarly, among patients with back pain, the level of functioning and severity of symptoms after treatment are worse in those who retain an attorney, initiate litigation, or become involved in worker compensation proceedings than in those who do not, even after adjustment for clinical findings (Trief and Stein, 1985; Atlas et al., 2000). Thus, while cases of workers' compensation represent a specific type of clinical problem, this observation highlights the fact that *patients present themselves for medical attention for a variety of reasons, of which the presence of disease is only one*—social and economic incentives may also be of considerable importance (Deyo, 2000).

It is possible to recognize a stereotyped behavior pattern in many patients demonstrating abnormal illness behavior, regardless of the specific diagnostic problem presented. Katon et al. (1991) studied frequent medical care users at a

Seattle health maintenance organization and found that 10% of the patients used about one-third of all services provided. Among this group of patients, one-half were psychologically distressed, suffering especially from major depression, panic disorder, or somatization disorder. The following attributes tend to characterize *chronic somatizers* (Benjamin and Bridges, 1992):

- They make excessive use of medical and surgical services.
- They are often not reassured by negative findings.
- They indulge in "doctor- and hospital-shopping."
- They resist the suggestion that psychological factors underlie their clinical problems.
- An atmosphere of mutual hostility often develops between them and their doctors.

The main categories of the *somatoform disorders*—somatization disorder and somatoform pain disorder, hypochondriasis, and conversion disorder—may also be considered examples of *abnormal illness behaviors* (Pilowsky, 1978). However, although *somatization* is defined as "symptoms without an organic basis," it is important to remember that it may coexist with demonstrable physical disease. Furthermore, it is important to note that the abnormal illness behaviors described in detail in later chapters do not in themselves represent psychiatric diagnoses, and not all patients with somatization have a diagnosable psychiatric disorder. Thus, when dealing with a particular psychosomatic condition such as chronic pain, irritable bowel, or chronic fatigue, a heightened sensitivity on the part of the physician to the true nature of the problem improves the chances of developing a satisfactory plan of treatment that will bring some respite from suffering.

The *hypochondriacal* patient tends to manifest a persistent fear of physical illness despite reassurance and the demonstration of medical evidence refuting physical illness. The patient is often in an agitated state and will try hard to convince the doctor of the existence or likelihood of disease. The DSM-IV (American Psychiatric Association, 1994) criteria also specify that the disturbance should have been present for at least six months and that the fear should not have a delusional quality (i.e., the patient can acknowledge the possibility that it is unfounded). In addition, the patient's preoccupation with the problem should be sufficient to cause clinically significant distress or impairment in social, occupational, or other important areas of functioning.

Somatoform pain disorder is characterized by a preoccupation with pain in the absence of adequate physical findings to account for the pain or its intensity. In about half of all cases the pain begins after physical trauma and characteristically persists long after clinical evidence of the trauma has resolved. Among patients with this disorder, a disproportionately large number began working at an unusually young age, hold either physically strenuous or overroutinized jobs, are "workaholics," and rarely take time off from work or for vacations. Typically, patients strongly deny the possibility of psychological factors causing the pain. The disorder is diagnosed almost twice as frequently in women as in men. Significantly, the same characteristics are said to be typical of patients suffering from the chronic fatigue syndrome (see Chapter 15).

Patients with *conversion disorder* suffer an alteration in or loss of physical function. The condition thus simulates a physical disorder but cannot be explained by any pathophysiological mechanism. The symptoms are *not intentionally produced*, that is, they do not reflect a deliberate intention to deceive, and invariably arise as the result of psychological conflict or stress. The most typical conversion symptoms are pseudoneurological, suggesting paralysis, aphonia, seizures, coordination disturbance, akinesia, dyskinesia, blindness, tunnel vision, anosmia, urinary retention, anesthesia, and paresthesia. Symptoms may also include seizures or convulsions. The more medically naive the patient, the more implausible the symptoms. The disorder may begin at any age, although it usually appears in adolescence or early adulthood. An important caveat relating to the diagnosis of conversion disorder is that some medical disorders may be clearly diagnosed only months or years after the symptoms first appear. Furthermore, conversion disorder may be superimposed on or follow a neurological or other general medical condition (American Psychiatric Association, 1994).

The definition of conversion disorder is unique in that it implies a specific mechanism to account for the disturbance (American Psychiatric Association, 1994). Primary gain is achieved when the individual, through the symptom, succeeds in keeping some internal conflict or need out of awareness. The conflict or need is "converted" into the symptom. In such cases, there is a temporal relationship between an environmental stimulus that is apparently related to a psychological conflict or need and the initiation or intensification of the stimulus. The symptom then acquires a symbolic value that is a representation and partial solution of the underlying conflict. As the clinical picture generally approximates the patient's naive idea of an appropriate disability, careful neurological examination usually confirms the nonneurological basis of the problem. For example functional vocal cord dysfunction may present as stridor, often being mistaken for an asthma attack, but laryngoscopy typically shows in these patients persistent adduction of the vocal cords during both inspiration and expiration. However, if the patient is asked to count during examination, the vocal cords will be found to move normally (Chapter 14). Secondary gain is achieved when the patient is able to avoid an activity that is particularly unpleasant or stressful or win a financial advantage such as workers compensation through development of the symptom. The clinical state may also be expected to lead to support from the environment that might not otherwise be forthcoming.

Various symptoms that may be defined as conversion symptoms according to the above definition occur in a fairly large number of people but usually as a short-lived and temporary experience. This may include a defined pattern of somatization, such as headache at a time of stress, or even a period of hypochondriacal concern following the death of a close friend or relative from a sudden and unexpected illness. What distinguishes the true conversion disorder, however, is that *it persists in a way that dominates the patient's thoughts and actions*, leading to repeated consultation, extensive investigation, and chronic dissatisfaction, in a manner similar to that of other somatoform disorders (Bass and Potts, 1993).

DIFFERENT FACES OF PSYCHOPHYSIOLOGICAL PROCESSES

We are constantly reacting to our environments, emotionally as well as physically. Although personality traits do not determine what disorder an individual will develop, they certainly influence the way in which the individual is affected by ill health or symptoms; that is, they influence how the individual perceives the experience and consequently the extent to which the clinical state induces a stress response. The spectrum of psychophysiological processes that may lead to impairment of health is extremely broad. In developed societies, they commonly reflect situations in our day-to-day existence, such as work or family life. In some individuals, longstanding symptoms date from a specific traumatic event. More often, the onset of symptoms occurs months or years after a stressful experience. This increases the physician's difficulty in linking the emotional impact of the experience to the ultimate development of a particular symptomatic physical state, and it strains the comprehension of the patient.

The Chronically Stressed Individual

To illustrate the protean expression of the processes under discussion, we consider cardiovascular disease, one of the potentially life-threatening physical expressions of chronic stress. Most people spend a substantial part of their lives, approximately one-third of the day, at work. Highly demanding work (such as repetitive factory work or dealing with a demanding public) with little latitude for decision making—little control (Karasek et al., 1981)—is considered to be particularly stressful.

In at least one study jobs considered as continuously stressful were associated over time with an increased left ventricle mass due to repeated blood pressure increases during the hours of stressful work each day (Schnall et al., 1990). The impact of such stress on the heart and circulatory system develops over a period of many years. The range of reaction to job stress is extremely broad, however, and may include behavior that attempts to alleviate the tension, such as cigarette smoking, excessive alcohol intake, or drug abuse. The physical disorders to which these habits contribute therefore represent the remote effects of the stress that prompted the habit in the first place. The effects of chronic stress on immune function as well as on the natural history of ischemic heart disease and diabetes mellitus are considered in detail in Chapters 6 and 7.

The Possible Outcome of Intense, Short-Lived Stress

Frequently, a short-lived experience arousing intense anxiety may have a profound influence on an individual's subsequent behavior. A common example is the experience of the elevator door not opening at the expected moment, or of actually being stuck in the elevator. The episode may last for less than a minute, but if it is associated with intense fear of being trapped in the confined space, a perception which may be strongly reinforced by the panic reaction of others in the elevator or possibly of being alone in this predicament, the individual may experience anxiety or even phobia when having to enter elevators thereafter. Similarly, the almost momentary sensation of a free fall and the intense fear it aroused when the airplane hit a sizable air pocket led to a subsequent fear of flying in a young patient.

In the case that follows, a short-lived experience—a fall down stairs—was associated by a mother with intense fear of irreparable brain damage to the infant held in her arms, resulting in a feeling of severe guilt in the mother. The outcome was a persistent migraine syndrome and an especially tense relationship with this daughter over 20 years.

CASE REPORT: TEN SECONDS OF STRESS
FOLLOWED BY MIGRAINE FOR 20 YEARS

The patient, a 39-year-old mother of five children, had suffered from recurrent migraine for more than 20 years. Over a five-year period attacks occurred with increasing frequency and intensity, and for at least two years she had spent from two to five days each month in bed with severe headaches. All recognized antimigraine medications were totally ineffective (sumatriptan and related drugs not yet available).

The migraine attacks had originally begun within a couple of weeks of the patient falling down stairs with her infant daughter, her first child, in her arms. This event had produced intense fear and apprehension that the infant had suffered brain injury from the fall. Despite repeated reassurance by the examining pediatrician that there was no injury, and subsequent evidence of normal development, the patient was plagued by a persistent feeling of guilt. The daughter, by now 20 years old, had a strained relationship with her mother. The mother was aware of the fact that her relationship with her four younger children was much less tense. She was happily married and appeared well adjusted to all the major aspects of her family and professional life.

The patient responded well to a course of relaxation therapy, during which she was taught deep relaxation (Chapter 19). While in that state she was encouraged to recall in as much detail as possible the original traumatic memory of the fall with the infant in her arms, a process that was repeated on a number of occasions. This resulted in a considerable reduction in the tension she felt when recollecting the event. Within a few weeks she reported relief of the headaches and an improved, more relaxed, relationship with her eldest daughter. Within six months of the patient's completion of treatment, her husband developed angina pectoris, suffered a myocardial infarction, was admitted to the coronary intensive care unit, and subsequently underwent coronary angiography and coronary artery bypass surgery. The potential implications and seriousness of her husband's illness were fully apparent to the patient, who might have been left at any stage to bring up a family of five children on her own. Thus all phases of his illness were extremely stressful for her. This ordeal lasted for about five months and despite her anxiety and numerous sleepless nights, there were no further migraine attacks during this time. Eight years have elapsed and the patient has remained migraine-free.

It seems likely that this patient had some physical predisposition to migraine, which developed in response to her anxiety over the fall. Beyond the question of physical predisposition, the extreme guilt reaction and persistent anxiety state followed her fall some 20 years earlier, despite both the doctor's repeated reassurances and the clearly visible evidence of her daughter's continued normal development. This unresolved facet of the problem presumably resided in her own personality structure. Yet the success of the behavioral intervention, after which the headaches disappeared and her relationship with her daughter improved, supports the view that a full exploration of the patient's personality was not a prerequisite for successful management of this clinical problem. Furthermore, this case illustrates that a significant state of anxiety may be triggered by a relatively minor event that is in no way life-threatening. The severity of the reaction is a function of the patient's perception of what the particular event meant at the time of its occurrence—in this case, intense fear of anticipated damage to her newborn infant.

IT COULD NEVER HAPPEN TO ME!

The naive perception that only certain personality types characterized by "hysterical" or anxious dispositions are likely to fall victim to debilitating psychophysiological processes is seriously in error. The corollary—those who are ostensibly best able to cope in their daily lives do not suffer from such problems—is also widely believed and is similarly erroneous. Any well-adjusted, nonanxious individual may be brought to a point of exhaustion, both physically and emotionally, through hard work and exaggerated demands of daily responsibility. This run-down condition may leave a person vulnerable to developing psychosomatic symptoms. The essential concept is that stress, whatever its source, may lead to a breakdown of normal emotional or physical integrity. It follows from this that psychophysiological processes encountered in general medicine are by no means the exclusive preserve of emotionally labile or unstable personalities. Every individual has a limit of tolerance to stressful situations; the appearance of unaccustomed emotional or physical symptoms may indicate that the limit has been reached. This is important because it needs to be recognized that even apparently emotionally stable individuals may manifest psychosomatic disorders.

SUMMARY

A central thesis of this book is that a large part of the physician's impact as a healer depends on, or is deeply colored by, her or his ability to correctly identify in clinical practice problems that are caused by psychophysiological processes. This means that for medical management to be most effective, the psychophysiological component of every clinical situation should be appraised for its potential contribution to the clinical state under consideration. The broad range of disorders having their origin in psychosomatic processes will be presented in later chapters. However, by using the therapeutic encounter to influence patients' attitudes and perceptions about the illness, doctors may help provide them with the resources to deal more effectively with the current clinical problem and to cope better with any stress in the future. This will involve:

1. A discussion of the importance of feeling in control and the manner in which the symptoms undermine the patient's feeling of control and self-confidence. The therapeutic encounter is presented as an educational package geared to help restore the feelings of control and therefore of self-confidence (Chapter 4).
2. A clearly understandable account of the particular clinical disorder with attention given to the patient's understanding and fears regarding the disorder. This is done both to enhance, through knowledge, the patient's sense of control and to correct mistaken or misplaced fears about the implications of the symptoms or disease (the cognitive aspect) (Chapter 18).
3. In cases where somatization is prominent, using clear explanation to create an awareness of the true significance of the symptoms as expressions of emotional distress and engaging the patient in behavioral interventions such as deep relaxation or meditation to enhance sensitivity to the somatic expression of emotional tension. This increased awareness assists in restoring feelings of control by providing the patient with techniques for counteracting the impact of the symptoms. Thus it helps convert a sense of help-

lessness into greater confidence that one is able to influence the intensity of the symptom. Even if the outcome of the therapeutic intervention is only partially effective, as it usually is, the positive impact of this knowledge and experience usually far exceeds its objective utility. This educational process, which forms the basis of the therapeutic encounter, is discussed in greater detail in Chapters 18 and 19.

REFERENCES

American Psychiatric Association (1994). Diagnostic and statistical manual of mental disorders, 4th ed. Washington, DC: Author.

Apley J, Nish N (1958). Recurrent abdominal pain: a field survey of 1000 school children. Arch Dis Child 33:165–170.

Atlas SJ, Chang Y, Kammann E, et al. (2000). Long-term disability and return to work among patients who have a herniated lumbar disc: the effect of disability compensation. J Bone Joint Surg Am 82:4–15.

Bass C, Potts S (1993). Somatoform disorders. In: Granville-Grossman K, ed. Recent Advances in Clinical Psychiatry, No. 8. New York: Churchill Livingstone, pp 143–163.

Benjamin S, Bridges K (1992). The special needs of chronic somatizers. In: Benjamin S, House A, Jenkins P, eds. Defining Needs and Planning Services. London: Gaskell Press, Royal College of Psychiatrists.

Blumer D, Heilbronn M (1982). Chronic pain as a variant of depressive disease: the pain-prone disorder. J Nerv Ment Dis 170:381–406.

Cassidy JD, Carroll LJ, Cote P, et al. (2000). Effect of eliminating compensation for pain and suffering on the outcome of insurance claims and whiplash injury. N Engl J Med 342:1179–1186.

Deyo RA (2000). Pain and public policy [editorial]. N Engl J Med 342:1211–1213.

Escobar JI, Burnam MA, Karno M, et al. (1987a). Somatization in the community. Arch Gen Psychiatry 44:713–718.

Escobar JI, Golding JM, Hough RL, et al. (1987b). Somatization in the community: relationship to disability and use of services. Am J Public Health 77:837–840.

Karasek R, Baker D, Marxer F, et al (1981). Job decision latitude, job demands, and cardiovascular disease: a prospective study of Swedish men. Am J Public Health 71:694–705.

Katon W, Lin E, Von Korff M, et al. (1991). Somatization: a spectrum of severity. Am J Psychiatry 148:34–40.

Kirmayer LJ, Robbins JM (1991). Introduction: concepts of somatization. In: Kirmayer LJ, Robbins JM, eds. Current Concepts of Somatization: Research and Clinical Perspectives. Washington, DC: American Psychiatric Press.

Kroenke K, Mangelsdorff AD (1989). Common symptoms in ambulatory care: incidence, evaluation, therapy, and outcome. Am J Med 86:262–266.

Lipowski ZJ (1988). Somatization: the concept and its clinical application. Am J Psychiatry 145:1358–1368.

Mechanic D (1961). The concept of illness behavior. J Chron Dis 15:189–194.

Mechanic D (1986). The concept of illness behavior: culture, situation and personal predisposition. Psychol Med 16:1–7.

Pilowsky I (1978). A general classification of abnormal illness behaviors. Br J Med Psychol 51:131–137.

Schnall PL, Pieper C, Schwartz JE, et al. (1990). The relationship between "job strain," workplace diastolic blood pressure, and left ventricular mass index. JAMA 263:1929–1935.

Sifneos PE (1973). The prevalence of alexithymic characteristics in psychosomatic patients. Psychother Psychosom 22:255–262.

Sifneos PE (1982). Comments on Blumer D and Heilbronn M. Chronic pain as a variant of depressive disease: the pain-prone disorder. J Nerv Ment Dis 170:420–421.

Trief P, Stein N (1985). Pending litigation and rehabilitation outcome of chronic back pain. Arch Phys Med Rehabil 66:95–99.

Urquhart J (1996). Patient compliance with crucial drug regimens: implications for prostatic cancer. Eur Urol 29(suppl 2):124–131.

World Health Organization (1994). International Classification of Disease. New York: Churchill Livingstone.

Chapter

3

CHALLENGES IN DOCTOR–PATIENT COMMUNICATION

This chapter covers two aspects of the doctor–patient relationship that are commonly problematic for both parties: the question of truth telling and the ability to allay anxiety effectively in the clinic. Often a direct, simple, accurate statement of the clinical problem as having a psychophysiological basis at best does nothing to allay existing anxiety and at worst actually succeeds in alienating the patient. In the doctor's mind, the act of telling it as it is means that the problem is being presented on the one hand truthfully and on the other in a way that should help eliminate or allay anxiety by excluding threatening diseases. The patient, however, having come to the doctor because of a physical complaint, may not be ready to accept that the problem has in essence an emotional basis. Furthermore, the news that the tests are all negative and that there is "nothing to worry about" does not provide an adequate explanation for the symptoms the patient knows he feels. In fact, the "don't worry" approach may be very alienating for the patient.

TRUTH TELLING

Truth and the Therapeutic Relationship

It would seem axiomatic that the doctor–patient relationship is based on trust in the physician's professional ability as well as the expectation of honesty and truthfulness in the physician's dealings with patients. In certain areas of clinical practice, however, the latter may be questionable. This is especially true in the case of either cancer or psychosomatic illness. Both of these areas oblige the physician to focus on issues that are highly charged in their potential implications for the patient, the first because of the ultimate prognosis and the second because of the implicit question of the patient's emotional stability.

Western societies, in their teaching of ethical concepts, tend to present the true–false dichotomy in absolute terms. This attitude is further reinforced in litigious countries where the importance of "having told the patient everything" could be taken to mean in a court of law that patients, forearmed with all relevant information, are in a position to exercise independent judgment in clinical decisions regarding their investigation or treatment. This presumably mitigates or absolves the treating physician of sole responsibility for the decision if things go badly for the patient.

Many physicians, when confronted with an oncological patient whose prognosis is poor, may balk at a frank statement of the situation and prefer instead an imprecise or even misleading presentation of the facts to the patient (although often a close family member will be told the truth). This can perhaps be justified as being in the patient's interest according to the Hippocratic tradition of *primum non nocere*. In discussing this common dilemma in clinical practice, Surbone (1992, 1994a) emphasizes the influence of doctors' cultural attitudes on their handling of the question of how much to tell their patients. In a study of 1171 breast cancer patients and their physicians and surgeons in general hospitals in Italy, designed to evaluate the frequency of disclosure of operable breast cancer, only 47% of the patients reported having been told that they had cancer and 25% of their physicians stated they had not given accurate information (Mosconi et al., 1991). Surbone points out that this has the undesirable effect of excluding the uninformed patients from the decision-making process regarding mastectomy or breast-conserving surgery, especially in those cases where outcomes are considered to be equivalent. Similarly, an inadequate presentation of a terminal state may lead patients to overestimate their survival chances and choose aggressive antineoplastic therapy. In the SUPPORT study (Study to Understand Prognoses for Outcomes and Risks of Treatment, 1995), patients who overestimated their prospects for survival and received aggressive antineoplastic therapy had exactly the same median survival as those who received palliative care and were 1.6 times more likely to have a hospital readmission, undergo attempted resuscitation, or die while receiving ventilatory support. As pointed out by Smith and Swisher (1998), surrogate decision makers not properly informed may also consent to far more aggressive treatment than they would want for themselves. Accurate end-of-life information could change a surrogate's role from doing everything to doing the right thing. Similarly, telling the patients the truth about their terminal cancer is an important step in the right direction.

After analyzing the difficulty that physicians have in understanding truth in the context of the doctor–patient interaction, Surbone (1994b) summarizes her viewpoint as follows:

> When perceiving truth as only the opposite or the absence of lie, we imply that truth is a fixed object merely needing to be described/verbalized. In medicine, truth equals information. When perceiving truth as a relational state, we simply imply that truth develops, in time and space, because of interactions: in medicine this happens between the patient, the disease, the doctor, the family, the society and the medications. Truth goes beyond information and reaches the level of communication, a bidirectional process by definition. Communication is the real goal.

The inference is that truthful communication presupposes a comprehensive view of patients, first as people, then as members of a family unit, and finally in the social context. The physician, while taking full professional responsibility for guiding patients along the most favorable path, sees the patients (and their families) as partners in the decision-making process; they therefore need to be given accurate information to help them reach a satisfactory decision. This humanistic, nondogmatic approach acknowledges that there are different ways of communicating, both verbal and nonverbal, and that what is not said may be as important as what is said. It also recognizes that the blunt delivery of unselected facts to the unprepared may convey a message as distorted and misleading in its impact as a frankly untruthful description of a patient's condition.

Truth and Psychophysiological Processes

In the field of psychosomatic medicine, the topics to be discussed with patients are usually not as highly charged as those encountered in oncology since they rarely represent life-or-death issues. Notable exceptions are the danger of suicide in depressed patients or death in unresponsive anorexia nervosa. But they are not less problematic with regard to the difficulty they cause the physician about being completely truthful. Many physicians confronted with patients who have psychosomatic problems will continue doing what they have been best trained to do, which is to doggedly pursue the search for disease states. This course of action is also common when patients have a prolonged clinical history of symptoms or serious inability to function despite an objectively satisfactory clinical state and consistently negative investigation results. This is clearly a situation in which emotional factors should be considered, yet the possibility of a psychophysiological explanation for the symptoms is often studiously disregarded by the physician—an attitude which is easier to maintain in this field than in oncology.

There are a number of possible explanations for the physician's failure to explore psychosomatic problems. One of these is simply that many people, including medical practitioners, have difficulty confronting or dealing with emotional problems in other people. This is especially true of those who feel themselves unqualified in this regard because of inadequate training. Surveys of practicing physicians reveal that they often feel inadequately trained to deal with commonly encountered psychiatric problems (Hyams et al., 1976; Fisher, 1978; Kantor and Griner, 1981) as well as psychiatric emergencies (Weissberg, 1990; Weissberg, 1991). This is supported by results in the field: it has been found that 30%–50% of significant psychiatric disorders such as depression and panic disorder are unrecognized or inadequately treated by primary (Moffic and Paykel, 1975; Knights and Folstein, 1977; Goldberg et al., 1982) or emergency room (Fleet et al., 1996) physicians. Fleet and colleagues (1996) studied 441 consecutive patients with chest pain on presentation to the emergency rooms of a number of Canadian hospitals. Of this group 25% were found to meet DSM criteria of panic disorder, but 98% of the panic patients were not recognized by attending emergency room cardiologists. Physicians may have similar difficulties in recognizing psychosocial and behavioral problems, such as major life stress and noncompliance, and in understanding their significance (Brody, 1980; Thompson, et al., 1982). In some cases, lack of attention to psychosomatic issues may result simply from neglect or from outright resistance on the part of the physician (Greenhill and Kilgore, 1950; Friedman and Cohen-Cole, 1981; Schwab, 1982).

Resistance by physicians to a recognition of these issues may be rooted in deeply personal reasons, but often it is based on simple misconceptions about the nature or significance of emotional problems in clinical practice. This in turn makes it more difficult for doctors to communicate their (often inaccurate) perceptions to patients. This applies in particular to the more common affective conditions that the physician is expected to manage, mainly depression and anxiety states associated with a disease or expressed through somatic symptoms. These patients are not necessarily seriously hampered by their clinical condition and may continue to work, manage a business or household, and relate to family and friends in a satisfactory manner.

If the physician suspects that emotional factors are implicated in a patient's clinical state, this possibility should be raised with the patient after a complete medical history has been taken and a full physical examination and relevant laboratory tests have been performed. Most patients are open to such a discussion. Many will express their appreciation that the subject has been raised, often admitting that they themselves had considered the possibility but had felt too embarrassed to mention it, and then explain why they had considered it. On the other hand, patients understandably resent having to contemplate a psychosomatic label before their clinical condition has received a thorough evaluation. When the subject is broached, some patients may persistently deny that emotion might be an important factor in their clinical condition. Even these patients, however, may respond positively to the suggestion that they participate in some form of behavioral intervention such as a stress management program, the principles of which are described in later chapters. As this is the most important part of management in practical terms, it makes no sense for the physician to insist on a diagnostic label that is discomforting to the patient. The physician may suggest deferring the diagnosis while the therapeutic program is being carried out and then evaluated. Once patients start responding to treatment the importance of a diagnostic label declines.

The point to be emphasized here is that telling the truth in the context of psychosomatic illness need not be an ordeal for either doctor or patient, provided that the physician creates the appropriate context for such a discussion by first thoroughly evaluating the patient's clinical state. It is usually possible to present the situation to patients as the kind of problem that affects many emotionally balanced, reasonably adjusted people, and for which a great deal can be done. Furthermore, it may be explained that everyone has limits in dealing with stress, especially when it relates to health. Thus, the experiencing of symptoms, especially when unexpected, may trigger a fear of serious life-threatening illness or a more general, ill-defined fear of "losing control" that results in anxiety. Except for a few conditions such as depression and panic disorder, specific diagnostic labels such as those provided by the DSM classification are best avoided. It is far preferable to use a general concept such as "stress reaction," which sounds familiar but not threatening and provides a suitable starting point for a serious discussion of the emotional aspects of the problem. It then becomes easier to plan proper management with the patient's willing cooperation.

IATROGENIC ANXIETY

The expression of emotional suffering as physical symptoms often presents diagnostic difficulties. The second major problem area in identifying and managing emotional difficulties relates to the impact of symptoms or disease processes on patients. The "stress of illness" is a concept that should be broadened to include the stress inherent in medical consultations, that is, the stress involved in talking to the doctor, undergoing diagnostic procedures, and in some cases undergoing treatment.

For the clinician, a stressed state has greatest relevance when it seems to be either the cause or the consequence of a particular clinical state. In either case it may be viewed as a contributory factor in the genesis of the patient's symptoms—for example, in hypertension (Schnall et al., 1990)—and possibly in preventing a satisfactory clinical response to treatment. Symptoms, particularly when associated with emotional distress, will often reinforce the fear of further attacks of these same symptoms, and this fear serves to perpetuate the anxiety–symptom cycle. Thus, anxiety caused by a symptom, whether it be asthma, migraine, angina pectoris, or diarrhea, may be the stimulus that triggers the next attack, a process also called "symptom anticipation" (Melmed et al., 1990). This cycle may cause a deterioration of the patient's condition, leading to the *mistaken assumption that the clinical course represents progression of an underlying pathological process*. The possibility that anxiety may be responsible for the physical deterioration even when the patient is suffering from an organic disease is often not considered by the treating physician.

Iatrogenic Induction of an Anxiety State

The physician may unwittingly play a major role in the genesis of a patient's anxiety state. Although in some cases it may not be possible for the doctor to reassure the patient because there is genuine suspicion of serious disease, unnecessary anxiety is often induced in the patient by inappropriate physician responses. The main sources of physician-induced anxiety are considered next.

Inadequate information or reassurance

This situation may arise when the doctor mistakenly assumes that the patient has been adequately reassured or deliberately holds back information because of the need to await test results. The former mistake is typically made when patients suffering from panic attacks present with a symptom such as palpitations or chest pain. After performing a complete physical examination as well as an electrocardiogram and chest x-ray, the doctor may quite reasonably reassure the patient that there is nothing wrong with his heart and that he should go home and forget about it. However, failure to address the patient's specific fears, which persist because the doctor has not explained why the *symptoms occurred in the first place*, permits the anxiety state to develop.

A failure to provide sufficient information often occurs when a doctor who is genuinely concerned about the presence of significant disease tries to avoid alarming the patient unnecessarily and thus says little while awaiting test results. More experienced physicians usually manage, without being brutally frank, to explain why a particular investigation may be desirable.

In addition to relieving anxiety, appropriate education of patients about their condition, especially when it is chronic, may substantially affect medication compliance and reduce overall utilization of medical services. This, for example, is the experience with asthma sufferers, many of whom feel that they lack adequate knowledge of their illness (Garfinkel et al., 1992; Lehrer et al., 1992). In general, attention to the psychoeducational aspects of the management of asthma and other chronic diseases seems to be highly cost-effective (Deter, 1986), as discussed in Chapter 14.

Over-reaction by the doctor to the discovery of abnormality

Patients may be subjected to unnecessary stress because of a doctor's inability to appraise correctly an abnormal physical sign or laboratory result in relation to an overall picture of good health. This can happen if discovery of the abnormality prompts the doctor to order additional investigations, many of them unnecessary. As an example, clinical examination might reveal a mild aortic incompetence murmur. This discovery might warrant noninvasive evaluation by electro- and echocardiography in order to establish a baseline for further evaluation and exclude clinically silent mitral valve disease, whereas an invasive procedure such as cardiac catheterization would be unnecessary in most cases. Similarly, abnormal laboratory results that contradict the clinical picture should be repeated (if necessary at a different laboratory) before being taken to reflect a genuine aberration. An apparently abnormal result may be obtained, for example, with a test procedure performed infrequently by the laboratory or a finding that the doctor has little experience interpreting.

In some cases, in order to coerce the patient into compliant behavior, the physician may demonstratively express surprise or even consternation on perceiving a particular abnormality. This type of behavior may produce a state of stress in the patient and may backfire badly in terms of its intended effects. I have seen an extremely severe anxiety state and panic disorder triggered by the doctor's exclamation in response to a patient's elevated blood pressure. The patient deduced that her life was in imminent danger and responded with intense anxiety. While it could be argued that particular personality factors would have predisposed the patient to an anxiety disorder at some stage of her life, there is no doubt that the doctor's behavior was the trigger for emotional problems that could have been avoided.

Failure to recognize an emotional cause of the symptoms

Failure or delay in diagnosing the real reason for a patient's clinical condition will naturally tend to perpetuate the problem, especially if the patient is alexithymic or a chronic somatizer. In some cases the absence of a diagnosis may lead to more invasive investigations or the prescription of drugs with more troubling side effects. The problem may be compounded by the patient's failure to recognize the underlying emotional reasons for the complaint; furthermore, aggressive denial by the patient of a possible psychological basis for the disorder may discourage the doctor from pursuing that line of inquiry. The ways in which this problem may be handled by the doctor are discussed further in Chapter 18.

Posttraumatic Stress Disorder Following Medical Events

Posttraumatic stress disorder (PTSD) is a psychiatric disorder that typically follows events "outside the range of usual human experience" (American Psychiatric Association, 1987). It is characterized by three types of symptoms:

- Repeatedly reliving the traumatic event.
- Avoiding cues reminding the patient of the event, together with a numbing of general responsiveness.
- Increased arousal.

These symptoms must be of at least one month's duration to justify the diagnosis of PTSD. Similar symptoms, lasting from two days to a month after a traumatic experience, are indicative of an acute stress disorder (American Psychiatric Association, 1994).

The severe, life-threatening stress associated with war, accidents, or natural disasters may lead to PTSD. Less well recognized is the fact that it may occur in the wake of medical or surgical events. While many physicians are aware of and sensitive to symptoms of anxiety and depression in their patients, the emotional impact of illness may be much more profound and the consequences far more serious than generally appreciated (Shalev et al., 1993).

Modern medicine and surgery often involve invasive procedures for which the patient has little or no preparation. Although the DSM-IV makes no mention of medical conditions or procedures as possible traumatic events, these may be associated with feelings of loss of control by the patient and a perceived threat to life, factors viewed as predisposing to the development of PTSD when they occur suddenly (Green et al., 1990). Thus, the possibility of PTSD should be considered in patients who have undergone a medical event associated with a feeling of intense and inescapable distress, lack of control, and perceived threat to life, as is likely to happen when given a diagnosis of cancer (Alter et al., 1996; Butler et al., 1996) or human immunodeficiency virus (HIV) positivity (Kelly et al., 1998). The delayed onset of this debilitating syndrome is also worthy of note. In a study of 61 HIV-positive patients, Kelly et al. (1998) found that 30% met the diagnostic criteria for PTSD, and in 10% the disorder had an onset more than six months after the initial HIV infection diagnosis. A similar delay in expression of PTSD has also been observed in patients with burn injuries (Yu and Dimsdale, 1999). Intense identification with a patient can also result in PTSD, as may occur in the mothers of children discovered to have cancer (Pelcovitz et al., 1996; Smith et al., 1999).

The prevalence of PTSD among medical patients is unknown. Kurtz et al. (1994) estimate that following myocardial infarction up to 16% of patients may show signs of chronic PTSD. While this figure may seem high, there are indications that PTSD does occur more often than has been realized in general medical practice (Bennett and Brooke, 1999). Cases have been recorded following myocardial infarction (Kurtz et al., 1988), spontaneous abortion (Fisch and Tadmor, 1989; Bowles et al., 2000), cardiac resuscitation, cranial surgery for the removal of a meningioma, and a large postoperative hemorrhage after tonsillectomy (Shalev et al. 1993), as well as in patients who have had intensive care management (usually with mechanical ventilation) of adult respiratory distress syndrome (Schelling et al., 1998). Common to most of these patients was the discrepancy between physical recovery on the one hand and poor psychological recovery and an avoidance of medical care on the other hand.

Unresponsiveness to seemingly adequate medical treatment together with persistence of symptoms and prolonged disability, as well as noncompliance in patients critically dependent on their medication, should alert the doctor to the possibility of a comorbid mental disorder. The failure of many successfully treated post–coronary artery bypass patients and postchemotherapy and postirradiation lymphoma patients to return to their former life-styles is well documented (Philip et al., 1981; Lloyd and Cawly, 1983; Delvin et al., 1987). It seems extremely likely that at least some of these patients are suffering from PTSD. Similarly, the noncompliance in taking immunosuppression medication (tacrolimus) of some juvenile liver transplant recipients has been attributed to PTSD with characteristic avoidance behavior (Shemesh et al., 2000). Once correctly diagnosed, such patients may receive substantial relief of their incapacitating symptoms through psychotherapy.

Among the cardinal signs that may help us recognize PTSD in medical patients are (after Shalev et al., 1993):

1. A history of a discrete medical/surgical event that was accompanied by an overwhelming experience of threat, pain, loss of control, or humiliation.
2. Unexplained delay in recovery and rehabilitation.
3. Persistent and distressing preoccupation with the illness, or the opposite, denying its consequences by disregarding advised limitations and engaging in life-threatening behavior (illustrated by the patient who, following a recent heart attack, insists on running up stairs).
4. Intrusive and distressing recollections of the event.
5. A persistent sense of threat to life unjustified by the medical condition.
6. Avoidance of medical care due to apprehension or denial of illness, or anxiety experienced on follow-up visits.
7. Loss of interest in previously enjoyable activities.
8. Nervousness, irritability, outbursts of anger, exaggerated startle response, and difficulty in concentrating.
9. Difficulty in falling or staying asleep, or frequent nightmares.

Management of Posttraumatic Stress Disorder

The considerable importance of doctors being alert to the possible existence of PTSD in medical patients coupled with the tendency of these patients to deliberately avoid medical contact may require that the doctor's concern be conveyed to the family (or significant other) in order to plan an effective intervention strategy. While clearly patients cannot be coerced into a treatment program, particularly of the kind needed here, this is one situation where the caring physician may need to initiate family pressure.

Management of PTSD usually requires the attentions of an experienced therapist. The generally poor outcome is hinted at by a large cross-sectional study in the United States which found that over a third of sufferers continued to satisfy the criteria for a diagnosis of PTSD six years after diagnosis (Kessler et al., 1995). The difficulty mentioned of avoidance of medical intervention may in part account for a significant number of patients who resist consulting a doctor and who therefore receive only partial treatment or even none at all. An additional problem with these patients is their tendency to suicide in the chronic situation (Amir et al., 1999).

A systematic review of 17 controlled trials of psychological treatment for 690 PTSD patients found that psychological treatment was associated with a greater improvement in treatment outcome as compared to supportive management or no intervention (Sherman, 1998). Ideally, patients with acute stress disorder should be actively treated with cognitive–behavioral therapy (CBT). Bryant et al. (1998) treated 24 subjects with acute stress disorder with five sessions of either CBT or supportive counseling within two weeks of their trauma. Fewer participants in CBT (8%) than in the counseling (83%) met criteria for PTSD following the interventions. Similarly, there were fewer cases of PTSD from the CBT group (17%) than from the counseling group (67%) six months after trauma. In addition, CBT has been shown to produce sustained improvement in sexually abused children suffering PTSD over a two-year follow-up period (Deblinger et al., 1999).

REFERENCES

Alter CL, Pelcovitz D, Axelrod A, et al. (1996). Identification of PTSD in cancer survivors. Psychosomatics 37:137–143.

American Psychiatric Association (1987). Diagnostic and Statistical Manual of Mental Disorders, 3rd ed, (DSM-IIIR). Washington, DC: Author.

American Psychiatric Association (1994). Diagnostic and Statistical Manual of Mental Disorders, 4th edition (DSM-IV). Washington, DC: Author.

Amir M, Kaplan Z, Efroni R, et al. (1999). Suicide risk and coping styles in posttraumatic stress disorder patients. Psychother Psychosom 68:76–81.

Bennett P, Brooke S (1999). Intrusive memories, post-traumatic stress disorder and myocardial infarction. Br J Clin Psychol 38:411–416.

Bowles SV, James LC, Solursh DS, et al. (2000). Acute and post-traumatic stress disorder after spontaneous abortion. Am Fam Physician 61:1689–1696.

Brody DS (1980). Physician recognition of behavioral, psychological and social aspects of medical care. Arch Int Med 140:1286–1289.

Butler RW, Rizzi LP, Handwerger BA (1996). Brief report: the assessment of posttraumatic stress disorder in pediatric cancer patients and survivors. J Pediatr Psychol 21: 499–504.

Deblinger E, Steer RA, Lippmann J (1999). Two-year follow-up study of cognitive behavioral therapy for sexually abused children suffering post-traumatic stress symptoms. Child Abuse Negl 23:1371–1378.

Delvin J, Maguire P, Phillips P, et al. (1987). Psychological problems associated with diagnosis and treatment of lymphomas. Br Med J 295:955–957.

Deter HC (1986). Cost–benefit analysis of psychosomatic therapy in asthma. J Psychosom Res 30:173–182.

Fisch RZ, Tadmor O (1989). Iatrogenic post-traumatic stress disorder [letter]. Lancet 2:1397.

Fisher JV (1978). What the family physician expects from the psychiatrist. Psychosomatics 19:523–527.

Fleet RP, Dupuis G, Marchand A, et al. (1996). Panic disorder in emergency department chest pain patients: prevalence, comorbidity, suicidal ideation, and physician recognition. Am J Med 101:371–380.

Friedman CP, Cohen-Cole SA (1981). The structure of internists' attitudes towards psychosocial factors in patient care. Gen Hosp Psychiatry 3:205–212.

Garfinkel SK, Kesten K, Chapman KR, et al. (1992). Physiological and nonphysiological determinants of aerobic fitness in mild to moderate asthma. Am Rev Respir Dis 145:741–745 [published erratum appears in Am Rev Respir Dis 1992; 146:269].

Goldberg D, Steele JJ, Johnson A, et al. (1982). Ability of primary care physicians to make accurate ratings of psychiatric symptoms. Arch Gen Psychiatry 39:829–833.

Green BL, Grace MC, Lindy JD, et al. (1990). Risk factors for PTSD and other diagnoses in a general sample of Vietnam veterans. Am J Psychiatry 147:729–733.

Greenhill M, Kilgore S (1950). Principles of methodology in teaching the psychiatric approach to medical house-officers. Psychosom Med 12:38–48.

Hyams L, Green ME, Maar E, et al. (1976). Varied needs of primary physicians for psychiatric resources. Psychosomatics 12:36–45.

Kantor SM, Griner PF (1981). Educational needs in general internal medicine as perceived by prior residents. J Med Educ 56:748–756.

Kelly B, Raphael B, Judd F, et al. (1998). Posttraumatic stress disorder in response to HIV infection. Gen Hosp Psychiatry 20:345–352.

Kessler RC, Sonnega A, Bromet E, et al. (1995). Posttraumatic stress disorder in the national comorbidity survey. Arch Gen Psychiatry 52:1048–1060.

Knights EB, Folstein MF (1977). Unsuspected emotional and cognitive disturbance in medical patients. Ann Intern Med 87:723–724.

Kurtz I, Garb R, David D (1988). Post-traumatic stress disorder following myocardial infarction. Gen Hosp Psychiatry 10:169–176.

Kurtz I, Shabtai H, Solomon Z, et al. (1994). Post-traumatic stress disorder in myocardial infarction patients: prevalence study. Isr J Psychiatry Relat Sci 31:48–56.

Lehrer PM, Sargunaraj D, Hochron S (1992). Psychological approaches to the treatment of asthma. J Consult Clin Psychol 60:639–643.

Lloyd GG, Cawly RH (1983). Psychological symptoms after myocardial infarction. Br J Psychiatry 142:120–125.

Melmed RN, Roth D, Edelstein E (1990). Symptom anticipation and the learned visceral response: a major neglected determinant of morbidity in functional and organic disorders. Isr J Med Sci 26:43–46.

Moffic HS, Paykel ES (1975). Depression in medical inpatients. Br J Psychiatry 126:346–353.

Mosconi P, Meyerowitz BE, Liberati MC, et al. (1991). Disclosure of breast cancer diagnosis: patient and physician reports. Ann Oncol 2:273–280.

Pelcovitz D, Goldenberg B, Kaplan S, et al. (1996). Posttraumatic stress disorder in mothers of pediatric cancer survivors. Psychosomatics 37:116–126.

Philip AE, Cay EL, Stuckey NH, et al. (1981). Multiple predictors and multiple outcomes after myocardial infarction. J Psychosom Res 25:137–141.

Schelling G, Stoll C, Haller M, et al. (1998). Health-related quality of life and posttraumatic stress disorder in survivors of the acute respiratory distress syndrome. Crit Care Med 26: 651–659.

Schnall PL, Pieper C, Schwartz JE, et al. (1990). The relationship between 'job strain', workplace diastolic blood pressure, and left ventricular mass index. JAMA 263:1929–1935.

Schwab JJ (1982). Psychiatric illness in medical patients: why it goes undiagnosed. Psychosomatics 23:225–232.

Shalev AY, Schreiber S, Galai T, et al. (1993). Post-traumatic stress disorder following medical events. Br J Psychol 32:247–253.

Shemesh E, Lurie S, Stuber ML, et al. (2000). A pilot study of posttraumatic stress and nonadherence in pediatric liver transplant recipients. Pediatrics 105:E29.

Sherman JJ (1998). Effects of psychotherapeutic treatments for PTSD: a meta-analysis of controlled clinical trails. J Trauma Stress 11:413–436.

Smith MY, Redd WH, Peyser C, et al. (1999). Post-traumatic stress disorder in cancer: a review. Psychooncology 8:521–537.

Smith TJ, Swisher K (1998). Telling the truth about terminal cancer. JAMA 279:1746–1748.

Support principal investigators (1995). A controlled trial to improve care for seriously ill hospitalized patients. JAMA 274:1591–1598.

Surbone A (1992). Truth telling to the patient. JAMA 268:1661–1662.

Surbone A (1994a). More on euthanasia [letter]. Ann Oncol 5:378–379.

Surbone A (1994b). Informed consent and truth in medicine. Eur J Cancer 30A:2189.

Thompson TL, Stoudemire A, Mitchell WD (1982). Under-recognition of patients' psychosocial problems by internists. Psychosom Med 44:127. Abstract.

Weissberg M (1990). The meagerness of physicians' training in emergency psychiatric intervention. Acad Med 65:747–750.

Weissberg MP (1991). Emergency psychiatry: a critical educational omission [editorial]. Ann Intern Med 114:246–247.

Yu BH, Dimsdale JE (1999). Posttraumatic stress disorder in patients with burn injuries. J Burn Care Rahabil 20:426–433; discussion 422–425.

Chapter

4

THE KEY QUESTION IN CLINICAL PRACTICE: WHO CONTROLS WHAT?

If I had to pinpoint the psychological concept with the most relevance and utility in medical practice, my choice would unquestionably be a proper understanding of control and its meaning in the clinical context. Like health, control is one of those fundamental conditions that is naturally so taken for granted that its substantial importance to any individual is defined almost solely by its absence. Problems of control are encountered by all practitioners of medicine, particularly as they relate to the doctor–patient relationship. Many of the worst shortcomings in patient management, in my experience, derive from an ignorance of this important issue. In the context of this discussion, "control" encompasses people's *feelings of control* over their own emotional and physical integrity as well as the external world. The *Oxford English Dictionary* defines control as "the fact of controlling or of checking and directing action; the function or power of directing and regulating; domination, command, sway."

Control may be perceived as a multilayered process, with each layer relating to different facets of our social and personal worlds. If we view it as a series of concentric circles, the outermost layer would comprise the general society in which we live; then our work and less intimate social interactions, then our more intimate social and family network; the next layer would include associations of increasing intimacy, with a marriage partner, constant companion, children, or parents, for example; and in the center, our perceptions and feelings about ourselves. The layers are interdependent, so that a serious disturbance at one level will reverberate through the rest. The sense of loss of control at any level will usually generate or increase anxiety, or it will give the individual a feeling of being stressed. Viewed in this context, the development of a disease or symptom may be an unexpected and sharp reminder that ultimately our health is mostly not directly under our own control.

THE IMPORTANCE OF CONTROL

The emotional impact of symptoms or disease appears to be strongly influenced by the patient's sense of control—or loss thereof—while experiencing the symptom. This notion has received substantial support from experiments in which potentially aversion-inducing stimuli were shown to be less threatening in situations where subjects felt that they had some measure of control (Pervin, 1963; Corah and Boffa, 1970; Staub et al., 1971; Glass and Singer, 1972). As Lefcourt (1973) claimed, "The perception of control would seem to be a common predictor of the response to aversive events regardless of species . . . the sense of control, the illusion that one can exercise personal choice, has a definite and positive role in sustaining life."

Control has been shown to be important in clinical and laboratory settings for both acute and chronic pain (Thompson, 1981; Chapman and Turner, 1986). Pain management—in particular, the inadequate treatment of pain—remains a vexing issue in the care of hospitalized patients (Marks and Sachar, 1973; Cohen, 1980). The system of patient-controlled analgesia (PCA) for the management of postoperative pain was introduced by Sechzer (1968), who observed that *patients decreased their demands for analgesics as the pain intensity decreased.* An instrument was then developed for the convenient administration of intravenous narcotics when the patient activated a button, in this way transferring the control of analgesic administration to the patient. The results of prospective, randomized trials during the 1990s point to several advantages of PCA over conventional analgesia in the early postoperative period. Although PCA does not always produce better pain relief, the reported benefits include less sedation, lower levels of narcotic consumption, fewer postoperative complications, and greater patient satisfaction (Smythe, 1992). These benefits have not all been supported by controlled trials, but PCA has, for example, been successfully used in the management of postoperative pain, following bone marrow transplantation (Hill et al., 1990; Zucker et al., 1998), and in cancer patients. In chronic cancer pain sufferers the use of this system was associated with a decrease in anxiety, reduced dependence on caregivers and sedation, and an increase in mobility (Kerr et al., 1988; Swanson et al., 1989). The findings have countered fears of addiction-inducing behavior and have also highlighted the substantial importance of control for patients and the extent to which it may influence pain perception.

The central role of feelings of loss of control in aggravating and perpetuating disease states is dramatically illustrated by the following case history.

CASE REPORT: ASTHMA OUT OF CONTROL

A 60-year-old woman with untreated chronic lymphocytic leukemia (mean total white blood cell count around 12,000 cells/mm^3) was referred for treatment of intractable asthma, which over the preceding four years had resulted in 34 hospital admissions in status asthmaticus as well as numerous emergency room visits for severe asthma attacks. With a past history of allergic bronchitis and rhinitis, her asthma had been of sufficient severity to warrant continuous steroid treatment for about 20 years and the patient showed clear clinical signs of iatrogenic Cushing's disease, including the typical facies, fragile atrophic skin, and marked osteoporosis with associated back pain. During the course of these four very difficult years the patient had been given the complete range of conventional medications used to treat asthma, including high doses of steroids. In addition, she had received numerous courses of broad-spectrum antibiotics during her hospital admissions, including a course of intravenous amphotericin B for a suspected monilia infection of the bronchi during one severe attack of asthma. She also underwent an extended trial during these four years of a salicylate-free diet, which had no impact on the course of her illness. The patient was referred for consultation and treatment at a point when the treating physicians felt that they had exhausted every therapeutic option and were at a loss to know how to proceed. There was considerable concern about the persistent and intractable course the asthma was following.

The patient readily conceded that she felt desperate about her condition and was very willing to try a program of deep relaxation exercises. She denied any other source of pressure or worry and regarded her family as being extremely supportive, an impression which was shared by the medical staff. The program of exercises invoked deep relaxation with the suggestion that she focus only on feelings of increased control during the relaxed state (see Chapter 19). No mention was made at any time about her breathing difficulties or her asthma attacks. Following a course of about six weekly meetings, she was given a tape made during one of the exercises and she then practiced independently. Occasional meetings for a follow-up report and reinforcement exercise were then held over a four-month period, but from the time of her first meeting until her death seven years later from a cerebrovascular accident, she was never admitted again to a hospital because of an asthma attack. Her emergency room visits gradually decreased too, and after about four months from the start of the program there were no further visits because of the asthma. Subsequently, her asthma remained well controlled on more modest doses of prednisone.

THE MAIN ASPECTS OF CONTROL
IN CLINICAL PRACTICE

We will consider in more detail the following aspects of control, all of which are important in clinical practice:

1. The concept of "locus of control," a component of personality, which helps define a subject's vulnerability to emotional pressure or stress in a particular clinical situation.
2. The sense of control, or lack of it, that patients may experience in the clinical context.
3. The notion of control in the doctor–patient relationship and its function in the unwritten "therapeutic contract."

Locus of Control

The locus of control in this context refers to a personality trait that contributes to a person's style in dealing with the environment (Rotter, 1966). An individual with an *internal locus of control* feels largely in control of herself or himself and the environment; that is, the person's own personal characteristics or behavior play a major role in influencing events important in her or his life. An individual with an *external locus of control* feels that the things that happen to him or her are controlled by unpredictable external forces which may be called fate, luck, or chance.

Of particular interest is the observation that individuals with an internal locus of control have fewer psychosomatic symptoms and are better at withstanding the stress of life events than are externally oriented persons (Hersch and Scheibe, 1967; Phares et al., 1968; Harrow and Ferrante, 1969). In a study of 116 adult outpatients with chronic anxiety disorder, those with an external locus of control were more depressed and had more severe anxiety, fatigue, and agoraphobia than those with an internal locus of control (Hoehn-Saric and McLeod, 1985). The former group also rated themselves as being more symptomatic than did the latter. In another study the effectiveness of PCA was found to correlate with the patient's locus of control (Johnson et al., 1989). An internal locus of control was predictive of increased satisfaction with PCA and lower pain scores. Furthermore, the greater prevalence of emotional and physical ill health (Strickland, 1978) in nonprofessionals (Ryckman and Malikiosi, 1974) and in the socioeconomically deprived has been attributed in part to the greater prevalence of an external locus of control among this population group (Husaini and Neff, 1981). This fundamental difference in coping styles between haves and have-nots, which may be an important contributor to the health gradient observed between these groups, is discussed in detail in Chapter 5.

Coping with and managing chronic diseases may similarly be affected by the patient's locus of control. Thus, among 312 adults with insulin-dependent diabetes mellitus, much more favorable metabolic control was observed in those patients with a strong internal locus of control (Stenstroem et al., 1998). Conversely, in a study of children, poor metabolic control and more hospitalizations were observed in boys with greater external locus of control (Lernmark et al., 1996).

While this does not suggest that locus of control is the sole factor influencing patient compliance and successful coping in a chronic disease such as diabetes mellitus, it does indicate that it may be a significant factor. Factors such as social support, however, are also of considerable importance (Tillotson and Smith, 1996; Aalto et al., 1997). A strong internal locus of control is considered a favorable trait in dealing with a broad variety of stressors, but an exaggerated sense of control, sometimes expressed as an exaggerated sense of responsibility, may create tensions that lead to a pain syndrome such as headache (Shulman, 1989) (see Chapter 10).

The way in which people relate to the environment may also be expected to influence their attitudes to the content and style of medical management. Thus, externally oriented patients are said to be amenable to a more directed treatment approach in which they adopt a passive attitude, and they may be more willing to accept treatment with medication. Conversely, it is claimed that patients with an internal locus of control prefer to play an active role in the therapeutic program (Frank et al., 1978). This does not mean that because a patient is assessed as having an external locus of control, the physician should adopt a more directive approach. Rather, it is prudent to assume that all symptomatic patients are struggling to maintain or regain their sense of control, regardless of where their locus of control may be. Accordingly, the therapeutic program must be directed toward helping patients to accomplish this and hence to achieve a sense of self-confidence in their ability to cope with their symptoms or disabilities. By educating patients to understand and manage their symptoms as independently and with as little anxiety as possible, the physician strives in the therapeutic encounter to make their orientation more "internal" and less "external." The objective is to reinforce those qualities that strengthen patients' feelings of self-reliance and help dispel feelings of dependency on the doctor and on medical institutions.

Control in the Clinical Context

Loss of control by patients is illustrated in the following three representative predicaments.

1. The patient is confronted by a situation that is, or is perceived to be, life-threatening. This could be a cardiac arrest, during which consciousness may be fully maintained for up to 15 or 20 seconds, or a diagnosis of cancer. In many cases, the gravity of the situation is reinforced by the demeanor of the attending physician, which may be one of unconcealed distress. Given the circumstances, the physician's response may be appropriate, but it will nevertheless serve to heighten the patient's apprehension. One might also argue that the patient's situation is so harsh, with death staring him in the face, that intense anxiety is the most normal response.

Receiving the diagnosis of a potentially fatal disease represents the ultimate loss of control, and strong emotional reactions by patients are predictable. Even in such life-threatening situations, however, the physician's appreciation of the importance of control may help the patients deal with the situation. Any distressed patient who knows that the physician truly understands the basis of her distress usually finds this helpful in dealing with the distress.

2. Patient may feel a loss of control when experiencing certain symptoms. It should be stressed that *any* symptom may be the precipitating experience. The idea that intense emotional reactions occur only in response to severe symptoms or life-threatening illness is misleading. The symptom may be trivial yet the emotional reaction severe—so severe as to even take the form of a posttraumatic stress disorder (Chapter 3).

Symptoms such as pain, dizziness, or palpitations may or may not have an organic basis, but if they are functional, the physician's verdict of "no organic disease" does not necessarily allay the patient's anxiety or symptoms. This is because the symptom experienced feels so real to the patient that dismissal of serious disease without further discussion of the likely cause of the symptom will not allay his anxiety. Nor is it helpful to explain that the symptom results simply from anxiety, as most patients are themselves able to make the link between the distress ascribed to the physical symptom and the presence of a background state of tension. This is the classical predicament of patients suffering from panic disorder: they rush to the emergency room because of the intense anxiety they feel with the symptom, whether it be chest pain, palpitations, or breathlessness, only to receive a negative evaluation. They are often informed by the treating physician that nothing has been found and that they should go home and "forget about it," advice that will tend to arouse antagonism and maybe even anger since, from the patient's point of view, the doctor has missed the point completely by not adequately explaining the symptom.

Recurrent symptoms such as finger pallor and numbness in Raynaud's disease, morning stiffness and joint pain in rheumatoid arthritis, or dyspnea in asthma may induce feelings of loss of control. This tends to produce anxiety and apprehension about the prospect of further attacks, leading to a state of anticipatory anxiety or symptom anticipation. Patients in whom the feeling of losing control is pronounced typically respond poorly to conventional medication and are often chronically dissatisfied with their management.

3. In some patients symptoms represent the somatic expression of an unrecognized or perhaps inadequately treated state of anxiety or depression. Its origin may be traceable to a stressful event or period, such as a sudden feeling of faintness or weakness, the sudden bleeding caused by an accidental abortion or after a therapeutic abortion (Neugebauer et al., 1992; Zolese and Blacker, 1992), or the nursing of a dying parent. Such an event may initiate a state of emotional distress that becomes progressively worse with time. If their emotional problems do not receive proper attention, the patients continue to suffer and are obliged to invest more and more emotional energy in maintaining their normal daily routine.

Patients' emotional responses to the development of symptoms are determined largely by their severity—that is, how much suffering they cause—and how they are interpreted by the sufferer—that is, whether they arouse fears of serious disease, disability, or death. The issue is further complicated by the fact that the severity of the symptom is frequently influenced by the patient's interpretation. Many patients experience considerably more anxiety over their symptoms than is objectively warranted. Some patients can independently describe their distress as resulting from a feeling of loss of control or are receptive to the physician's suggestion that their distress is rooted in a feeling of having lost control at the time of the symptoms.

Frequency of attacks is another factor in determining patients' sense of control. The more frequent the attacks of pain (as with headaches or irritable bowel syndrome), dyspnea (as in asthma), morning stiffness (as in rheumatoid arthritis), digital vasospasm (Raynaud's phenomenon), or other symptoms, the more the feeling of loss of control is reinforced. It is probably for this reason that repeated attacks of any symptoms often are associated in time with an increase in their intensity. Furthermore, the shorter the interval between attacks, the more pronounced is this tendency. A typical sequence in such cases, therefore, is apprehension of serious illness while experiencing a symptom, feeling of loss of control, anxiety around the possibility of further attacks (anticipatory anxiety), increase in the frequency of attacks, reinforced feelings of loss of control, increase in the intensity of the attacks, reinforced feelings of loss of control, increased anxiety, more frequent and more intense symptoms, and so on.

To put things in perspective, however, it should be emphasized that most patients take their illness fairly well, cope with the attendant disappointments and frustrations, and recover without physical and emotional scars. Moreover, even in tertiary medical referral centers, most consultations are for medical problems that are neither life-threatening nor crippling. It is not for the management of such patients that my comments on control are intended. The concepts developed in this chapter are meant to be applied to those suffering and dissatisfied patients who remain symptomatic despite apparently adequate treatment or after their practitioner's extensive investigation and reassurance they have no disease. Focusing on feelings of control in such patients helps us to appreciate an important determinant of the ability to cope with ill health or symptoms of any kind. Understanding this and responding appropriately to it are important in the management of the problem. The principles elaborated in Chapters 18 and 19 were developed especially to strengthen feelings of control in such patients.

The Physician's Feeling of Control and the Therapeutic Contract

Few professions allow one as direct access to people's private worlds as does medicine. Problems of health often generate feelings of vulnerability that increase a patient's dependence on the treating physician. Such patients may regress to an attitude toward the doctor reminiscent of parent–child relationships, with feelings of passivity on the patient's part. The physician's role in Western medicine has traditionally been an authoritarian one. The doctor–patient relationship is therefore likely to compound the patients' feelings of loss of control if the doctor's attitude is paternalistic or autocratic. Where the illness is short-lived this may not matter, but in the patients who most concern us here, the issue gains considerable importance.

Things are happening to most patients over which they have no control. Up to the time of the illness, they have lived independently, choosing their activities and acquaintances according to inclination. Now they depend on external support. They must accommodate themselves to doctors, nurses, physiotherapists, hospital clerks, secretaries, medications, dialysis, and so on. A sensitive doctor can help patients cope with these unwelcome feelings of dependence by treating them as active partners in the planning and execution of whatever has to be done. The situation clearly demands a certain amount of role playing and the control which patients are permitted to exercise may be illusory, at least to some extent. Nevertheless, its importance to the patient should not be underestimated. Restoring to the patient even a modest level of perceived control is almost invariably the first step in the alleviation or resolution of any condition of stress.

The point is well illustrated by the case of a liaison psychiatrist who was called to advise on the management of a patient admitted to the medical wards in advanced cardiac failure. The patient, described by the ward staff as "totally uncooperative," was refusing to take his medication as instructed. On observing the patient's state of complete dependence, the psychiatrist advised that the patient be given all his tablets each morning with the suggestion that he divide the doses during the day at his own convenience. The patient's attitude and compliance changed immediately. Having been permitted to exercise even such minimal autonomy, he felt he was partly in control of his life once again.

HOW TO IDENTIFY LOSS OF CONTROL

In all branches of clinical practice, each major disorder has easily recognizable aspects. Thus even the inexperienced practitioner can recognize a condition, but it takes more experience and clinical astuteness to recognize the more subtle, partial, or mixed presentations. Psychophysiological problems in clinical practice may appear even more complicated because of the diversity of personalities and apparently limitless number of individual characteristics that can influence a person's emotional response to illness. In a patient who is unresponsive to what one considers adequate therapy, the clinician's predicament may be expressed as follows: does persistence or exacerbation of symptoms represent intractability and progression of the pathological process underlying the disorder, or does it represent the interplay of emotional distress with the underlying disorder?

The population we are considering consists of those patients in whom an emotional reaction causes the physical symptoms or contributes significantly to their intensification. These patients may be identified both by the clinical context of their disorder and by a characteristic thought process that will be described below. The natural history of their medical state has the following typical patterns, a course which should arouse the suspicion of emotional causation:

1. Symptoms that prove intractable and unresponsive to apparently adequate anagement.
2. Suffering over a long period that cannot be accurately diagnosed despite extensive investigation.
3. Chronic or recurrent pain syndromes that are often given diagnostic labels such as fibrositis, lower back pain, osteoporosis, osteoarthritis, and cholelithiasis.

The thesis offered here is that clinical conditions may be perpetuated or exacerbated by the attendant emotional reaction even though the patients do not necessarily suffer from specific psychopathology. Indeed, a number of studies have failed to demonstrate a difference in the psychopathology of patients suffering from certain chronic pain syndromes, regardless of whether they are functional or organic in origin (Castelnuovo-Tedesco and Krout, 1970; Woodforde and Merskey, 1972; Sternbach et al., 1973; Raymer et al., 1984).

In the clinical circumstances just described, the recognition of patients who have lost control is considerably aided by the identification of two characteristic responses:

1. A marked loss of self confidence, to the extent that the loss of self-confidence and the loss of control are wholly interchangeable concepts. Thus, if a patient talks about losing self-confidence, he or she will always admit to feeling as well a loss of control, and vice versa. The two concepts are tightly integrated in practice and the presence of one indicates the presence of the other.
2. A typical pattern of thought called "intrusive," "obsessive," or "repetitive" thinking.

Intrusive thinking has been defined as "repetitive, unwanted, intrusive thoughts of internal origin" (Rachman and de Silva, 1978). Intrusive thoughts are a normal occurrence and most people are likely to experience them from time to time (Freeston et al., 1994). Their content in normal people may not differ from that in obsessional individuals who are seeking psychiatric help for the problem (Rachman and de Silva, 1978), although there is a tendency in the psychology literature to distinguish between worry, more typical of an anxiety state, and obsessive intrusive thoughts, which typify obsessive-compulsive disorder (Langlois et al., 2000). The essential differences lie in the frequency, duration, intensity, and consequences of the thoughts. In obsessional patients, the intrusive thinking causes marked anxiety. They recognize their preoccupations as being beyond their control and not the kinds of thoughts they would expect to have (American Psychiatric Association, 1994).

Intrusive thinking was first described by Freud and Breuer in neurotic patients as a process reflecting previous traumatic experiences. Subsequent authors have confirmed this association with traumatic and stressful experiences of various kinds (Horowitz, 1975; Rachman, 1980; Horowitz et al., 1983), and especially with posttraumatic stress disorder (see Chapter 3). A special questionnaire, "The Impact of Event Scale", was developed to evaluate both intrusion and avoidance as measures of a stress response (Horowitz et al., 1979). The intrusive thinking of patients typically seen in psychiatric clinics, unlike that of patients typically seen in medical clinics, is often manifested as well in nightmares, repetitive involuntary attacks of emotion, and compulsive behavior such as repeated hand washing or checking to see whether a particular door is locked, expressions of posttraumatic stress disorder and obsessive-compulsive behavior, respectively (American Psychiatric Association, 1994). In nonpsychiatric patients, the process usually is less intense and is quickly forgotten with effective reassurance or resolution of the underlying problem. In the medical clinic the presence of intrusive thinking, nevertheless, gives the physician a clear indication of psychological distress in the patient.

The main advantages of inquiring about both loss of self-confidence and intrusive thinking is that the patient does not immediately understand the significance of the question and seldom if ever becomes evasive or defensive about the answer, as happens with many patients when asked directly about their emotional state. Furthermore, a high level of intrusivity and/or loss of self-confidence alerts the physician to the certain presence of psychological distress in the patient, regardless of any denials.

In persistently suffering patients the tendency toward intrusive thinking may be pronounced, occupying a considerable part of their waking hours. This can be determined simply by asking patients how much of their undistracted or free time during the day—when they are *not* busy with specific activities—they spend thinking or worrying about their symptoms. A widespread misconception in clinical practice holds that distractibility can distinguish psychophysiologically induced, that is, functional, symptoms, especially pain, from symptoms of organic origin. This is incorrect. Any symptom from any cause, including pain from cancer or from surgery, may be alleviated or eliminated by distraction.

The idea is to obtain an approximate indication of the intrusive thinking, expressed as a percentage. Almost all patients in significant distress give figures ranging from 50% to 100%. However, from a systematic evaluation of 100 consecutive patients in a cardiac outpatient clinic, it appears that any figure above 20% is associated with clinically significant anxiety or depression (Yatziv and Melmed, 1998), suggesting that the phenomenon is much more prevalent in the medical clinic than has been appreciated. In this study the presence of intrusivity was checked against the Zung Anxiety and Depression questionnaires. In a study of 283 women diagnosed with early stage breast cancer, Baider and Kaplan De-Nour (1997) found a strong relationship between thought intrusion and psychological distress, and they suggested that the phenomenon be regarded as indicative of an adjustment disorder with intrusive symptoms.

RELIGION AND CONTROL

While the concepts of control and locus of control discussed above appear to have considerable validity in the clinical context, religious beliefs must also be mentioned as a relevant influence in clinical practice. On the face of it, belief in the "almighty" or "a higher power" clearly represents the giving up of control in a very substantial way to a considerable force distinct from oneself. In a sense it is the ultimate external locus of control state because a truly religious person would believe that all aspects of her or his existence and fate are ordained by an external, supernatural power. Yet many studies of stress or suffering have found that religion, particularly as it pertains to intrinsic spiritual beliefs and/or personal devotion, has a significant buffering effect (Miller et al., 1997; Kendler et al., 1999). This may express itself, for instance, as improved life satisfaction (Levine et al., 1995; Ayele et al., 1999), less depression or more rapid recovery from depression in old age (Wolinsky et al., 1996; Braam et al., 1997; Koenig et al., 1998), or in elderly patients with cancer (Fehring et al., 1997). Shams and Jackson (1993) found that religious conviction buffered the negative psychological impact of unemployment.

These studies suggest that a profound belief in an all-powerful and benevolent force does in fact constitute a significant exception to the general rule of enhanced emotional vulnerability associated with an external locus of control. Levine et al. (1995) examined the impact of religious belief on health status and life satisfaction among African-Americans, a group suggested to be especially vulnerable to the impact of stress through widespread socioeconomic hardship and a generally external locus of control (Husaini and Neff, 1981). They obtained their data from the National Survey of Black Americans, a nationally representative sample of blacks at least 18 years old. The findings showed a statistically significant positive effect of organizational religion on both health and life satisfaction, for nonorganizational religion on health, and for personal religion on life satisfaction. This association of religion on well-being was consistent over an extended range of ages from under 30 years to over 50 years.

REFERENCES

Alto AM, Uutela A, Aro AR (1997). Health related quality of life among insulin-dependent diabetics: disease-related and psychosocial correlates. Patient Educ Couns 30:215–225.

American Psychiatric Association (1994). Diagnostic and Statistical Manual of Mental Disorders, 4th ed. Washington, DC: Author.

Ayele H, Mulligan T, Gheorghiu S, et al. (1999). Religious activity improves life satisfaction for some physicians and older patients. J Am Geriatr Soc 47:453–455.

Baider L, Kaplan De-Nour A (1997). Psychological distress and intrusive thoughts in cancer patients. J Nerv Ment Dis 185:346–348.

Braam AW, Beekman AT, Van Tilburg TG, et al. (1997). Religious involvement and depression in older Dutch citizens. Soc Psychiatry Psychiatr Epidemiol 32:284–291.

Castelnuovo-Tedesco P, Krout BM (1970). Psychosomatic aspects of chronic pelvic pain. Int J Psychiatry Med 1:109–126.

Chapman CR, Turner JA (1986). Psychological control of acute pain in medical settings. J Pain Symptom Manage 1:9–20.

Cohen FL (1980). Postsurgical pain relief: patients' status and nurses' medication choices. Pain 9:265–274.

Corah N, Boffa J (1970). Perceived control, self-observation, and response to aversive stimulation. J Pers Soc Psychol 16:1–4.

Fehring RJ, Miller JF, Shaw C (1997). Spiritual well-being, religiosity, hope, depression, and other mood states in elderly people coping with cancer. Oncol Nurs Forum 24:663–671.

Frank JD, Hoehn-Saric R, Imber SD, et al. (1978). Effective Ingredients of Successful Psychotherapy. New York: Brunner-Mazel, pp 35–42.

Freeston MH, Gagnon F, Ladouceur R, et al. (1994). Health-related intrusive thoughts. J Psychosom Res 38:203–215.

Glass DC, Singer JE (1972). Behavioral aftereffects of unpredictable and uncontrollable aversive events. Am Scient 60:457–465.

Harrow M, Ferrante A (1969). Locus of control in psychiatric patients. J Consult Clin Psychol 33:582–589.

Hersch PD, Scheibe KE (1967). Reliability and validity of internal–external control as a personality dimension. J Consult Psychol 31:609–613.

Hill HF, Chapman CR, Kornell JA, et al. (1990). Self-administration of morphine in bone marrow transplant patients reduces drug requirements. Pain 40:121–129.

Hoehn-Saric R, McLeod DR (1985). Locus of control in chronic anxiety disorders. Acta Psychiatr Scand 72:529–535.

Horowitz MJ (1975). Intrusive and repetitive thoughts after experimental stress: a summary. Arch Gen Psychiatry 32:1457–1463.

Horowitz M, Wilner N, Alvarez W (1979). Impact of Event Scale: a measure of subjective stress. Psychosom Med 41:209–218.

Horowitz MJ, Simon N, Holden M, et al. (1983). The stressful impact of news of risk for premature heart disease. Psychosom Med 45:31–40.

Husaini BA, Neff JA (1981). Social class and depressive symptomatology: the role of life change events and locus of control. J Nerv Ment Dis 169:638–647.

Johnson LR, Magnani B, Chan V, et al. (1989). Modifiers of patient-controlled analgesia efficacy. 1. Locus of control. Pain 39:17–22.

Kendler KS, Gardner CO, Prescott CA (1999). Clarifying the relationship between religiosity and psychiatric illness: the impact of covariates and the specificity of buffering effects. Twin Res 2:137–144.

Kerr IG, Sone M, DeAngelis C, et al. (1988). Continuous narcotic infusion with patient controlled analgesia for chronic cancer pain in outpatients. Ann Intern Med 108:554–557.

Koenig HG, George LK, Peterson BL (1998). Religiosity and remission of depression in medically ill older patients. Am J Psychiatry 155:536–542.

Langlois F, Freeston MH, Ladouceur R (2000). Differences and similarities between obsessive intrusive thoughts and worry in a non-clinical population: study 1. Behav Res Ther 38:157–173.

Lefcourt HM (1973). The function of the illusions of control and freedom. Am Psychol 28:417–425.

Lernmark B, Dahlqvist G, Fransson P, et al. (1996). Relations between age, metabolic control, disease adjustment and psychological aspects in insulin-dependent diabetes mellitus. Acta Paediatr 85:818–824.

Levine JS, Chatters LM, Taylor RJ (1995). Religious effects on health status and life satisfaction among black Americans. J Gerontol B Psychol Sci Soc Sci 50:S154–S163.

Marks RM, Sachar EJ (1973). Undertreatment of medical inpatients with narcotic analgesics. Ann Intern Med 78:173–181.

Miller L, Warner V, Wickramaratne P, et al. (1997). Religiosity and depression: ten-year follow-up of depressed mothers and offspring. J Am Acad Child Adolesc Psychiatry 36:1416–1425.

Neugebauer R, Kline J, O'Conner P, et al. (1992). Depressive symptoms in women in the six months after miscarriage. Am J Obstet Gynecol 166:104–109.

Pervin LA (1963). The need to predict and control under conditions of threat. J. Personality 31:570–587.

Phares EJ, Ritchie DE, Davis WL (1968). Internal–external control and reaction to threat. J Pers Soc Psychol 10:402–405.

Rachman S (1980). Emotional processing. Behav Res Ther 18:51–60.

Rachman S, de Silva P (1978). Abnormal and normal obsessions. Behav Res Ther 16:233–248.

Raymer D, Weininger O, Hamilton JR (1984). Psychological problems in children with abdominal pain. Lancet 1:439–440.

Rotter JB (1966). Generalized expectancies for internal versus external control of reinforcement. Psychol Monograph 80 (Whole No. 609):1–28.

Ryckman RM, Malikiosi M (1974). Differences in locus of control orientations for members of selected occupations. Psychol Rep 34:1224–1226.

Sechzer PH (1968). Objective measurement of pain. Anesthesiology 29:209–210.

Shams M, Jackson PR (1994). The impact of unemployment on the psychological well-being of British Asians. Psychol Med 24:347–355.

Shulman BH (1989). Psychological factors affecting migraine. Clin J Pain 5:23–28.

Smythe M (1992). Patient-controlled analgesia: a review. Pharmacotherapy 12(2):132–143.

Staub E, Tursky B, Schwartz GE (1971). Self-control and predictability: their effects on reactions to aversive stimulation. J Pers Soc Psychol 18:157–162.

Stenstroem U, Wikby A, Andersson P-O, et al. (1998). Relationship between locus of control beliefs and metabolic control in insulin-dependent diabetes mellitus. Br J Health Psychol 3:15–25.

Sternbach RA, Wolf SR, Murphy RW, et al. (1973). Traits of pain patients: the low back "loser." Psychosomatics 14:226–229.

Strickland BR (1978). Internal–external expectancies and health related behaviors. J Consult Clin Psychol 46:1192–1211.

Swanson G, Smith J, Bulich R, et al. (1989). Patient controlled analgesia for chronic cancer pain in the ambulatory setting: a report of 117 patients. J Clin Oncol 7(12): 1903–1908.

Thompson SC (1981). Will it hurt less if I can control it? A complex answer to a simple question. Psychol Bull 90:89–101.

Tillotson LM, Smith MS (1996). Locus of control, social support, and adherence to the diabetes regimen. Diabetes Educ 22:133–139.

Wolinsky FD, Stump TE (1996). Age and the sense of control among older adults. J Gerontol B Psychol Soc Sci 51:S217–S220.

Woodforde JM, Merskey H (1972). Personality traits of patients with chronic pain. J Psychosom Res 16:167–172.

Yatziv O, Melmed RN (1998). Unpublished observations.

Zolese G, Blacker CVR (1992). The psychological complications of therapeutic abortion. Br J Psychiatry 160:742–749.

Zucker TP, Flesche CW, Germing U, et al. (1998). Patient-controlled versus staff-controlled analgesia with pethidine after allogeneic bone marrow transplantation. Pain 75:305–312.

Chapter

5

STRESS: THE BROADER CONTEXT

This chapter examines processes that, as stressors, challenge the physical and psychological health of the individual. To the extent that stressful events often precede or accompany psychosomatic illness, it is helpful to understand which personal experiences tend to be widely regarded as stressful and why. We are now able to define those events in the lives of most people that, on the psychological level, are likely to be interpreted as stressful. Extensive research has helped elucidate the nature of stress and determine its biological impact. Questions about what constitutes a stressful experience and why it is stressful, and about the role of stress in the causation and natural history of disease, are among the issues considered here.

In addition to personal behavior and life-style, we consider socioeconomic factors that may buffer or aggravate stress and significantly influence health: income and the material environment, education, social support, employment, and so on. In industrialized countries we see consistently that socioeconomic inequalities parallel inequalities of health and that mortality from all causes increases progressively as one descends the social ladder (Acheson, 1999). Consequently, an awareness of the influence of social factors on health in general and disease outcome in particular helps provide a multidimensional perspective for the practitioner charged with the assessment and care of the individual patient.

Although some may find the grouping of issues presented here under the rubric of stress a too facile representation of complex topics, I believe that it does accurately reflect current understanding of the essence of the stress response as originally conceived by Selye (1946). Namely, multiple factors lead to a final common pathway of psychophysiological responses which, when sustained, will have a deleterious effect on the health of the individual. The behavioral responses to stress become a central issue in accounting for and in managing many of the injurious effects of chronic stress, so we consider these as well.

DEFINING STRESS AND DESCRIBING ITS CONSEQUENCES

The normal steady state of organ and tissue function is known as *homeostasis*, and any force that works to disturb homeostasis may be considered a *stressor*. Each organ and body system has its normal range of function, as well as the adaptive resources (i.e., reserve capacity) to restore homeostasis in the event of its being disturbed. A stressed state is likely to occur when an individual's adaptive resources are taxed or exceeded by the stressor.

On a day-to-day basis, the adverse circumstance, or stressor, may simply be described as "any [life] event that causes change or demands readjustment in one's normal routine" (Kobasa and Hilker, 1982). In the psychological sphere, the limits of functional normality may be difficult to determine, though a stressed state usually expresses itself clinically through negative thoughts and feelings. On a personal level, however, we may recognize not only that stress is part of our normal lives, but that for the most part we cope without undue mental or physical discomfort. Indeed, the manageable stresses of daily life may be extremely important for personal growth and the development of creative potential. In general, our powers of adaptation are well developed and the mental processes that govern our adaptability to emotionally uncomfortable or threatening events or situations may be considered analogous to the biological systems that help ensure our physical survival. In both situations, there is a measure of reserve function that enables us to respond to unusual demands, thus ensuring our adaptation and survival in extraordinary or stressful situations.

In recent years the concept of allostatic (adaptive) systems has been developed to describe body mechanisms that are activated especially in response to stressful situations that may, in varied ways, perturb body homeostasis (Sterling and Eyer, 1988). Examples of such stressors include noise, crowding, isolation, hunger, extremes of temperature, and infections (McEwen, 1998). The allostatic response to such situations includes activation of the sympathetic nervous system and the hypothalamic–pituitary–adrenal (HPA) axis, which in turn leads to the secretion of catecholamines from sympathetic nerves and the adrenal medulla as well as glucocorticoids from the adrenal cortex. In situations where the stressor is maintained (persistent noise, crowding, isolation, hunger, etc.) or frequently repeated (work stress), it is reckoned that over time, exposure to increased secretion of stress hormones may produce an allostatic load with pathophysiological consequences (McEwen and Stellar, 1993). Allostatic load refers to the cumulative, multisystem effects of repeated fluctuations of physiological and metabolic responses to stress that may predispose the organism to disease.

Positive and Negative Effects of Stress

Many people are aware of the role that stress can have in positively influencing performance of a particular task. This beneficial effect of stress appears to be most evident when we are well prepared for the task (usually mentally but also often physically) and especially when we have a sense of being firmly in control of its execution, through familiarity and practice. But in situations where the stress is sustained over a long period or is of unusual intensity, and especially where the stressful experience is associated with *feelings of loss of control*, the stress is likely to be manifested as tension, anxiety, depression, or panic (Dohrenwend and Dohrenwend, 1974).

In clinical medicine, stress is generally considered for its negative effects on the health of the individual. These effects may be clinically silent, as in hypertension, or they may be expressed as somatic symptoms. The spectrum of circumstances to be considered varies from the sustained negative influence of a socioeconomically disadvantaged life on the health of the individual to the precipitation of a health crisis by an identified stressor that is not necessarily remarkable in itself.

Socioeconomic Factors and Stress-Related Illness

For those with lives of unremitting stress, which in Western societies means especially the socioeconomically deprived population groups in large cities, morbidity is increased and life expectancy is reduced (Syme and Berkman, 1976; McCord and Freeman, 1990; Pappas et al., 1993). In particular, the relation between low income and poor health is well established (Lynch, 1996), and this generalization is valid even after the exclusion of suicide, homicide, and drug- and accident-related events, all of which are more prevalent in deprived communities.

Many factors have been considered in the attempt to explain these disturbing facts, and it is widely accepted that the causes are multifactorial. They include personality factors such as locus of control as well as social isolation, learned helplessness, unhealthy eating habits, smoking, inefficient use of medical services, and poor compliance in drug taking, to name but a few. Even if each of these factors proves to be significantly more prevalent among the socioeconom-ically deprived, however, it may be appropriate to apply Occam's Razor and re-gard sustained *stress* as the common element in this population. Many of the so-cial and personal factors listed above are thought to predispose the individual to a state of increased stress or to result from it. Thus, some people may take to ha-bitual smoking, excessive alcohol consumption, and drug abuse to reduce the sense of personal distress.

While most studies have tended to evaluate the relationship of socioeconomic status and health in a particular community at a particular moment in time, Lynch et al. (1997) addressed the impact of economic hardship (defined as a total house-hold income of less than 200% of the federal poverty level) over a 29-year pe-riod. Compared to subjects without economic hardship, those with economic hardship in 1965 (less than $6634 annually; 6982 respondents), 1974 (less than $11,000 annually; 4864 respondents), and 1983 (less than $20,356 annually; 1799 respondents) were much more likely to have difficulties in 1994 with activities of daily living such as cooking, shopping, and managing money; other indepen-dent activities such as walking, eating, dressing, and using the toilet; and clini-cal depression. The authors found little evidence of reverse causation, that is, that episodes of illness might have caused subsequent economic hardship (see below).

It has become apparent in recent years, however, that economic hardship per se, and the associations of hunger and want that this usually conjures up, cannot adequately explain the impact of social gradient on health and mortality within industrialized societies. This is because true hunger and more extreme degrees of physical deprivation resulting from poverty actually affect only a small sec-tor of the economically disadvantaged in industrialized countries.

To illustrate this point, note that although inadequate access of the socioeco-nomically deprived to satisfactory medical care could be one possible explana-tion of stress-related illness in the United States (Institute of Medicine, 1988), this does not appear to be universally true. In Britain, for example, the gap in disease outcome according to socioeconomic status appears to have widened over the last 30 years despite the establishment of the National Health Service, which was specifically created to respond to the needs of the socioeconomically de-prived (Blaxter, 1987). In addition, such patients may undergo more procedures and interventions than patients from higher socioeconomic groups, but with poorer outcome (Marmot and McDowall, 1986). It follows that the poorer out-come does not necessarily result from the lesser use of costly modern techniques of evaluation or treatment in this sector of the population.

Alter et al. (1999) studied the effects of socioeconomic status on access to in-vasive cardiac procedures and on mortality after myocardial infarction of 51,591 patients in Ontario, Canada. These patients, as Canadian citizens, have a health care plan that covers all medically necessary services without any user fee and is based on the principle of access according to need rather than income. It was found that, with respect to coronary angiography, increases in neighborhood income from the lowest to the highest quintile were associated with a 23% increase in rates of use and a 45% decrease in waiting times. The lowest quintile corresponded to a median personal income ranging from $12,508 to $17,930, whereas the highest quintile corresponded to a range of $26,300 to $44,409 (one Canadian dollar equivalent to 68 U.S. cents). There was a strong inverse relation between income and mortality at one year ($P < 0.001$), a fact which is likely to reflect the disproportionate number of patients with acute myocardial infarction in the lower income quintiles.

Although Canada's universal health insurance programs have promoted greater equity in access to medical care (Enterline et al., 1973), several studies have shown continuing income differences in the rates of use of specific services (Anderson et al., 1993; Katz and Hofer, 1994; McIsaac et al., 1997). The study by Alter et al. (1999) shows that these inequities persist for a cohort of persons who were hospitalized for the same condition and who should have been treated similarly. These authors emphasize that while access to coronary angiogram was strongly influenced by whether the index admission took place in or near a hospital with on-site facilities for invasive procedures, income-related differences in mortality were found within groups of hospitals with different types of on-site facilities.

The British civil service can be used to illustrate the same point. It has a strong hierarchical structure with four defined grades, professional and executive, administrative, clerical, and support staff, in descending order of seniority. Studies show that within this hierarchy, there is a clear stepwise gradient of mortality (North et al., 1993). As this is a population group that can in no way be considered to be economically impoverished, some other explanation must be sought. In the absence of material deprivation, one's position in a social hierarchy apparently may impose a degree of psychosocial deprivation and stress that can seriously damage health (Acheson, 1999). This implies that lack of control over one's work and life decisions may, over time, prove to be a significant stressor.

Two aspects of research in this field that warrant special consideration are the health implications of the number of years of formal education and in the role of social isolation in the predisposition to and outcome of disease states.

Formal education level as a risk factor for morbidity and mortality

The number of years of formal education has emerged, from numerous studies, as the most sensitive social indicator for determining both morbidity and mortality in a given population. This measure has a number of obvious advantages: it is quantitative, it is much more easily determined than any of the psychological constructs for which it may be a marker, and it is not affected by diseases that normally begin after age 25, as are parameters such as income, occupation, and many of the behaviors referred to as detrimental to health (Pincus, 1988). In relation to the central observation of a connection between mortality and socioeconomic status, the Adult Morbidity and Mortality Project in Tanzania has shown that those with eight years of education have half the mortality experienced by those who have four years (quoted by Acheson, 1999). In nonindustrialized countries, the implications of education are likely to extend beyond the individual's welfare, as indicated by the observation that the general educational level for women in developing countries has greater effects on family health than any other single factor (Caldwell, 1993). It is easier to intuitively understand how education influences population health and survival in nonindustrialized countries than the similar relationship observed in industrialized countries. In a study of 6321 adolescents aged 12 to 17 years, as the educational level of the responsible adult increased, cigarette smoking, sedentary life-style and insufficient consumption of fruits and vegetables decreased among the dependent adolescents (Lowry et al., 1996). This must mean that here too the impact of years of education on health cannot solely be due to economic deprivation.

Epidemiological studies in Britain (Marmot and McDowall, 1986; Blaxter, 1987), Italy (LaVecchia et al., 1987), and the United States (Liu et al., 1982: Pincus et al., 1987) indicate that the frequency of many common diseases—including back pain, arthritis, hypertension and other cardiovascular diseases, peptic ulcer, diabetes mellitus, and chronic lung disease—varies inversely with the number of years of formal education. Just how significant this factor might be is shown by the fact that the chance of developing any of these diseases increases from 6:1 to 3:1, or doubles, when the number of years of formal education drops from 12 to 9. This increase is not explained by age, sex, race, or smoking (Pincus et al., 1987). The severity of chronic, nonalcoholic liver disease has also been found to be similarly significantly related to years of education, patients with a more severe progression on average having fewer years of education (Davis et al., 1998). These studies support the contention that the level of formal education is correlated with higher incidence, or prevalence, of morbidity and mortality for many chronic diseases.

In three common diseases in particular—low back pain, coronary heart disease, and rheumatoid arthritis—there is convincing evidence of an association between low formal education level and poor outcome which is independent of recognized physiological variables. Deyo and Diehl (1988) found that the outcome of lower back pain was most strongly influenced by the patient's perception of whether he or she "always feels sick," by previous episodes of back pain, and by the level of formal education. The outcome was not predicted by sophisticated imaging procedures, laboratory tests, or physical examination. In studies of rheumatoid arthritis, formal education level appeared to have a substantial impact on morbidity and mortality over a nine-year period (Pincus and Callahan, 1985; Callahan and Pincus, 1988), but age, duration of disease, the number of joints involved, functional measures, and medication did not. The patient's clinical status was assessed by the number of joints involved, erythrocyte sedimentation rate, grip strength, walking time, and questionnaire self-assessment measures.

Although the precise mechanism mediating the influence of years of education on health is not known, a number of possible explanations are appropriate to the differing circumstances mentioned above. In Third World and nonindustrialized countries one would expect virtually any education to favorably influence such behavioral domains as personal hygiene, nutrition, and participation in immunization programs, with beneficial effects on health. In the industrialized nations, the extent of education fundamentally touches two major health-related areas. It influences both life-style factors and the degree of control any individual is ultimately able to exercise in many critical facets of life, personal or occupational. To this end even a three-year deficit in school education, as stated above, could make a profound difference regarding eligibility for employment. Decision-making latitude would accordingly be much reduced in the nonskilled work sector, possibly leading to a state of chronic stress with its negative effects on the individual's emotional and physical health.

The broader social impact of education, while outside the scope of this text, should receive some mention because it appears to have health consequences too. Thus, children of deprived single-parent families were randomly assigned to either attend or not attend nursery school. Evaluation up to 27 years of age indicated that those who did attend nursery school had consistently better health, higher educational achievements, higher earnings, and lower rate of crime (NHS Center for Reviews and Dissemination, 1997; Zoritch and Roberts, 1998). The socialization value of early school experience would appear to profoundly influence later social performance, educational achievement, and health status, although the main determinant of the health status is not clear. Higher, more favorable economic status, life-style factors linked to this, and a greater measure of effective control over work and other life events may all be operative.

Social support and stress

Social support may play an important role as a buffer or modifier of life's stresses. Cassel (1976) and Cobb (1976) suggested that social activity, as well as psychological coping styles, reduces the deleterious effects of stress in a nonspecific way by buffering the individual from "noxious" (i.e., potentially health harming) stimuli. This hypothesis has received substantial support from a series of well-executed epidemiological studies (Marmot et al., 1975; Medalie and Goldbourt, 1976; Berkman and Syme, 1979; Mueller, 1980).

Yet it has been argued that the association between social network and mortality may be spurious, resulting rather from the tendency of sick people (particularly when solitary) to drift downward in socioeconomic status and also to lose contact with relatives and friends. This is the so-called drift, or vulnerability, hypothesis (Lawrence, 1958; Cassel, 1976). In a prospective study of 989 middle-aged men followed for nine years, however, the extent of their social network (including persons per household unit, home activities, activities outside the home, and social activities) was found to correlate significantly with mortality (Welin et al., 1985). This association held even when health status at entry to the study, age, and the presence of risk factors for coronary artery disease were taken into account. The authors concluded that an active social life protects middle-aged men against premature death. In their comprehensive evaluation of the impact of sustained economic hardship over 29 years on health and social functioning, Lynch et al. (1997) found little evidence for reverse causation in this context, that is, that episodes of illness might have led to subsequent economic hardship.

An extensive body of literature, dating back to the nineteenth century, shows that married persons have lower death rates from a variety of diseases than single persons (Berkson, 1962). Similarly, a relationship between marital status and survival after the diagnosis of cancer has been documented. A study of population-based data on 27,779 cancer cases, for example, revealed that married persons with cancer had a five-year survival that was comparable with being in an age category 10 years younger (Goodwin et al., 1987). This improved survival rate was evident even after allowing for the fact that married people tend to have their cancer diagnosed at an earlier stage than single people, and that they more frequently receive optimal treatment. It should be noted that the association between social network and mortality seems to be much more significant for men than for women (House et al., 1982).

Another social factor, unemployment, seems to have a significant impact on health, although it is complex and often difficult to investigate. The term "unemployment" may imply very different processes. It may refer to a community's aggregate unemployment rate or to an individual's unemployment experience of either losing a job or entering the workplace and being unable to find one. The effects of unemployment on health are usually categorized in relation to physical health, mental health, and well-being, or role functioning (Dooley et al., 1996). An additional complication is that certain types of employment are intrinsically stressful and leaving a stressful job might be beneficial to one's health (Wheaton, 1990).

Most studies of the health consequences of unemployment reveal substantial effects on health in general and on life expectancy (Smith, 1985a; Smith, 1985b). For example, changes in the unemployment rate and business failure rate in nine countries have been positively correlated with increases in heart disease mortality two to five years later. The correlation persisted even after adjustments were made for consumption of alcohol, cigarettes, and animal fats and for other factors (Brenner, 1987). A Swedish study showed a similar tendency for unemployment to be higher in localities with above-average male mortality from ischemic heart disease (Starrin et al., 1988), while in a British study heart disease mortality was elevated among unemployed men (Moser et al., 1987). In another prospective cohort study called the British Regional Heart Study, 1779 men experienced some unemployment or retired during the five years after their initial screening, while 4412 remained continuously employed during the same period (Morris et al., 1994). The men in the former group were twice as likely to die during the following 5.5 years as men who remained continuously employed. Even men who retired early for reasons other than illness and who appeared to be relatively advantaged and healthy had a significantly increased risk of mortality compared with men who remained continuously employed. Of the 309 men who died during follow-up, 186 died from cardiovascular disease (156 from ischemic heart disease) and 142 from cancer (43 from lung cancer). Thus, although most of the studies that examine specific causes of mortality tend to focus on ischemic heart disease, the effect of unemployment on health is not disease-specific.

Other studies indicate that deleterious effects on health may occur in workers who know that they are about to lose their jobs, that is, *in anticipation* of unemployment. Ferrie et al. (1995) compared the health of 666 members of a government office threatened with privatization to that of members of 19 other departments containing 9642 respondents. They found that the health status of the employees facing privatization tended to deteriorate when compared to the rest of the cohort and that this deterioration was not associated with a change in health-influencing behaviors such as alcohol drinking, smoking, and exercise patterns. Similarly, a study of shipyard workers in Sweden threatened with unemployment showed an increase in serum cholesterol concentration (mean 0.25 mmol/L) in 439 of 976 workers, which also correlated with an increase in blood pressure (Mattiasson et al., 1990). The cholesterol change was more pronounced in those who reported sleep disturbance. As risk factors for ischemic heart disease, these changes may ultimately contribute to increased morbidity and mortality among the unemployed.

Parenthetically, it is clear that sleep disturbance is a possible consequence of psychosocial stress. A six-year follow-up study of adults showed mortality to be high among men with sleep disturbance (Kripke et al., 1979). Epidemiological studies also showed an increased mortality among adults sleeping less than seven hours and more than nine hours even when a large number of confounding variables were taken into consideration (Wingard and Berkman,1983).

Not all studies are as categorical about the deleterious effects of unemployment on health as those cited above. A Finnish study examined census records for all 20- to 64-year-old economically active men in 1985 and then evaluated information on unemployment and deaths in this population from 1987 through 1993 (Martikainen and Valkonen, 1998). Mortality was about the same in occupation groups with differing unemployment rates. These relationships were similar for all age groups and for mortality from diseases as well as accidents and violence, suggesting to the authors that unemployment does not seem to cause mortality in the short term. However, in a society where unemployment benefits provided by the state buffer the economic hardship and uncertainties caused by unemployment in less socialized countries, the negative impact of unemployment on health may also be softened.

Mental health also is not affected in a uniform manner by employment status. In a community sample of 1026 people, Cleary and Mechanic (1983) found that employed women who were married and had children had higher rates of psychological distress than housewives, presumably reflecting the strain of pursuing a career and responding at the same time to the often exhausting demands of child rearing. Cheng (1989) also found higher rates of minor psychiatric morbidity among women in employment than out of it. Similarly, perfectionism and superefficiency may play roles as personality characteristics of working women who suffer from chronic fatigue syndrome (see Chapter 15). Thus, it would seem that if employment simply imposes more demands, the role of psychological stress may be substantial.

IDENTIFYING STRESS IN CLINICAL PRACTICE

While familiarity with the foregoing issues may be important in planning health policy from a community to a national level, the process of dealing with any particular patient in the clinic is not necessarily enhanced by such knowledge. For example, we may be well aware that a state of unemployment is negatively affecting a patient's health but practically unable to influence the situation. The same will be true of the patient's level of education. Thus, we now turn to the challenge of evaluating the role of stress in precipitating or perpetuating a particular clinical state, beginning by enumerating those situations or experiences that most people experience as stressful. It is useful to consider four major categories of stressful experience:

1. *Life events*, which include events that may occur in the lives of all individuals and often cause significant tension or anxiety. Such events are of three main types:
   a. *Major life events.* These are life experiences of a kind that everyone may undergo at some time, including death of a close family member or

friend, divorce, losing a job, or moving. All of these events are stressful to some degree in most people.

b. *Physiological changes.* Some physiological processes, such as adolescence or menopause, signify major transitions in the course of life, each with its own challenges. Changes in physiology, and the development of secondary sexual characteristics in the case of adolescence, herald entry into a new phase of life. This may be stressful because of its real or assumed implications. Another category of physiological stressors involves situations in which basic needs and daily routines of living are drastically changed, such as sleep deprivation.

c. *Catastrophic experiences.* Some events are of such magnitude that they would seriously stress all individuals regardless of their mental status or physical health. These are beyond the range of normal experience and include natural or man-made disasters such as earthquakes, flooding, hurricanes, fires, explosions, terrorist attacks, and war (see discussion of PTSD in Chapter 3).

2. *Symptom-related* stress in the context of a medical disorder. This subject is treated in detail in Chapter 7.

3. *Personality factors* of a kind that especially predispose the individual to stress. For example, a person with strongly obsessional characteristics, in whom a sense of order and personal control are of paramount importance, may be especially vulnerable to the stress of dealing with the unexpected, particularly if this is associated with a feeling of not being in control. In some people, however, stress may result from an unusual vulnerability to the usual pressures of daily life. These are often individuals with "trait" or "free-floating" anxiety who are chronically anxious and respond to many of the inevitable daily frustrations with exaggerated emotional reactions (World Health Organization,1994, p 158).

4. *Stressful life-style,* which negatively affects the physical and emotional condition of the individual. This could be a consequence of excessive work demands or of unemployment. Included here are the consequences of work stress which appears to be the most significant chronic stressor in our 24-hour routine such as that associated with boredom or limited decision-making latitude.

Life Events as Stressors

There are certain life experiences over which we have little control and which may be very stressful. Bereavement, divorce, loss of job, and similar events, particularly when they occur together, may be predisposing factors in the expression of disease processes as well as psychiatric symptoms. In the landmark study of Holmes and Rahe (1967), the development of psychiatric complaints or physical illness in 5000 subjects was evaluated in relation to a number of stressful life events. According to these authors, the cumulative impact of a sequence of stressful life events made the development of physical or emotional illness more likely. Among the most stressful of the 43 items on the list were death of a spouse, divorce, marital separation, marriage, death of a close family member, jail detention, major personal injury or illness, and being fired from work. The authors emphasized that only some of the events on their list are negative or stressful in the conventional sense of being socially undesirable. Many of them, such as marriage, marital reconciliation, or gain of a new family member, are considered socially desirable but may nevertheless be stressful.

An important criticism of this approach, however, centers on the widespread tendency of people to attribute physical symptoms or illness retrospectively to particular events—in other words, to find a reason for their illness, an attitude referred to as "effort after meaning" (Creed, 1985). In the Schedule of Recent Experiences devised by Holmes and Rahe, the subject (respondent) decides on the criteria for inclusion of an event and may in this way bias reporting of events in the direction of their assumed importance. Furthermore, the subject may include life events that are the result rather than the cause of the disease. These limitations were addressed by the Life Events and Difficulties Schedule (LEDS) of Brown and Harris (1978), in which the timing and definition of events and illness are determined by an observer and not by the respondent. In addition, all symptoms and illness-related events are excluded. A review of studies utilizing the LEDS approach provides suggestive evidence that major life events lead to or precipitate physical or psychiatric illness (Creed, 1985), a conclusion similar to that reached by Holmes and Rahe.

What makes life events stressful?

Holmes and Rahe (1967) offer the following analysis of what makes an event stressful:

> One theme was common to all these life events. The occurrence of each usually evoked or was associated with some adaptive or coping behavior . . . Thus, each item has been constructed to contain life events whose advent is either indicative of or requires a significant change in the ongoing life pattern of the individual. The emphasis is on change from the existing steady state and not on psychological meaning, emotion, or social desirability.

This view is supported by others who see "stressfulness" as a function of life change rather than the undesirability of life events (Dohrenwend, 1973). However, some workers consider the social undesirability of life events, and especially the way this affects the individual, to be of greater importance in determining stressfulness (Mueller et al., 1977). Common sense suggests that both factors are important. Clearly, a socially undesirable event will almost inevitably be a stressful experience. Nevertheless, not all stressful events are socially undesirable.

The delay in the development of physical illness

Creed (1985) emphasizes the importance of considering the timing of the physical consequences of life events. He points out that much more than one month may elapse between the event and the onset of illness. The significance of this observation is a subject for discussion in its own right. However, it is precisely because of this separation of events that the possible connection between the onset or exacerbation of symptoms and the stressful experience is often not appreciated by either the patient or the treating physician.

In a study of the adverse effects of stress on 160 members of the management staff of a large public utility situated in a major metropolitan area, Kobasa et al. (1979) found that illness symptoms lagged behind stressful experience (in work, family, social, and personal lives) by approximately six months. However, the somatic expression of a particularly stressful and prolonged life event may sometimes be delayed even by years. Examples of this may be found among patients who have nursed a parent or very close relative or companion over a long period. Months or even years later an anxiety state or even panic disorder may develop around the patient's interpretation of bodily sensations of little or no pathological significance, where the symptoms are assumed by the patient to represent a sinister disease similar to that suffered by the patient's parent. Reports of posttraumatic stress disorder occurring up to 17 years after childhood abuse similarly illustrate this delay phenomenon (Lindberg and Distad, 1985).

Does Stress Cause Disease?

The question of whether stress causes disease has now been evaluated from two very different perspectives. The earlier approach, described in some detail above, was to try to evaluate the additive contribution of stressful life events to the breakdown of normal mental or physical health. In prospective studies of the role of life events predisposing individuals to significant disease, the evidence favoring such an association is at best weak (Theorell et al., 1975; Goldberg and Comstock, 1976). Masuda and Holmes (1967) concluded that "this clustering of social or life events achieved etiological significance as a necessary but not sufficient cause of illness and accounted, in part, for the time of onset of illness." Social stressors and life events may therefore be considered important in promoting or unmasking disease processes, mental or physical, in individuals who are predisposed to the development of the disorder.

The second approach seems more promising, although it has not yet been extensively evaluated. Here individuals are categorized according to the presence or absence of physiological and metabolic parameters of stress—sustained stress in particular—and these groups are followed in order to evaluate their continued mental and physical functioning. This approach emphasizes the distinctive biological response patterns of individuals to stressors of any kind without trying to determine the nature of the particular stressor. This point may be illustrated by the way people respond to public speaking, an unusual stressor but a useful example for our purposes. In most people the challenge of public speaking produces a rise in cortisol secretion through activation of the HPA axis. After repeated public speaking, however, most people adapt and fail to show a cortisol increase when challenged. However, about 10% of subjects continue to find public speaking stressful, and their cortisol secretion increases each time they speak in public (Kirschbaum et al., 1995). Thus, any individual for whom public speaking is a very regular occurrence and in whom increased cortisol secretion represents the usual response might well ultimately show the negative health effects of sustained increased cortisol secretion.

Evaluating the allostatic load (above) formed the basis of a prospective study by Seeman et al. (1997a) as part of the MacArthur studies of aging. A cohort of 1189 men and women, aged 70–79 years, was followed over a 2.5-year period. All subjects were assessed as to their allostatic load. The measures were designed to summarize levels of physiological activity across a range of systems pertinent to disease risk (McEwen and Stellar, 1993) and were considered by the authors "to reflect parameters of regulatory systems whose activity contributes importantly to wear and tear on the body." They included systolic and diastolic blood pressure (indexes of cardiovascular activity); waist-to-hip ratio (an index of long-term levels of metabolism and adipose tissue deposition thought to be influenced by glucocorticoid activity); serum high-density lipoprotein (HDL) and total cholesterol levels (indexes of long-term atherosclerosis risk); blood plasma levels of total glycosylated hemoglobin (an integrated measure of glucose metabolism over several days); serum dehydroepiandrosterone sulfate (DHEA-S; a functional HPA antagonist); and 12-hour urinary cortisol excretion (an integrated measure of 12-hour HPA axis activity); and 12-hour urinary norepinephrine and epinephrine excretion levels (integrated indexes of 12-hour sympathetic nervous system activity). The results of this study indicated that higher allostatic load scores were associated with poorer cognitive and physical functioning and with a significantly increased risk of cardiovascular disease, independent of demographic and other health status risk factors (Seeman et al, 1997b).

This approach to the evaluation of the health consequences of stress suffers from the limitation of evaluating physiological and metabolic parameters that are not solely indicators of the stressed condition. For example, the levels of cholesterol and glucose in the blood, while influenced by stress, are regulated mainly by constitutional factors or disease processes totally unrelated to stress of any kind. Similarly, increases in body fat are associated with a sedentary life-style and a high calorie intake from food and alcohol. Thus, the "allostatic load" might be more accurately conceptualized as the sum of stress-induced metabolic and physiological changes in the body as well as life-style factors deleterious to health. Although the latter are clearly often associated with chronic stress, they are not synonymous with it.

Life-Style Factors and Stress Evaluation

Health behavior is a central issue when assessing the health consequences of chronic stress, whether in the affluent or the socioeconomically disadvantaged. In the 1990 Youth Risk Behavior Survey, 11,631 high school students gave information on physical activity, diet, substance use, and other negative health behaviors (Pate et al., 1996). Two groups of students, high-active (2652 subjects) and low-active (1641 subjects), were then evaluated for health behavior styles. The low-active group was characterized by cigarette smoking, marijuana use, lower fruit and vegetable consumption, greater television watching, failure to wear a seat belt, and low perception of academic performance. There was a significant association with race/ethnicity in the latter group, confirming that sociocultural factors are also important. Similarly, in a study of 6321 adolescents aged between 12 to 17 years, as the education level of the responsible adult and the family income increased, the adolescents were less likely to be sedentary and to engage in heavy smoking or in episodic heavy drinking (Lowry et al., 1996).

In a survey of physical activity in a diverse, randomly chosen sample of 5000 women, Sternfeld et al. (1999) revealed that the least inclination to exercise was found especially in women who were older, overweight, or married and with young children at home, and who perceived themselves as having little time for physical activity. They also tended to have no more than a high school education and to be current smokers. Because psychosocial factors are modifiable in a way that most demographic factors are not, interventions designed to promote physical activity have focused on behavioral strategies for increasing self-efficacy (in effect, strengthening the internal locus of control), social support, and positive attitude toward exercise behavior (King et al., 1995). Changing long established habits, however, may be a particularly difficult assignment in the absence of additional factors that provide a strong incentive for change such as potentially life-threatening ill health or debilitating symptoms. Educating 120 previously sedentary females to exercise regularly, Marcus and Stanton (1993) observed a very substantial attrition rate, which averaged 72% at the end of an 18-week program.

The Ultimate Challenge: Stress and the Individual

After the foregoing detailed discussion, we are still left with the challenge of creating order of these topics so that we may utilize the information in a practical way. We have come a long way in defining and understanding what in society constitutes stress for many people. The demographic, social, and economic factors discussed here should be viewed as risk factors in evaluating holistically any particular clinical problem, though our ability to influence these factors at the level of the individual patient is strictly limited. These are essentially issues of social policy that belong to the arena of public debate and which may have important consequences for the mental and physical health of the society's members. We have learned too that change of any kind, including physiological processes such as puberty or menopause or supposedly desirable social events such as marriage or the birth of a child, may similarly be significantly stressful for certain individuals.

We have been particularly unsuccessful, on the other hand, in being able to predict either from life events or the newer approach of allostatic load evaluation how any particular individual will fare from a health point of view in the face of stress. This is mainly because, as indicated, the ultimate impact of stress and its consequences in any person mostly depends on particular personality characteristics. This conclusion, suggested by a review of a large body of literature, is essentially that formulated by Cassileth et al. (1984): "Adaptation represents not the demands of a particular stress, such as a specific diagnosis, but rather the manifestations of enduring personality constructs and capacities." As recognized by the ancient Greek philosopher Epictetus, our reactions are determined less by events themselves than by the way we perceive them. Goldberg and Huxley (1992) spelled out the operational implications of this important realization: "It is time to move away from the current emphasis upon stressful life events, and turn attention to vulnerability . . . Some individuals destabilize with very small stressors, and some even develop symptoms in the absence of discernible acutely stressful events . . . One needs to study factors such as coping styles . . . and locus of control. It is of great interest to document the methods of psychological restitution that spontaneous restituters have used, as these may be useful to others."

In this spirit we may reflect on our knowledge of people who have experienced exceptional hardship or suffering and yet have remained mentally and physically healthy. Likewise, most patients with a chronic medical disorder are able to adjust well to their illness. In a study by Cassileth et al. (1984), patients stressed by chronic physical illness (arthritis, diabetes, cancer, renal disease, dermatological disorders) were found to be indistinguishable from healthy subjects with regard to their mental health status. This study supports the widespread current belief that there are no unique emotional traits which predispose an individual to specific diseases and that emotional status seems largely independent of diagnosis. Other studies suggest that it is the severity rather than the type of disability that is associated with psychological distress among patients with a variety of chronic illnesses (Viney and Westbrook, 1981; Viney and Westbrook, 1982). For example, patients suffering from cancer, one of the most feared of diseases, approximate the general public in terms of general mental health (Schmale et al., 1983) and the prevalence of psychiatric disorders, excluding adjustment disorder (Derogatis et al., 1983; Glass, 1983) and depression (Plumb and Holland, 1977). It is interesting to note that in the study by Cassileth et al. (1984) as well as that of Earle et al. (1979), the older the patients, the better their mental health scores.

Though most people withstand the stress of illness well, some are remarkable for their resilience. The personality characteristics of such "hardy" individuals—those who remained healthy physically and mentally despite severe stress—were described by Kobasa et al. (1979; 1985) as follows:

1. *A sense of personal commitment in life.* "Committed persons possess the sense of purpose and of active involvement which minimizes the threat of otherwise stressful events, and provides a basis for continual grappling with problems and setbacks. In contrast, the alienated person considers the world rather worthless and finds insufficient value in stressful events to justify any effort to cope with them" (Kobasa et al.,1979).

2. *Personal sense of control* in relation to life events. "Persons who feel in control of their lives [i.e., who have a stronger internal locus of control] experience less threat in stressful life events because they believe in their ability to transform situations cognitively and to respond flexibly enough to be effective. In contrast, persons who believe that they are externally controlled are overwhelmed by stress because they feel powerless to cope, to influence, and to transform, and nihilistic in the face of the presumed power arrayed against them" (see Chapter 4).

3. *Ability to seek novelty and challenge in change* rather than always to seek the familiar and secure. Underlying this is the idea that such individuals would be practiced at dealing with change and consequently better able to handle stress. Conversely, those who constantly seek security and familiarity will be uneasy with change and therefore less able to cope with stress.

From the perspective of the medical practitioner, this analysis complements the views of Goldberg and Huxley (1992) quoted earlier, offering us a much more optimistic perspective. Although we may have no resources as doctors to directly influence the major socioeconomic stressors discussed above, we are often able to assist the individual in crisis. We are able, for instance, to undertake an intervention in most suffering patients which, by utilizing the principles of cognitive management, behavioral therapy, and life-style counseling, can assist motivated individuals to understand better the nature of stress and its impact on them as well as provide resources to modify their response. The "enduring personality constructs and capacities" referred to by Cassileth et al. (1984), while possibly leading the individual into crisis, are often modifiable. Clinical experience appears to support this contention, and among the principal objectives of this book is an elaboration of the principles and processes involved in achieving this end.

REFERENCES

Acheson D (1999). Equality of health: dream or reality? J R Coll Physicians Lond 33:70–77.

Alexander F (1950). Emotional factors in metabolic and endocrine disturbances. In: Psychosomatic Medicine: Its Principles and Application. New York: WW Norton.

Alter DA, Naylor D, Austin P, et al. (1999). Effects of socioeconomic status on access to invasive cardiac procedures and on mortality after acute myocardial infarction. N Engl J Med 341:1359–1367.

Anderson GM, Grumbach K, Luft HS, et al. (1993). Use of coronary artery bypass surgery in the United States and Canada: influence of age and income. JAMA 269:1661–1666.

Berkman LF, Syme SL (1979). Social networks, host resistance, and mortality: a nine-year follow-up study of Alameda County residents. Am J Epidemiol 109:186–204.

Berkson J (1962). Mortality and marital status: reflections on the derivation of etiology from statitistics. Am J Public Health 52:1318–1329.

Blaxter M (1987). Evidence of inequality in health from a national survey. Lancet 1:30–33.

Brenner MH (1987). Economic change, alcohol consumption and heart disease mortality in nine industrialized countries. Soc Sci Med 25:119–132.

Brown GW, Harris T (1978). The Social Origins of Depression: A Study of Psychiatric Disorder in Women. London: Tavistock Publications; New York: Free Press.

Caldwell JC (1993). Health transition: the cultural, social and behavioral determinants of health in the Third World. Soc Sci Med 36:125–135.

Callahan LF, Pincus T (1988). Formal education level as a significant marker of clinical status in rheumatoid arthritis. Arthritis Rheum 31:1346–1357.

Cassel J (1976). The contribution of the social environment to host resistance: the Fourth Wade Hampton Frost Lecture. Am J Epidemiol 104:107–123.

Cassileth BR, Lusk EJ, Strouse TB, et al. (1984). Psychosocial status in chronic illness: a comparative analysis of six diagnostic groups. N Engl J Med 311:506–511.

Cheng TA (1989). Psychosocial stress and minor psychiatric morbidity: a community study in Taiwan. J Affect Disord 17:137–152.

Cleary PD, Mechanic D (1983). Sex differences in psychological distress among married people. J Health Soc Behav 24:111–121.

Cobb S (1976). Presidential Address 1976. Social support as moderator of life stress. Psychosom Med 38:300–314.

Creed F (1985). Life events and physical illness. J. Psychosom. Res 29:113–123.

Davis H, Shuval D, Kaplan A, et al. (1998). A psychological study of patients with uncomplicated, nonalcoholic, chronic liver disease. J Psychosom Res 44:547–554.

Derogatis LR, Morrow GR, Fetting J, et al. (1983). The prevalence of psychiatric disorders amongst cancer patients. JAMA 249:751–757.

Deyo RA, Diehl AK (1988). Psychosocial predictors of disability in patients with low back pain. J Rheumatol 15:1557–1564.

Dohrenwend BS (1973). Events as stressors: a methodological inquiry. J Health Soc Behav 14:167–175.

Dohrenwend BS, Dohrenwend DP (1974). Stressful Life Events: Their Nature and Effects. New York: Wiley.

Dooley D, Fielding J, Levi L (1996). Health and unemployment. Annu Rev Public Health 17:449–465.

Earle JR, Perricone PJ, Maultsby DM, et al. (1979). Psycho-social adjustment of rheumatoid arthritis patients from two alternative treatment settings. J Rheumatol 6:80–87.

Enterline PE, Salter V, McDonald AD, et al. (1973). The distribution of medical services before and after "free" medical care: the Quebec experience. N Engl J Med 289:1174–1178.

Ferrie JE, Shipley MJ, Marmot MG, et al. (1995). Health effects of anticipation of job change and non-employment: longitudinal data from the Whitehall II study. Br Med J 311:1264–1269.

Glass RM (1983). Psychiatric disorders among cancer patients. JAMA 249:782–783.

Goldberg D, Huxley P (1992). Common Mental Disorders: A Bio-Social Model. New York: Routledge, pp 144–145.

Goldberg EL, Comstock GW (1976). Life events and subsequent illness. Am J Epidemiol 104:146–158.

Goodwin JS, Hunt WC, Key CR, et al. (1987). The effect of marital status on stage, treatment, and survival of cancer patients. JAMA 258:3125–3130.

Holmes TH, Rahe RH (1967). The Social Readjustment Rating Scale. J Psychosom Res 11:213–218.

House JS, Robbins C, Metzner HL (1982). The association of social relationships and activities with mortality: prospective evidence from the Tecumseh Community Health Study. Am J Epidemiol 116:123–140.

Institute of Medicine (1988). The future of public health. Washington, DC: National Academy Press.

Katz SJ, Hofer TP (1994). Socioeconomic disparities in preventive care persist despite universal coverage: breast and cervical screening in Ontario and the United States. JAMA 272:530–534.

King AC, Haskell WL, Young DR, et al. (1995). Long-term effects of varying intensities and formats of physical activity on participation rates, fitness and lipoproteins in men and women aged 50, 60, 65 years. Circulation 91:2596–2604.

Kirschbaum C, Prussner JC, Stone AA, et al. (1995). Persistent high cortisol responses to repeated psychological stress in a subpopulation of healthy men. Psychosom Med 57:468–474.

Kobasa SC, Hilker RR (1982). Executive work perceptions and the quality of working life. J Occup Med 24:25–29.

Kobasa SC, Hilker RR, Maddi SR (1979). Who stays healthy under stress? J Occup Med 21:595–598.

Kobasa SC, Maddi SR, Puccetti MC, et al. (1985). Effectiveness of hardiness, exercise and social support as resources against illness. J Psychosom Res 29:525–533.

Kripke DF, Simons RN, Garfinkel L, et al. (1979). Short and long sleep and sleeping pills: is increased morbidity associated? Arch Gen Psychiatry 36:103–116

LaVecchia C, Negrl E, Pagano R, et al. (1987). Education, prevalence of disease, and frequency of healthcare utilization: the 1983 Italian National Health Survey. J Epidemiol Comm Health 41:161–165.

Lawrence PS (1958). Chronic illness and socioeconomic status. In: Jaco EG, ed. Patients, Physicians and Illness. New York: Free Press.

Lindberg FH, Distad LJ (1985). Post-traumatic stress disorders in women who experienced childhood incest. Child Abuse Negl 9:329–334.

Liu K, Cedres LB, Stamler J, et al. (1982). Relationship of education to major risk factors and death from coronary heart disease, cardiovascular diseases, and all causes: findings of three Chicago epidemiologic studies. Circulation 66:1308–1314.

Lowry R, Kann L, Collins JL, et al. (1996). The effect of socioeconomic status on chronic disease risk behaviors among US adolescents. JAMA 276:792–797.

Lynch JW (1996). Social position and health. Ann Epidemiol 6:21–23.

Lynch JW, Kaplan GA, Shema SJ (1997). Cumulative impact of sustained economic hardship on physical, cognitive, psychological, and social functioning. N Engl J Med 337:1889–1895.

Marcus BH, Stanton AL (1993). Evaluation of relapse prevention and reinforcement interventions to promote exercise adherence in sedentary females. Res Q Exerc Sport 64:447–452.

Marmot MG, McDowall ME (1986). Mortality decline and widening social class inequalities. Lancet 2:274–276.

Marmot MG, Syme SL, Kagan A, et al. (1975). Epidemiologic studies of coronary heart disease in Japanese men living in Japan, Hawaii and California; prevalence of coronary and hypertensive heart disease and associated risk factors. Am J Epidemiol 102:514–525.

Martikainen PT, Valkonen T (1998). The effects of differential unemployment rate increases of occupation groups on changes in mortality. Am J Public Health 88:1859–1861.

Masuda M, Holmes TH (1967). Magnitude estimates of social readjustments. J Psychosom Res 11:219–225.

Mattiasson I, Lindgarde F, Nilsson JA, et al. (1990). Threat of unemployment and cardiovascular risk factors: longitudinal study of quality of sleep and serum cholesterol concentrations in men threatened with redundancy. Br Med J 301:461–466.

McCord C, Freeman HP (1990). Excess mortality in Harlem. N Engl J Med 322:173–177.

McEwen BS (1998). Protective and damaging effects of stress mediators. N Engl J Med 338:171–179.

McEwen BS, Stellar E (1993). Stress and the individual: mechanisms leading to disease. Arch Intern Med 153:2093–2101.

McIsaac W, Goel V, Naylor CD (1997). Socioeconomic status and visits to physicians by adults in Ontario, Canada. J Health Serv Res Policy 2:94–102.

Medalie JH, Goldbourt U (1976). Angina pectoris among 10,000 men. II. Psychosocial and other risk factors as evidenced by a multivariate analysis of a five year incidence study. Am J Med 60:910–921.

Morris JK, Cook DG, Shaper AG (1994). Loss of employment and mortality. Br Med J 308:1135–1139.

Moser KA, Goldblatt PO, Fox AJ, et al. (1987). Unemployment and mortality: comparisons of the 1971 and 1981 longitudinal census sample. Br Med J 294:86–90.

Mueller DP (1980). Social networks: a promising direction for research on the relationship of the social environment to psychiatric disorder. Soc Sci Med 14A:147–161.

Mueller DP, Edwards DW, Yarvis RM (1977). Stressful life events and psychiatric symptomatology: change or undesireability? J. Health Soc Behav 18:307–317.

NHS Center for Reviews and Dissemination (1997). Mental health promotion in high risk groups. Effect Health Care 3.

North F, Syme SL, Feeney A, et al. (1993). Explaining socioeconomic differences in sickness absence: the Whitehall II study. Br Med J 313:1177–1180.

Orth-Gomer K, Unden A-L, Edwards M-E (1988). Social isolation and mortality in ischemic heart disease: a 10-year follow-up study of 150 middle-aged men. Acta Med Scand 224:205–215.

Pappas G, Queen S, Hadden W, et al. (1993). The increasing disparity in mortality between socioeconomic groups in the United States, 1960 and 1986. N Engl J Med 329:103–109.

Pate RR, Heath GW, Dowdam, et al. (1996). Associations between physical activity and other health behaviors in a representative sample of US adolescents. Am J Public Health 86:1577–1581.

Pincus T (1988). Formal educational level—a marker for the importance of behavioral variables in the pathogenesis, morbidity, and mortality of most diseases? [editorial] J Rheumatol 15:1457–1460.

Pincus T, Callahan LF (1985). Formal education as a marker for increased mortality and morbidity in rheumatoid arthritis. J Chronic Dis 38:973–984.

Pincus T, Callahan LF, Burkhauser RV (1987). Most chronic diseases are reported more frequently by individuals with fewer than 12 years of formal education in the age 18–64 United States population. J Chronic Dis 40:865–874.

Plumb MM, Holland J (1977). Comparative studies of psychological function in patients with advanced cancer. I. Self-reported depressive symptoms. Psychosom Med 39:264–276.

Schmale AH, Morrow GR, Schmitt MH, et al. (1983). Well-being of cancer survivors. Psychosom Med 45:163–169.

Seeman TE, Singer BH, Rowe JW, et al. (1997a). Price of adaptation-allostatic load and its health consequences. Arch Intern Med 157:2259–2268.

Seeman TE, McEwen BS, Singer BH, et al. (1997b). Increase in urinary cortisol excretion and memory declines: MacArthur studies of successful aging. J Clin Endocrinol Metab 82:2458–2465.

Selye H (1946). The general adaptation syndrome and the diseases of adaptation. J Clin Endocrin Metab 6:117–230.

Smith R (1985a). "He never got over losing his job": death on the dole. Br Med J 291:1492–1495.

Smith R (1985b). "I'm just not right": the physical health of the unemployed. Br Med J 291:1626–1629.

Starrin B, Larsson G, Brenner SO (1988). Regional variations in cardiovascular mortality in Sweden: structural vulnerability in the local community. Soc Sci Med 27:911–917.

Sterling P, Eyer J (1988). Allostasis: a new paradigm to explain arousal pathology. In: Fisher S, Reason J, eds. Handbook of Life Stress, Cognition and Health. New York: John Wiley, pp 629–649.

Sternfeld B, Ainsworth BE, Quesenberry CP (1999). Physical activity patterns in a diverse population of women. Prev Med 28:313–323.

Syme SL, Berkman LF (1976). Social class, susceptibility and sickness. Am J Epidemiol 104:1–8.

Theorell T, Lind E, Floderus B (1975). The relationship of disturbing life changes and emotions to the early development of myocardial infarction and other serious illnesses. Int J Epidemiol 4:281–293.

Viney LL, Westbrook MT (1981). Psychological reactions to chronic illness-related disability as a function of its severity and type. J Psychosom Res 25:513–523.

Viney LL, Westbrook MT (1982). Coping with chronic illness: the mediating role of biographic and illness-related factors. J Psychosom Res 26:595–605.

Welin L, Tibblin G, Svardsudd K, et al. (1985). Prospective study of social influences on mortality: the study of men born in 1913 and 1923. Lancet 1:915–918.

Wheaton B (1990). Life transitions, role histories, and mental health. Am Sociol Rev 55:209–223.

Wingard DL, Berkman LF (1983). Mortality risk associated with sleeping pattern among adults. Sleep 6:102–107.

World Health Organisation (1994). International Classification of Disease 10. London: Churchill Livingstone.

Zoritch B, Roberts I (1998). The health and welfare effects of preschool day care: a systematic review of RCTs. Cochrane Library, issue 2. Oxford:Update Software.

Chapter

6

STRESS AND IMMUNE FUNCTION

The idea that stress may impair immune function is not new. In the first half of the twentieth century, stress was considered to be important in the development of pulmonary tuberculosis (Ishigami, 1919; Holmes et al., 1957; Kissen, 1958). Sanitoriums for tuberculosis existed long before the antibiotic era, testifying to the belief that a relaxed environment, good nutrition, and a fair measure of sunshine would provide the body with its best chance of combating the dreaded infection. While this belief was sustained over the years on little more than clinical impression, our present understanding of the impact of stress on immune function supports the soundness of this approach. Today we have a much clearer idea of how and why sanatorium measures may have favorably influenced immune function in combating diseases like tuberculosis.

The role of stress in predisposing particularly to viral infections has been supported by epidemiological studies. Kasl et al. (1979) prospectively followed 1400 West Point cadets over a four-year period and found that their tendency toward seroconversion to the Epstein-Barr virus (EBV) and their susceptibility to infectious mononucleosis (IM) were related to psychosocial factors such as a high level of motivation for a military career, poor academic progress, and having a father who was an overachiever. Two-thirds of the entering cadets were found to be immune, one-fifth of the susceptible seroconverted each year, and one-fourth of those infected each year developed clinical IM. The coexistence of strong motivation for academic success with poor academic performance appeared to increase susceptibility to EBV. A study by Glaser et al. (1999) on West Point military cadets showed that it was the stress of examination rather than the impact of the stress of training that modulated the expression of EBV immunoglobulin (IgG) antibodies, which showed a rise in titer during the examination week.

In a well-designed study carried out with a large group of volunteers, Cohen et al. (1991) showed that susceptibility to infection caused by each of three different common cold viruses (rhinovirus, coronavirus, and respiratory syncytial virus) was significantly related to stress. The degree of stress was evaluated from the number of major stressful life events judged by the subjects to have had a negative impact on their psychological state in the past year, the degree to which current demands were perceived to exceed their ability to cope, and an index of current negative affect. The increased risk of infection found in subjects with higher stress index scores was not due to associations between stress and either exposure to virus or health practices. Unlike other researchers who have documented an association between psychological stress and the risk of acute infectious respiratory illness (e.g., Meyer and Haggerty, 1962; Boyce et al., 1997; Graham et al., 1986), Cohen and colleagues controlled for the possible effect of stressful events on exposure to infectious agents and also provided evidence of the biological mechanism through which stress might influence a person's susceptibility to infection: suppression of host resistance that leaves the person vulnerable to multiple infectious agents. In addition to broad alterations in immune function, local respiratory mucosal factors (the portal of entry of the infecting virus), which are important for host defense, might be compromised in the stressed state.

In a prospective three-year study of recurrent herpes labialis (RHL) in 149 student nurses (Friedman et al., 1977), about 50%–60% of the RHL episodes were not preceded by any recorded trauma, sunburn, or upper respiratory infection (URI). Of the identifiable factors associated with an attack, 80%–90% of the variance was related to antibody titer to herpes simplex virus and to RHL frequency by history and during the first six months of study. About 6%–10% of the variance could be explained by social factors (social class and social assets) and mood. Attacks were unrelated to the menstrual cycle. Clearly, stress may be operating to induce attacks of RHL in all these categories of identifiable antecedents. Certainly, the first six months of nursing study may be assumed to represent a period of stress. In addition, the frequency of RHL by history may also be influenced by antecedent stress factors in the subjects' lives.

In a study of immune changes in 71 caregivers of dementia sufferers and 58 control subjects, Glaser and Kiecolt-Glaser (1997) found a significantly higher antibody titer to total viral antigen of herpes simplex type 1 (HSV-1) and a poorer HSV-1–specific T-cell response than controls. These changes, induced by the stress of a particularly difficult occupation, reflect a shift in T helper (Th) cells from a Th1 to a Th2 immune response (see below) and indicate a weakening of cellular immunity, a condition likely to facilitate activation of the herpes virus.

STRESS-MEDIATED CHANGES IN IMMUNE FUNCTION

The largest body of information on stress-associated infections relates to conditions (many of them viral) that primarily affect the oral cavity and respiratory system. To some extent this simply reflects the most prevalent, contagious, community-acquired infections, as well as the fact that the oral cavity is normally colonized by microorganisms. The studies cited thus far appear to indicate, however, that stress does alter, in some way, the normal barrier function of the oral and respiratory mucosa. Could an altered state of mucosal defense be explained simply by the observed reduction in salivary immunoglobulin A (IgA) secretion in stressed subjects (Jemmott et al., 1983)? Immunoglobulin is the predominant class of immunoglobulin found in saliva and is involved in defense against infections, particularly those of the respiratory and gastrointestinal tracts (South et al., 1969; Rossen et al., 1970; Tomasi and Grey, 1972). The uncertain clinical implication of its reduced secretion in defined stressed populations, such as in students before examinations, represents a predicament common to most of the work in this field.

The question raised may be stated as follows: If stress plays a role in predisposing the individual to the development of a particular inflammatory process, whether of infective (e.g., herpes simplex, common cold) or noninfective (e.g., aphthous ulcers) etiology, do the observed aberrations of immune function (such as reduction in salivary IgA) provide a sufficient basis for this predisposition? The oronasal cavities are protected by a substantial mass of lymphatic tissue (Waldeyer ring, which includes the tonsils and adenoids), pointing to the importance of local cellular activity in the effective maintenance of the barrier function. In stressed states, cellular immunity appears to weaken and humoral defense mechanisms such as antibody production tend to become more active, a change in immune function that may promote vulnerability to the gamut of respiratory infections discussed above. Reduced IgA secretion in saliva in stressed states should therefore be viewed as part of a broader state of impaired cellular immunity, the nature of which is described in this chapter.

THE Th1–Th2 HYPOTHESIS: THE BASIS OF STRESS-INDUCED IMMUNE MODULATION

The Th1–Th2 hypothesis is based on the experimental observation that broadly speaking, the immune system fluctuates normally between two cardinal functional states. These states are termed Th1 (T helper 1) and Th2 (T helper 2) based on *in vitro* measurement of cytokines produced by antigen- and mitogen-stimulated peripheral blood mononuclear cells. The cytokines characteristic of the Th1 state are interleukins IL-2 and IL-12 and an interferon, IFN-γ, (pro-inflammatory cytokines) and these are considered to promote cellular immunity. The Th2 state is characterized by the presence of other cytokines, such as IL-4, IL-6, and IL-10, and a reduced secretion of the former cytokines which promote cellular immunity. Thus, the Th2 state is considered to be a state of diminished cellular immunity and in general a disease-susceptible condition, although it promotes B-cell maturation and antibody production. While the name suggests that these different cytokines are T helper cell products, they are in fact produced by a number of cell types including CD4$^+$ Th cells, CD8$^+$ T cells, accessory cells, B cells, and natural killer (NK) cells. For this reason, some workers prefer to designate the states according to the main function of the immunoregulatory cytokines (i.e., type1/type2), rather than on the basis of the cell types, as above (Clerici and Shearer, 1994).

In brain-injured human subjects and rats, sympathetic discharge associated with the brain injury was accompanied by rapid systemic release of IL-10, a powerful monocyte-derived anti-inflammatory cytokine (Woiciechowsky et al., 1998). In the rat model, propranolol prevented the increase in plasma interleukin levels following brain injury, confirming that its secretion is mediated by monocyte β-adrenergic receptor stimulation. Although they normally function to prevent overresponsiveness of the immune system, cytokines such as IL-10 and IL-1RA (IL-1 receptor antagonist), when secreted in excess, shift the balance toward a state of relative immunosuppression. The IL-10 inhibits the monocytic production of pro-inflammatory cytokines, such as tumor necrosis factor (TNF-α), and is an inducer of the anti-inflammatory IL-1 receptor antagonist (IL-1Ra) (de Waal Malefyt et al., 1991). In addition, it is a major depressor of specific cellular immunity through its reduction of monocytic MHC (major histocompatibility complex) class II (HLA-DR [human lymphocyte antigen degeneration reaction]) expression and antigen-presenting capacity as well as its suppression of monocytic production of IL-12 (a cytokine that promotes cellular immunity by activation of NK cells, inducing interferon [IFN]-γ production and Th1 cell differentiation). Low HLA-DR expression on monocytes indicates their functional deactivation.

There is in addition another level of reciprocal regulatory control of immune function between the Th1 and Th2 states. For example, the secretion of interferon-γ by Th1 cells inhibits Th2 cells, and the secretion of interleukin-10 by Th2 cells reciprocally inhibits Th1 cells (Mosmann and Sad, 1996).

In many respects glucocorticoids play a very similar role to that of the cytokines in the normal processes of immune modulation. The basal levels of glucocorticoids regulate the normal expression of hormonal effects and optimize the adaptive responses of tissues and organs to unusual demands imposed by stress. The cytokines may similarly be viewed as mostly modulating and optimizing immune function, particularly in the face of the most common challenge to the integrity of the organism, namely, infection. In mice that are genetically unable to produce IL-6, certain basal immune functions are affected (Manfredi et al., 1998), for instance, natural killer activity and IL-2 production are lower in splenocytes of IL-6–deficient animals. These animals nevertheless show a normal degree of immunosupression with restraint stress, suggesting that IL-6 plays a permissive rather than essential role in immune modulation, as it does with glucocorticoids. Similarly, as described above for IL-10, a cytokine with an immunoinhibitory function assumed to prevent overresponsiveness of the immune system in response to an antigenic challenge (de Waal Malefyt et al., 1991), when secreted in excess immune dysregulation results (Woiciechowsky et al., 1998).

Glucocorticoids also inhibit pro-inflammatory cytokine production. *In vitro*, physiological levels of glucocorticoids diminish the production of IL-2 and INF-γ (Th1 state) and promote the production of IL-4 and IL-10 (Th2 state) (Daynes and Araneo, 1989; Rook et al., 1994). Other reported stress-induced immune changes indicative of impaired Th1 responses are reduced natural killer cell activity (see below), reduced production of interferon-γ by mitogen-stimulated peripheral blood leukocytes and of IgA secretion in saliva, and a reduced mitogen-stimulated lymphoproliferative response (Jemmott et al., 1983; Kiecolt-Glaser et al., 1984; Kiecolt-Glaser et al., 1986).

Studies of immune function in stressed states that have been associated with reactivation of viruses are compatible with a shift from a Th1 to a Th2 state, reflecting an impairment of cellular immunity and resulting in an increase in the viral antibody titers (Glaser et al., 1985; Glaser et al., 1991). In analyzing the main immune effects of stress in HIV-positive individuals, Cole and Kemeny (1997) argue that immune function shifts from a Th1 to Th2 condition in most situations that negatively influence the natural history of HIV infection, including situations of stress (Clerici and Shearer, 1994; Kemeny, 1994). Such a shift toward a Th2 state would also explain the tendency toward elevated titers of antibodies to the Epstein-Barr virus (EBV) and human herpes virus 6, among others, in chronic fatigue syndrome (CFS; Chapter 15), possibly stimulated by IL-6, a Th2 cytokine that promotes B cell maturation and antibody production. It was this observation of raised antibody titers, essentially a secondary consequence of CFS inducing a predominantly Th2 state in immune function, that gave rise to the erroneous idea that CFS resulted from a recrudescence of Epstein-Barr infection. Also, depressed patients have increased antibody titers to herpes simplex virus (HSV-1) and cytomegalovirus compared with other hospitalized or healthy controls (Lycke et al., 1974) as well as a marked decline in varicella-zoster virus–specific cellular immunity (Irwin et al., 1998).

We are now in a much better position to understand the soundness of the principles underlying the sanatorium treatment of tuberculosis in the preantibiotic era. By ensuring good nutrition and rest and minimizing stress the immune system was shifted toward an optimal Th1 state of enhanced cellular immunity to combat the dreaded tuberculous infection. Experimentally it has been shown in mice that reactivation of mycobacterial growth through activation of the hypothalamic–pituitary–adrenal axis, as may occur in stress or depression, resulted in a shift from a Th1 to a Th 2 cytokine pattern in both CD4 and CD8 T cells (Howard and Zwilling, 1999).

Studies by Glaser et al. (1998) confirm the need for a distinction between the immune processes involved in the acquisition of immunity to an unrecognized antigen such as the antibody response to a vaccine and situations where the individual is already immunized and producing antibodies to a recognized antigen as occurs with persistent viral infection such as the Epstein-Barr virus. The former mainly requires an active T cell response and the secretion of IL-2, a Th1 cytokine, the latter an expression of enhanced Th2 activity. Glaser et al. (1998) showed that a stressed state impairs the immune response to vaccines. In their studies, caregivers of Alzheimer's disease patients showed a poorer antibody response and virus-specific T cell response following vaccination with influenza virus vaccine compared to the control subjects. Similar findings occurred in medical students immunized with hepatitis B vaccine at examination time. Those students reporting greater social support and lower anxiety and stress levels demonstrated a higher antibody response to the vaccine and more vigorous T cell responses to the hepatitis virus surface antigen.

A significant increase in serum IL-6 (pro-inflammatory, type 2 cytokine) was also found in patients suffering from posttraumatic stress disorder (PTSD), a condition characterized by frequent intense bouts of anxiety and autonomic activation (Maes et al., 1999), as discussed in Chapter 3. This increase was potentiated by the concurrence of PTSD and major depression. The secretion of interleukin-4 by Th2 cells stimulates the production of IgE, and this is likely to be the mechanism underlying the high incidence of atopy in depression (see Chapter 16). Thus, in a condition of chronic stress, as exemplified by CFS, chronic PTSD, and depression, the ongoing antigenic stimulation of any persistent viral infection will provide the basis for an enhanced antibody response, as well as predisposing to atopy, through the mediation of Th2 cytokines.

Neuroimmune Interactions

Neural or neuroendocrine modulation of immune function is an active area of research (Ader et al., 1995). Peripheral nerves and the autonomic nervous system innervate lymphatic, splenic, and thymic tissue (Bellinger et al., 1990; Tollefson and Bulloch, 1990; Muller and Weihe, 1991). Experiments have shown that both the disruption of neural innervation *in vivo* and the addition of humoral sympathetic effectors *in vitro* lead to changes in the immune response (Besedovsky et al., 1979). Lymphocytes and macrophages contain receptors for and respond functionally to neurotransmitters, neuropeptides, and neurohormones; moreover, they are capable of producing many of these substances (Payan, 1989; Sreedharan et al., 1989; Galin et al., 1990; Heagy et al., 1990; Wenger et al., 1990).

The classical experimental studies of Ader and Cohen (1975), which demonstrated that humoral and cell-mediated immune responses could be suppressed by behavioral conditioning techniques, represent the clearest and most dramatic experimental study of immune modulation by the nervous system. Conditioned immunosuppression was achieved by pairing the consumption of saccharin-sweetened water—the conditioned stimulus (CS)—with an immunosuppressive drug, cyclophosphamide—the unconditioned stimulus (US). When later subjected to antigen challenge and allowed to drink sweetened water, conditioned animals reexposed to the CS had attenuated immune responses. The authors further showed that in the New Zealand mouse, which is genetically predisposed to develop an autoimmune illness with the clinical characteristics of systemic lupus erythematosis, proteinuria development and mortality were significantly retarded in conditioned mice compared with untreated controls and nonconditioned animals that received unpaired treatment with saccharine and cyclophosphamide (Ader and Cohen, 1982). This study demonstrated that, by modifying the natural history of the disease, the conditioned immunosuppression was of definite biological significance. The same conditioning technique prolonged the survival of foreign tissue grafted onto mice (Gorczynski, 1990). A limited study in 10 multiple sclerosis patients paired four intravenous treatments of cyclophosphamide with a conditioned stimulus (Giang et al., 1996). Eight of the ten subjects subsequently displayed a decrease in peripheral blood leukocytes following the conditioned stimulus ($P = 0.04$), suggesting that humans may be similarly conditioned.

Recurrent Herpes Labialis

Recurrent herpes labialis (RHL) is a particularly interesting model because in addition to the epidemiological evidence that stress is an important precipitator of recurrent infection, there is good experimental evidence pointing to the primacy of immunological mechanisms in its occurrence. Furthermore, I would speculate here that as herpes labialis is a persistent infection of nerves, neurological mechanisms may also be involved.

In the quiescent phase, viral genomic material has been found in sensory ganglionic neurons, especially the trigeminal ganglion, but also in the sacral and vagal nuclei (Bastian et al., 1972; Baringer and Swoveland, 1973). Early viral products are formed within the neuron but final replicative assembly of the intact virus occurs in the buccal epithelial cells, leading to an inflammatory as well as an immune response. During the active phase of infection, the herpes virus mainly infects the epithelial cells of the lips and circumoral skin and it is from these sites that viral shedding occurs. Two distinct mechanisms, one immune and one neural, could theoretically be involved, although the tendency to recurrence in approximately one-half of infected individuals seems increasingly to be mediated by changes in immune function.

The immune response

The immune changes following recovery from primary herpes simplex virus (HSV) infection appear to be of three major types:

1. Development of delayed-type hypersensitivity (DTH), a persistent response indicative of the establishment of immune memory (Lausch et al., 1966).
2. Lymphoproliferation, an *in vitro* response that correlates with HSV-specific DTH and is widely accepted as indicative of previous exposure to antigen (Rosenberg et al., 1972; Jacobs et al., 1976; Morahan et al., 1978).
3. Antigen-driven cell-mediated effector responses that can be measured *in vitro*, such as the generation of cytotoxic lymphocytes (Pfizenmaier et al., 1977) and the production of cytokines (Bell et al., 1978).

Experimental studies *in vivo* in mice and *in vitro* have assisted in defining the primary role of macrophages and T cells (γ/δ T cell receptor positive) in repressing herpesvirus infection of the trigeminal ganglion throught the secretion of antiviral molecules such as interferon-γ, TNF-α, and nitric oxide (Cantin et al., 1999; Kodukula et al., 1999). Cytokines Il-4 and Il-6 (Th2-type cytokines), produced under hyperthermic stress or UV irradiation, were associated with reactivation of the herpesvirus (Noisakran et al., 1998; Shimeld et al., 1999).

The development of recrudescent HSV-2 lesions (genital herpes) in humans coincides with depressed levels of virus-specific cell-mediated immunity as measured *in vitro* by lymphokine production (Glaser and Kiecolt-Glaser, 1997). This depression is also correlated with a change in the homeostatic balance of immunoregulatory T lymphocyte subsets characterized by a significant increase in $T8^+Ia^+$ cells, which appear to possess suppressor activity (Sheridan et al., 1982). Patients with impaired cell-mediated immunity often suffer severe herpetic infections (Korsager et al., 1975). Furthermore, Glaser et al. (1987) have demonstrated significant impairment of lymphokine leukocyte migration-inhibition factor in medical students at times of examination stress, a finding compatible with the type of immune change known to predispose individuals to RHL (O'Reilly et al., 1977).

The neurological response

The unusual propensity of the herpes virus to recur on the lips and genitalia, and to a certain extent the cornea (herpes infections of the finger nailfold, called herpetic whitlow, usually do not recur), suggests that other factors in addition to immune suppression are operative. Herpes varicella-zoster infections of the skin (where the latent virus is located within the dorsal root ganglion) may occasionally be recurrent and here too a similar nonimmune mechanism may be involved. The recurrence of an inflammatory and often painful process in the anatomical location of the lips, which have a rich cortical representation, may have the effect of recruiting additional sensory fibers that innervate this area, as well as elements of the sensory pathway right up to the cerebral cortex, as described Chapter 8.

We may speculate that the presence of viral components in the sensory ganglion of particular nerves could alter the nerve sufficiently for the process to be registered at a higher level of the nervous system. These factors, in addition to the element of anticipation likely to follow a known precipitator of an attack of herpes, whether it be a fever, exposure to sunlight, or stress, may serve in some way to facilitate recurrence (Melmed et al., 1990). Virus shedding is known to occur in the absence of overt lesions; thus, reactivation does not necessarily result in clinical symptoms. However, it seems that clinical activation is an expression of an immune-mediated process.

STRESS AND CANCER

Studies in humans suggest that psychosocial factors are capable of influencing the natural history of some common malignancies. A prospective five-year study of 69 consecutive female patients with early breast cancer indicated that the psychological response to the diagnosis of cancer appeared to influence the outcome (Greer et al., 1979). Patients' psychological responses, assessed three months postoperatively, were examined in relation to outcome five years after mastectomy. Recurrence-free survival was significantly more frequent among patients who had initially reacted to the diagnosis by denial or who had shown a "fighting spirit" (15/20, 75%) than in patients who had shown either stoic acceptance or a helpless/hopeless response (13/37, 35%). The pattern was similar when the early psychological response was related to mortality: an initial reaction of stoic acceptance or helplessness/hopelessness was shown by 88% (14/16) of the women who eventually died of the disease but only 46% (13/28) of those who remained alive and well respectively ($P < 0.025$).

Earlier studies had indicated that feelings of hopelessness, higher scores on the Minnesota Multiphasic Inventory (MMPI) Depression Scale, and loss of close personal relationships are associated with occurrence of cancer (LeShan and Worthington, 1956; Schmale and Iker, 1966; Greene, 1966; Thomas and Duszynski, 1974). In a prospective study of 2020 men, Schekelle et al. (1981) found that depression, as measured with the MMPI scale, was associated with a twofold increase in the chances of death from cancer during 17 years of follow-up. This association persisted even after adjustments for age, cigarette smoking, alcohol consumption, family history of cancer, and occupational status, and it was not specific for any particular site or type of cancer. These authors concluded that depression seems to impair mechanisms, presumably immunological, for preventing the onset and spread of cancer.

The importance of marital state and social support was underlined by the findings of Goodwin et al. (1987), who used population-based data on 27,779 cancer patients to examine the effects of marital status on diagnosis, treatment, and survival. Unmarried persons with cancer had a decreased overall survival. The authors identified both biological (site, morphological type, and extent of disease at time of diagnosis) and nonbiological factors (access to medical care, compliance with therapy) likely to influence survival. Although all of these factors, after correcting for the influence of age and gender, played a part in determining the poorer survival of the unmarried persons, a significant relationship was demonstrated between marital status and survival from cancer. Being married was associated with an increase in five-year survival comparable with being in an age group 10 years younger. Reynolds and Kaplan (1990) also found that women who were socially isolated were at substantially elevated risk for dying of cancer. Those who had few social contacts and felt isolated had an almost fivefold increase in relative risk for dying of cancer. In addition, men with few social connections showed significantly poorer survival rates.

Survival of cancer patients increases with socioeconomic status (Linden, 1969; Lipworth et al., 1970; Syme and Berkman, 1976; Dayal et al., 1982) and part of the beneficial effect of being married may be the generally higher socioeconomic status of married persons (Wilder, 1976). The effects of socioeconomic status on survival, ranging from a 20% to 40% increase, are comparable with the effects of marital status reported by Goodwin et al. (1987).

Data like those just cited, pointing to the very significant negative health effects of social isolation, have formed the basis of several intervention studies aimed at ameliorating these effects. The impact of psychosocial intervention on the survival time of 86 patients with metastatic breast cancer was prospectively evaluated by Spiegel et al. (1989). The intervention lasted for a year, during which time both control and intervention groups (which were randomly selected) received routine oncological care. The intervention group in addition met weekly for 90 minutes with a psychiatrist or social worker and a therapist with breast cancer in remission. The focus of the discussion was on coping mechanisms and patients were encouraged to express their feelings about the illness and its effects on their lives. The objective was to reduce anxiety, depression, and pain. Social isolation was countered by the development of strong relationships within the group, and patients were encouraged to be more assertive with doctors. In addition, patients were encouraged to extract meaning from tragedy by using their experience to help other patients and their families. Survival was 36.6 months on average (SD 37.6 months) in the intervention group, compared with 18.9 months (SD 10.8 months) in the control group, a highly significant difference ($P < 0.0001$).

Two additional randomized studies similarly indicated that psychotherapeutic interventions aimed at enhancing both social support and emotional expression enhance survival in patients with cancer (Richardson et al., 1990; Fawzi et al., 1993). These two studies focused on patients with lymphoma or leukemia and melanoma. However, two other studies failed to find any relationship between psychosocial intervention and cancer survival (Gellert et al., 1993; Ilnyckj et al., 1994). Thus, three randomized prospective studies found an increased survival of cancer patients given psychosocial treatment as compared to controls, whereas one matching and one randomized study did not show such a difference.

Potential Mechanism for Enhanced Survival by Psychosocial Intervention in Cancer Patients

Although it is clear that more studies are needed to determine the likely benefits of psychosocial intervention in cancer patients, the foregoing carefully executed studies reporting a positive outcome suggest that it does help in some patients. Concerning a likely mechanism, Spiegel et al. (1998) argue: "There is good reason to believe that stress caused by the diagnosis of medical illness (i.e. cancer), uncertainty about the future, loss of control, and social isolation may adversely affect immune capabilities for tumor resistance with clinically relevant consequences. Conversely, enhanced psychosocial support via group therapy or other means may plausibly improve medical outcome by buffering the consequences of such stress and therefore ameliorating immune function." The same authors then suggest that natural killer (NK) cells may be important mediators of the impact of psychosocial intervention on the natural history of cancer because

1. Abnormalities of NK cell function and numbers have been associated with a wide array of human diseases, including increased risk for various cancers (Whiteside and Herberman, 1995).
2. Natural killer cells kill a variety of tumor cells both *in vitro* and in animal studies (Whiteside and Herberman, 1995).
3. Psychosocial factors may impair NK cell function.

The third point has been demonstrated for depression (Stein et al., 1991) (see Chapter 16) and anxiety, whereas social support and interpersonal relationships seem to mitigate the effects of stress on NK cells (Kiecolt-Glaser et al., 1984; Kennedy et al., 1988).

The mechanism underlying the cytotoxic attack by NK cells of cancer cells as well as some virally transformed cells is that these are two categories of cell types that may lack expression of MHC class I molecules. Normally the MHC class I molecule on the cell surface functions to inhibit NK cell induced cytotoxicity. With failure to recognize this molecule on the target cell surface, the NK cell responds by inserting the pore-forming molecule perforin into the membrane of the target cell and then injecting it with cytotoxic enzymes (Moretta et al., 1997).

The clinical relevance of psychosocial effects on NK cell function is suggested by an observed relationship between social factors, higher NK cell function, and slower disease progression in two studies of cancer patients (Levy et al., 1991; Fawzi at el., 1993). Regardless of whether the interplay of cancer with the immune system is mediated by a single cell type (which does not seem likely to me) or by a more complex system of interactions, however, the probable centrality of NK cell activity in this process puts the emphasis again on a mechanism mediated through cellular immunity, that is, on a Th1 type of reaction. This fits well the general thesis about changes in the normal Th1/Th2 balance in the direction of a weakening of Th1-associated processes (above) and perhaps an enhamcement of Th2 associated processes, mediating the effects of stress on immune function.

Toward a Universal Mechanism of Stress-Induced Immunomodulation

If stress indeed impairs immune surveillance or immune responses in otherwise healthy subjects, as accumulating scientific evidence suggests, then it does so by modulating immune function rather than producing a truly immunocompromised state. Thus, stress has not been noted to lead to opportunistic infections or Kaposi's sarcoma, diseases that characterize the immunocompromised individual, such as patients receiving chronic high-dose glucocorticoid therapy or those with HIV infection. On the other hand, modulation of immune function by neuropsychological influences through an effect on lymphokine and cytokine production, as suggested above, would help explain how stress could influence a wide range of pathological processes.

The Th1/Th2 hypothesis of immune responses appears to go a substantial way in providing a physiological explanation for a number of seemingly disparate observations, both clinical and experimental, and makes it easier to understand why stress-induced immune changes may have such different effects on different individuals. Just as immune surveillance of the body in the case of autoimmune disease, a viral infection, cancer, or tuberculosis is likely to involve different components of the immune system, so the effects of stress may influence a variety of pathological processes by modulating the secretion of common mediators which control the diverse elements of the different immunological processes. Significantly, though, all the pathological processes listed in this chapter appear to be dependent on cell-mediated immune processes for their optimal control (suppression), and it is precisely this facet of immune function that appears to be most susceptible to the deleterious effects of stress.

REFERENCES

Ader R, Cohen N (1975). Behaviorally conditioned immunosuppression. Psychosom Med 37:333–340.

Ader R, Cohen N (1982). Behaviorally conditioned immunosuppression and murine systemic lupus erythematosis. Science 215:1534–1536.

Ader R, Cohen N, Felten D (1995). Psychoneuroimmunology: interactions between the nervous system and the immune system. Lancet 345:99–103.

Baringer JR, Swoveland P (1973). Recovery of herpes-simplex virus from human trigeminal ganglions. N Engl J Med 288:648–650.

Bastian FO, Rabson AS, Yee CL, et al. (1972). Herpesvirus hominis: Isolation from human trigeminal ganglion. Science 178:306–307.

Bell RB, Aurelian L, Cohen GH (1978). Proteins of herpes virus type 2. IV. Leucocyte inhibition responses to type common antigen(s) in cervix cancer and recurrent herpetic infections. Cell Immunol 41:86–102.

Bellinger DL, Lorton D, Romano TD, et al. (1990). Neuropeptide innervation of lymphoid organs. Ann NY Acad Sci 594:17–33.

Besedovsky HO, Del Rey A, Sorkin E, et al. (1979). Immunoregulation mediated by the sympathetic nervous system. Cell Immunol 48:346–355.

Boyce WT, Jensen EW, Cassel JC, et al. (1977). Influence of life events and family routines on childhood respiratory tract illness. Pediatrics 60:609–615.

Cantin E, Tanamachi B, Openshaw H (1999). Role for gamma interferon in control of herpes simplex virus type 1 reactivation. J Virol 73:3418–3423.

Clerici M, Shearer GM (1994). The Th1–Th2 hypothesis of HIV infection: new insights. Immunol Today 15:575–581.

Cohen S, Tyrrell DA, Smith AP (1991). Psychological stress and susceptibility to the common cold. N Engl J Med 325:606–612.

Cole SW, Kemeny ME (1997). Psychobiology of HIV infection. Crit Rev Neurobiol 11:289–321.

Dayal HH, Power RN, Chiu C (1982). Race and social economic status in survival from breast cancer. J Chron Dis 35:675–683.

Daynes RA, Araneo BA (1989). Contrasting effects of glucocorticoids on the capacity of T cells to produce the growth factors interleukin 2 and interleukin 4. Eur J Immunol 19:2319–2325.

De Waal Malefyt R, Abrams J, Bennet B, et al. (1991). Interleukin 10 (IL-10) inhibits cytokine synthesis in human monocytes: an autoregulatory role of IL-10 produced by moncytes. J Exp Med 174:1209–1220.

Fawzi FI, Fawzy W, Hyun CS, et al. (1993). Malignant melanoma: effects of an early structured psychiatric intervention, coping, and affective state on recurrence and survival 6 years later. Arch Gen Psychiatry 50:681–689.

Friedman E, Katcher AH, Brightman VJ (1977). Incidence of recurrent herpes labialis and upper respiratory infection: a prospective study of the influence of biologic, social and psychological predictors. Oral Surg Oral Med Oral Pathol 43:873–878.

Galin FS, LeBoeuf RD, Blalock JE (1990). Characteristics of lymphocyte-derived proopiomelanocortin-related mRNA. Ann NY Acad Sci 594:382–384.

Gellert GA, Maxwell RM, Siegel BS (1993). Survival of breast cancer patients receiving adjunctive psychosocial support therapy: a 10-year follow-up study. J Clin Oncol 11:66–69.

Giang DW, Goodman AD, Schiffer RB, et al. (1996). Conditioning of cyclophosphamide-induced leukopenia in humans. J Neuropsychiatry Clin Neurosci 8:194–201.

Glaser R, Friedman SB, Smyth J, et al. (1999). The differential impact of training stress and final examination stress on herpesvirus latency at the United States Military Academy at West Point. Brain Behav Immun 13:240–251.

Glaser R, Kiecolt-Glaser JK (1997). Chronic stress modulates the virus-specific immune response to latent herpes simplex virus type 1. Ann Behav Med 19:78–82.

Glaser R, Kiecolt-Glaser JK, Malarky WB, et al. (1998). The influence of psychological stress on the immune response to vaccines. Ann NY Acad Sci 840:674–683.

Glaser R, Kiecolt-Glaser JK, Speicher CE, et al. (1985). Stress, loneliness, and changes in herpesvirus latency. J Behav Med 8:249–260.

Glaser R, Pearson GR, Jones JF, et al. (1991). Stress-related activation of Epstein-Barr virus. Brain Behav Immun 5:219–232.

Glaser R, Rice J, Sheridan J, et al. (1987). Stress-related immune suppression: health implications. Brain Behav Immun 1:7–20.

Goodwin JS, Hunt WC, Key CR, et al. (1987). The effect of marital status on stage, treatment, and survival of cancer patients. JAMA 258:3125–3130.

Gorczynski RM (1990). Conditioned enhancement of skin allografts in mice. Brain Behav Immun 4:85–92.

Graham NM, Douglas RM, Ryan P (1986). Stress and acute respiratory infection. Am J Epidemiol 124:389–401.

Greene SM (1989). The relationship between depression and hopelessness: implication for current theories of depression. Br J Psychiatry 154:650–659.

Greene WA (1966). The psychosocial setting of the development of leukemia and lymphoma. Ann NY Acad Sci 125:794–801.

Greer S, Morris T, Pettingale KW (1979). Psychological response to breast cancer: effect on outcome. Lancet 2:785–787.

Heagy W, Laurance M, Cohen E, et al. (1990). Neurohormones regulate T cell function. J Exp Med 171:1625–1633.

Holmes TH, Hawkins NG, Bowerman CE, et al. (1957). Psychosocial and physiological studies of tuberculosis. Psychosom Med 19:134–143.

Howard AD, Zwilling BS (1999). Reactivation of tuberculosis is associated with a shift from type 1 to type 2 cytokines. Clin Exp Immunol 115:428–434.

Ilnyckyj A, Farber J, Cheang M, et al. (1994). A randomized controlled trial of psychotherapeutic intervention in cancer patients. Ann R Coll Physicians Surg Can 27:93–96.

Irwin M, Costlow C, Williams H, et al. (1998). Cellular immunity to varicella-zoster virus in patients with major depression. J Infect Dis 178(suppl 1):S104–S108.

Ishigami T (1919). The influence of psychic acts on the progress of pulmonary tuberculosis. Am Rev Tuberculosis 2:470–484.

Jacobs RP, Aurelian L, Cole GA (1976). Cell-mediated immune response to herpes simplex virus: type-specific lymphoproliferative responses in lymph nodes draining the site of primary infection. J Immunol 116:1520–1525.

Jemmott JB III, Borysenko JZ, Borysenko M, et al. (1983). Academic stress, power motivation, and decrease in salivary secretory immunoglobulin A secretion rate. Lancet I:1400–1402.

Kasl SV, Evans AS, Niederman JC (1979). Psychosocial risk factors in the development of infectious mononucleosis. Psychosom Med 41:445–466.

Kemeny ME (1994). Stressful events, psychological responses, and progression of HIV infection, In: Glaser R, Kiecolt-Glaser JK, eds. Handbook of Human Stress and Immunity. New York: Academic Press.

Kennedy S, Kiecolt-Glaser JK, Glaser R (1988). Immunological consequences of acute and chronic stressors: mediating role of interpersonal relationships. Br J Med Psychol 61:77–85.

Kiecolt-Glaser JK, Garner W, Speicher CE, et al. (1984). Psychosocial modifiers of immunocompetence in medical students. Psychosom Med 46:7–14.

Kiecolt-Glaser JK, Glaser R, Strain EC, et al. (1986). Modulation of cellular immunity in medical students. J Behav Med 9:5–21.

Kissen DM (1958). Emotional Factors in Pulmonary Tuberculosis. London: Tavistock Publications.

Kobasa SC, Hilker RR (1982). Executive work perceptions and the quality of working life. J Occup Med 24:25–29.

Kodukula P, Liu T, Rooijen NV, et al. (1999). Macrophage control of herpes simplex virus type 1 replication in the peripheral nervous system. J Immunol 162:2895–2905.

Korsager B, Spencer ES, Mordhurst CH, et al. (1975). Herpesvirus hominis infections in renal transplant recipients. Scand J Infect Dis 7:11–19.

Lausch RN, Swyers JS, Kaufman HE (1966). Delayed hypersensitivity to herpes simplex virus in the guinea pig. J Immunol 96:981–987.

LeShan L, Worthington RE (1956). Some recurrent life history patterns observed in patients with malignant disease. J Nerv Ment Dis 124:460–465.

Levy SM, Herberman RB, Lippman M, et al. (1991). Immunological and psychosocial predictors of disease recurrence in patients with early-stage breast cancer. Behav Med 17:67–75.

Linden G (1969). The influence of social class in the survival of cancer patients. Am J Public Health 59:267–274.

Lipworth L, Abelin T, Connelly RR (1970). Socioeconomic factors in the prognosis of cancer patients. J Chron Dis 23:105–115.

Lycke E, Norrby R, Roos B-E (1974). A serological study on mentally ill patients with special reference to the prevalence of herpes virus infections. Br J Psychiatry 124:273–279.

Maes M, Lin AH, Delmeire L, et al. (1999). Elevated serum interleukin-6 (IL-6) and IL-6 receptor concentrations in posttraumatic stress disorder following accidental manmade traumatic events. Biol Psychiatry 45:833–839.

Manfredi B, Sacerdote P, Gaspani L, et al. (1998). IL-6 knock-out mice show modified basal immune functions, but normal immune response to stress. Brain Behav Immun 12:201–211.

Melmed RN, Roth D, Edelstein EL (1990). Symptom anticipation and the learned visceral response: a major neglected determinant of morbidity in functional and organic disorders. Isr J Med Sci 26: 43–46.

Meyer RJ, Haggerty RJ (1962). Streptococcal infections in families. Pediatrics 29:539–549.

Morahan PS, Breinig MC, McGeorge MB (1978). Immune responses to vaginal or systemic infection of BALB/c mice with herpes simplex virus type 2. IARC Sci Publ. 24:759–763.

Moretta A, Biassoni R, Bottino C, et al. (1997). Major histocompatibility complex class I-specific receptors on human natural killer and T lymphocytes. Immunol Rev 155:105–117.

Mosmann TR, Sad S (1996). The expanding universe of T-cell subsets: Th1, Th2 and more. Immunol Today 17:138–146.

Muller S, Weihe E (1991). Interrelation of peptidergic innervation with mast cells and ED1-positive cells in rat thymus. Brain Behav Immun 5:55–72.

Noisakran S, Halford WP, Veress L, et al. (1998). Role of the hypothalamic pituitary adrenal axis and IL-6 in stress-induced reactivation of latent herpes simplex virus type 1. J Immunol 160:5441–5447.

O'Reilly RJ, Chibbaro A, Anger E, et al. (1977). Cell-mediated responses in patients with recurrent Herpes Simplex infections. II. Infection-associated deficiency of lymphokine production in patients with recurrent herpes labialis or progenitalis. J Immunol 118:1095–1102.

Payan DG (1989). Neuropeptides and inflammation: the role of substance P. Ann Rev Med 40:341–352.

Pfizenmaier KH, Jung H, Starzinski-Powitz A, et al. (1977). The role of T cells in anti-herpes simplex virus immunity. I. Induction of antigen-specific cytotoxic T lymphocytes. J Immunol 119:939–944.

Reynolds P, Kaplan GA (1990). Social connections and risk for cancer: prospective evidence from the Alameda County Study. Behav Med 16:101–110.

Richardson JL, Shelton DR, Krailo M, et al. (1990). The effect of compliance with treatment on survival among patients with hematological malignancies. J Clin Oncol 8:356–364.

Rook GAW, Hernandez-Pando R, Lightman SL (1994). Hormones, peripherally activated prohormones and the regulation of the Th1/Th2 balance. Immunol Today 15:301–303.

Rosenberg GL, Farber PA, Notkins AL (1972). In vitro stimulation of sensitized lymphocytes by herpes simplex virus and vaccinia virus. Proc Natl Acad Sci 69:756–760.

Rossen RD, Butler WT, Waldman RH, et al. (1970). The protein of nasal secretions. II. A longitudinal study of IgA and neutralizing antibody levels in nasal washings from men infected with influenza virus. JAMA 211:1157–1161.

Schekelle RB, Raynor WJ, Ostfeld AM, et al (1981). Psychological depression and 17-year risk of death from cancer. Psychosom Med 43:117–125.

Schmale AH, Iker HP (1966). The affect of hopelessness and the development of cancer. Psychosom Med 28:714–721.

Sheridan JF, Donnenberg AD, Aurelian L, et al. (1982). Immunity to herpes simplex virus type 2. IV. Impaired lymphokine production during recrudescence correlates with an imbalance in T-lymphocyte subsets. J Immunol 129:326–331.

Shimeld C, Easty DL, Hill TJ (1999). Reactivation of herpes simplex virus type 1 in the mouse trigeminal ganglion: an in vitro study of virus antigen and cytokines. J Virol 73:1767–1773.

South MA, Copper MD, Wollheim FA, et al. (1969). The IgA system: II. The clinical significance of IgA deficiency. Am J Med 44:168–178.

Spiegel D, Bloom JR, Kraemer HC, et al. (1989). Effect of psychosocial treatment on survival of patients with metastatic breast cancer. Lancet 2:888–891.

Spiegel D, Sephton SE, Terr AI, et al. (1998). Effects of psychosocial treatment in prolonging cancer survival may be mediated by neuroimmune pathways. Ann NY Acad Sci 840:674–683.

Sreedharan SP, Kodama KT, Peterson KC, et al. (1989). Distinct subsets of somatostatin receptors on cultured human lymphocytes. J Biol Chem 264:949–952.

Stein M, Miller AH, Trestman RL (1991). Depression, the immune system, and health and illness. Findings in search of meaning. Arch Gen Psychiatry 48:171–177.

Syme SL, Berkman LF (1976). Social class, susceptibility and sickness. Am J Epidemiol 104:1–8.

Thomas CB, Duszynski KR (1974). Closeness to parents and the family constellation in a prospective study of five disease states: suicide, mental illness, malignant tumor, hypertension and coronary heart disease. Johns Hopkins Med J 134:251–270.

Tollefson L, Bulloch K (1990). Dual-label retrograde transport: CNS innervation of the mouse thymus distinct from other mediastinal viscera. J Neurosci Res 25:20–28.

Tomasi TB, Grey HM (1972). Structure and function of immunoglobulin A. Prog Allergy 16:81–213.

Wenger GD, O'Dorisio MS, Goetzl EJ (1990). Vasoactive intestinal peptide. Messenger in a neuroimmune axis. Ann NY Acad Sci 594:104–119.

Whiteside TL, Herberman RB (1995). The role of natural killer cells in immune surveillance of cancer. Curr Opin Immunol 7:704–710.

Wilder MH (1976). Differentials in health characteristics by marital status, United States, 1971–1972, Vital and Health Statistics Series 10, No.104, data from the National Heath Survey. Rockville, Md: National Center for Health Statistics.

Woiciechowsky C, Asadullah K, Nestler D, et al. (1998). Sympathetic activation triggers systemic interleukin-10 release in immunodepression induced by brain injury. Nat Med 4:808–813.

Chapter

7

CLINICAL CONSEQUENCES OF STRESS

A psychosocial factor potentially relates psychological phenomena to the social environment and to pathophysiological changes (Hemingway and Marmot, 1999). This chapter attempts to show how psychosocial factors may act as stressors to promote disease occurrence or to aggravate existing diseases. The stressors that we consider vary, but all essentially represent conditions in which the individual's sense of control is seriously challenged or even lost. Whether the problem is called an "adjustment disorder," the "stress of illness," or any other name, the point is that the physician is often led into psychosomatic considerations by the patient's suffering, an unexpected deterioration of the clinical state, or poor clinical response despite seemingly adequate treatment.

In addition, there may be indications in the patient's emotional state or behavior that should arouse the suspicion that he or she is not coping adequately with disease. These indicators may vary from depression to apathy (especially an inappropriate detachment), from avoiding contact with medical personnel to inappropriately excessive physical activity (e.g., a patient with proven ischemic heart disease running up stairs), from lack of compliance in taking medications to heavy smoking or other substance abuse. Although physicians often refer to these behavioral patterns, with resignation, as "self-destructive," it is important to realize that looking beyond them to the question of loss of control and its management may help patients respond to the emotional demands of the situation and also protect them from the dangerous consequences of their behavioral response. It is by effectively attending to the patient's distress that we may best be able to produce changes in undesirable (i.e., damaging) patterns of behavior. As we will see in Chapter 8, the various mechanisms often are better appreciated when considered in a specific context. For this reason, the phenomena discussed in this chapter, while relating to common diseases, help illustrate some of the multiplicity of psychosocial influences and their pathophysiological consequences that are seen in different clinical situations.

PSYCHOSOCIAL ASPECTS OF
CORONARY HEART DISEASE

Psychosocial and demographic factors, particularly level of education and extent of social isolation (Ruberman et al., 1984; Orth-Gomer et al., 1988), have a substantial impact on morbidity and mortality in coronary heart disease. In a study of 1739 male survivors of myocardial infarction, the risk of sudden coronary death over a three-year period, for those with little education (up to eight years of schooling) who had complex ventricular premature beats in a one-hour standard 12-lead electrocardiogram monitoring session, was more than three times higher than the risk for better educated men with the same arrhythmia (cumulative mortality rate of 33% and 9%, respectively). No such difference appeared in the absence of this particular arrhthymia, and there was no relationship between education level and risk of recurrent infarct (Weinblatt et al., 1978). Five years after the infarct, the risk of death for the patients with little education was more than twice that of their better educated counterparts (Ruberman et al., 1981).

The same group of investigators conducted psychosocial interviews with 2320 male survivors of acute myocardial infarction and found that, with adequate controls for other important prognostic factors, the risk of cardiac death in patients classified as being socially isolated and having a high degree of life stress was more than four times greater than in patients with low levels of both stress and social isolation. High levels of stress and social isolation were most prevalent among the least educated men and least prevalent among the best educated (Ruberman et al., 1984). The same inverse relationship between mortality from coronary heart disease and education has been reported in a number of studies (Hinkle et al., 1968; Shekelle, 1969). A study comparing 100 consecutive sudden deaths with 100 nonfatal myocardial infarctions found that the fatal events were related to socioecononic status (Myers and Dewar, 1975). Prospective studies have also shown education and socioeconomic status to be inversely related to cardiac mortality of all types (Rose and Marmot, 1981; Liu et al., 1982).

One might ask whether the findings in these studies may not simply reflect a poorer standard of medical care in socioeconomically deprived and poorly educated groups. The best-known studies were done in Britain where the National Health Service provides all citizens with access to satisfactory medical care. The cumulative research experience derived from different approaches (see Chapter 5) convincingly points to the conclusion that socioeconomic disadvantage, social isolation, and lack of education are linked to increased mortality in patients suffering from heart disease and other causes.

Depression as a Risk Factor for Coronary Artery Disease

Hemingway and Marmot (1999) reviewed 11 prospective studies published between 1986 and 1997 that investigated depression or anxiety in the etiology of coronary heart disease and found all of them positive. Several studies have shown that depression is an independent predictor of poor outcome after the onset of clinical coronary artery disease (Carney et al., 1988; Frasure-Smith et al., 1995; Barefoot et al., 1996). Frasure-Smith et al. (1993) found that depression was associated with a greater than fourfold increased risk of fatal outcome during the first six months following acute myocardial infarction after adjusting for relevant covariates, including left ventricular dysfunction. In patients with ischemic heart disease and heart failure, the presence of depression is a better predictor of functional capacity than is the left ventricular ejection fraction (Skala et al., 1995).

Prospective studies controlled for socioeconomic status, cardiovascular risk factors, and preexisting heart disease have also shown depressed affect and hopelessness to be independent risk factors for fatal and nonfatal coronary heart disease. Similarly, in a sample of older adults participating in a clinical trial, an increasing level of depression over time, but not the extent of baseline depressive symptoms, was a predictor for cardiovascular events (Wassertheil-Smoller et al., 1996).

The question of whether depression can be considered a risk factor for the development of coronary heart disease was investigated in the Johns Hopkins Precursor Study (Ford et al., 1998). This was a prospective study of 1190 male medical students who were enrolled between 1948 and 1964 and from whom information was collected on family history, health behaviors, and clinical depression. The cumulative incidence of clinical depression in the medical students at 40 years of follow-up was 12%. Those who developed depression did not differ from the nondepressed subjects in terms of cardiovascular risk factors such as baseline blood pressure, serum cholesterol levels, smoking status, physical activity, obesity, or family history of coronary artery disease. The men who reported clinical depression were at a significantly greater risk for subsequent coronary artery disease and myocardial infarction (relative risk 2.12 for both). Perhaps most remarkable was the finding that the increased risk associated with clinical depression was present even for myocardial infarctions occurring 10 years after the onset of the first depressive episode. This tendency has been noted by others as well (Barefoot et al., 1996).

Also relevant to this discussion is the observation that giving up hope—"hopelessness," defined as negative expectations about oneself and the future—has adverse physical and mental health consequences (Everson et al., 1996). While it may seem probable that most individuals exhibiting an attitude of hopelessness are depressed, Greene (1989) pointed out that not all depressed individuals experience hopelessness. Anda et al. (1993) reported that hopelessness significantly predicted fatal and nonfatal ischemic heart disease (IHD) after 12 years of follow-up in a cohort of more than 2800 initially healthy men and women from the National Health Examination Follow-Up Survey. Similarly, Everson et al. (1996) found that a high level of hopelessness was associated with increased risk of myocardial infarction and cardiovascular mortality, as well as other adverse health outcomes, after six years of follow-up in middle-aged men from eastern Finland. In both studies, controlling for traditional cardiovascular risk factors had relatively little impact on the observed associations between hopelessness and cardiovascular morbidity and mortality. A separate study of 942 participants in the Kuopio Ischemic Heart Disease Study (middle-aged men from eastern Finland) revealed a relationship between hopelessness and the progression of carotid atherosclerosis (Everson et al., 1997). Carotid ultrasonography was performed at baseline and four years later. Men reporting high levels of hopelessness at baseline had faster progression of carotid atherosclerosis than men reporting low to moderate levels of hopelessness.

Although the mechanism for the adverse effects of depression or hopelessness on the coronary arteries has not been elucidated, sympathetic nervous activity is increased in patients with major depression (Gold et al., 1988; Veith et al., 1994). If sustained, this might predispose to life-endangering ventricular arrhythmias (Podrid et al., 1990) or coronary artery spasm (Yeung et al., 1991). This important clinical association has not yet been clearly explained, but it is worth noting that catecholamine β receptor blockers (e.g., atenolol, propranolol) as well as angiotensin-conversion inhibitors (e.g., convertin), drugs that diminish sympathetic effects on the heart and blood vessels, are of proven efficacy in prolonging life after a myocardial infarct. They are consequently recommended for secondary prevention (i.e., the prevention of further heart attack or other ischemic complications) in patients with coronary artery disease (Krumholz et al., 1998; Freemantle et al., 1999; Frishman and Cheng, 1999).

Job Stress and Cardiovascular Disease

Since a large part of our lives is spent working, a stressful job could be expected to have a physiological impact. In this section we examine some aspects of the work environment that induce stress and thus could contribute to the development of coronary artery disease.

A very important reason for the impact of stress on the cardiovascular system is the sensitive dependence of cardiovascular responses on nervous stimulation and control. In a review entitled "An Essay on the Circulation as Behavior," Engel (1986) described the cardiovascular responses as an integral component of the animal's behavior. There are continuous responses to the numerous behavioral changes that occur in any 24-hour period, and in day-to-day living there is no stress without a cardiovascular response. In other words, emotional stress and the cardiovascular response to it are part of the same integrated condition. Engel's view is based on decades of research in many laboratories. Moreover, it is central to understanding what happens physiologically to an individual under stress.

The impact of job stress

The correlation between blood pressure measurements and specific morbid events is poorly documented in the literature, despite a strong association between increased blood pressure and increased risk of disease and death. Searching for the basis of this association, Devereux et al. (1983) studied blood pressure changes by the continuous monitoring of hypertensive subjects during their routine activities over 24 hours. The best correlation between left ventricular mass index (g/m^2, as an objective indicator of mean blood pressure levels) and blood pressure was obtained in subjects whose blood pressure was monitored while they were at work. The correlation between left ventricular mass index and blood pressure readings taken in the clinic, at home, or during sleep was significantly weaker. These findings indicate that in hypertensive individuals, a rise in blood pressure is of greatest physiological significance in the work situation.

Is it possible to identify those elements that can make work stressful? The landmark study in this field was performed by Karasek et al. (1981), who examined the relationship between specific job characteristics and subsequent cardiovascular disease in a large random sample of the Swedish male working population. The authors postulated that tension results from the combined effects of the work situation, that is, the stressors (especially the demands of the job and boredom) and the environmental modulators of stress, particularly the degree of decision-making freedom (control) available to the worker in coping with those demands. Jobs such as assembly-line work, which are both *psychologically demanding* and characterized by *low decision latitude* (i.e., little or no control), proved to be significantly associated with coronary heart disease.

Other studies have focused on the association between work stress and cardiovascular disorders in selected occupational groups that are assumed to be stressful, such as bus drivers and air traffic controllers. What the Swedish study set out to do, however, was to provide a theoretical framework for identifying stress-related job characteristics which could be applied to the entire work force, permitting as well the generation of specific hypotheses for testing. More recent analysis of the Karasek model has suggested that a third factor, *skill discretion* (choice of activity), in addition to decision authority and the psychological demands of the job, would increase the model's validity (Schreurs and Taris, 1998). In a subsequent study of American workers, Karasek et al. (1988) confirmed that high-stress jobs as defined in their Swedish study are associated with an increased prevalence of myocardial infarction.

Schnall et al. (1990) used criteria similar to those of Karasek et al. (1981) for the classification of high-stress jobs in a study that showed a definite tendency of stressed workers to develop both hypertension and hypertensive disease as manifested by an increased left ventricular mass index. Six of ten studies performed between the years 1984 to 1997 that utilized criteria similar to those of Karasek et al. (1981) were similarly positive, although it appears that lack of control could be more critical than psychological demands as a stress that impairs health (Hemingway and Marmot, 1999). An alternative model of psychosocial work characteristics suggested to be important in generating significant stress in the worker involves an imbalance between work effort and rewards received (Bosma et al., 1998).

The predisposed worker: mechanism of stress-induced cardiac ischemia

Here we consider the effects of job stress on individuals with established coronary artery disease. For such persons the likelihood that stress will induce ischemia is much higher. Few studies have specifically evaluated the effects of stressful or emotional events on cardiac activity during ambulatory Holter monitoring, that is, long-term electrocardiogrpahic monitoring. One revealed that the duration of ambulatory recorded ST segment depression was longer per unit time spent in mentally stressful activities than in routine physical activities or during rest (Barry et al., 1988). It also indicated that in coronary patients, ischemia induced by mental stress occurs at a lower level of myocardial work requirements (as reflected by heart rate and blood pressure changes) than it does in exercise-associated ischemia (Schiffer et al., 1980; LeVeau et al., 1989). Myocardial ischemia induced by mental stress and recorded as characteristic changes on the electrocardiogram may often be clinically "silent," meaning without pain (Deanfield et al., 1984; Rozanski et al., 1988; Bairey et al., 1992). These observations suggest that coronary vasoconstriction mediated by increased sympathetic activity, causing decreased blood flow and therefore reduced oxygen delivery, may be the mechanism of stress-induced myocardial ischemia. Stressful experiences may lower the threshold for ischemia by promoting coronary artery spasm, and this could be a mechanism of acute myocardial infarction triggered by emotional stress in a patient with only mild (<30%) coronary artery stenosis (Yeung et al., 1991; Gellernt and Hochman, 1992).

In the presence of coronary artery disease, stress may suffice to precipitate ischemia and could therefore predispose the patient to a possibly lethal arrhythmia or myocardial infarction. Mittleman et al. (1995) interviewed 1623 patients, on average within four days of a myocardial infarction. They identified 39 patients with episodes of anger in the two hours preceding the onset of myocardial infarction and concluded that anger may indeed precipitate myocardial infarction. Given the relationship between mental stress and myocardial ischemia quoted above, however, it was perhaps surprising that anger proved to be such an uncommon precipitant of myocardial infarction. In addition, reversible cardiogenic shock precipitated by emotional distress has been reported in the total absence of coronary artery disease (Hachamovitch et al., 1995), an exceedingly rare occurrence.

Is personality a risk factor?

Both the personality and the social network of the individual play a role in the development of stress. While common sense suggests that a type A personality (time-pressured, competitive, impatient, intensely motivated) may be particularly vulnerable to job stress, does the personality structure itself predispose the individual to coronary artery disease? The literature is equivocal on this subject, but after an initial tendency toward an affirmative answer (Rosenman et al., 1976; Haynes et al., 1980), a systematic review of prospective cohort studies clearly indicated that type A personality does not *of itself* lead to coronary artery disease (Hemingway and Marmot, 1999). This is supported as well by the evaluation of the role of personality (particularly type A) in the Multiple Risk Factor Intervention Trial (MRFIT) study (Hollis et al., 1990). After prospectively evaluating more than 3000 participants, the authors concluded that *the impact of life events on cardiovascular risk did not differ by behavior type category.* This conclusion has also received support from numerous other studies (Ray, 1991). This could be explained by the work of Karasek and colleagues (1981, 1988) cited earlier. The stress of a job's high psychological demands in combination with the individual's own self-demanding standards may well be moderated by a substantial degree of control (decision making) in the job (Kobasa and Hilker, 1982).

Summary

The available epidemiological evidence supports the conclusion that sustained job stress increases the likelihood of developing coronary artery disease. Although a number of interacting factors contribute to the negative outcome of such stress, including level of education, sex, cigarette smoking, and social isolation, job stress itself appears to be an independent determinant of the lower health status of the socioeconomically deprived sector of the population in Western societies. The more comprehensive understanding, during the last decade, of factors that make a job stressful should help us identify high-risk occupations, or aspects of specific work situations, and formulate intervention programs aimed at modifying their impact.

STRESS AND METABOLIC CONTROL IN DIABETES MELLITUS

To be informed that one is suffering from diabetes mellitus, particularly of the insulin-dependent type (IDDM), is to be confronted with an exceptionally stressful situation. The realization that one's very survival, from the moment of diagnosis, depends on the daily self-administration of at least one or two subcutaneous injections of insulin, as well as a stringent dietary regime, is a challenge to human adaptability. In addition, most patients probably learn that the condition will ultimately lead to significant vascular complications that may include heart disease, renal failure, and blindness. The disturbing impact of this reality, particularly on the young patient, has been discussed in the clinical literature (Benedek, 1948; Mirsky, 1948; Jacobson, 1996). The unremitting demands of the diabetic state exact a substantial price from the patient in terms of emotional adaptation, and this is all too frequently underappreciated by physicians. As diabetes mellitus is the most common of the serious metabolic diseases, the part played by the stress of the illness in influencing the quality of metabolic control has been extensively reviewed (Burch and Phillips, 1962; Johnson, 1980; Barglow et al., 1984; Helz and Templeton, 1990).

The so-called brittle diabetes, which occurs most commonly in younger people with insulin-dependent diabetes (Gill et al., 1985), is characterized by glycemic instability leading to the disruption of life from repeated hospital admissions for hypoglycemic attacks and/or diabetic ketoacidosis. Among diabetologists in the United Kingdom, 93% consider psychosocial factors, including the patient's manipulation of insulin therapy, as the most common underlying cause (Gill et al., 1996). Studying 89 patients with a mean age of 16 years, Morris et al. (1997) found much evidence of poor compliance with insulin therapy and poor glycemic control, including diabetic ketoacidosis. A substantial body of clinical experience supports the need for detailed psychosocial evaluation of all diabetic patients, particularly young insulin-dependent diabetics, where there are management difficulties due to instability of metabolic control or problems of patient compliance (White et al., 1984).

Psychiatric disorders are underdiagnosed in diabetic patients. Popkin et al. (1988) studied 75 patients who underwent evaluation for pancreatic transplantation and found that about half of them met the criteria for one or more psychiatric diagnoses. The lifetime prevalence of major depression in this group was 25%. Others have also found an increased prevalence of depression in adults with IDDM (Gavard et al., 1993). A history of depression is associated with substantially worse glycemic control and more serious retinopathy than are seen in patients without psychiatric disorders (Lustman et al., 1986). Anxiety symptoms may also be associated with poor glycemic control, and the symptoms of anxiety may mimic those of hypoglycemia (Lustman, 1988).

Effects of Stress on Carbohydrate and Fat Metabolism

The main stress hormones, including corticosteroids, catecholamines, glucagon, and growth hormone, are all able to raise the level of glucose production, either by enhancing gluconeogenesis or by stimulating glycogenolysis. A variable combination of hormones is secreted in any stressed individual and this is substantially more potent in raising blood glucose than any single hormone alone. In dogs, glucagon, epinephrine, or cortisol alone produced only mild elevations in plasma glucose concentrations, whereas the increase in plasma glucose caused by combined infusion of any two of these hormones was 50%–215% more than the sum of the corresponding individual infusions (Eigler et al., 1979). This synergistic interaction of hormones in raising blood glucose explains the phenomenon of *stress hyperglycemia*.

Both in humans and in animals, all ketotic states, whether physiological or pathological, are characterized by a relative or absolute deficiency of insulin (McGarry and Foster, 1977). In contrast to their effects on blood glucose, physiological increments of epinephrine, cortisol, and glucagon, either individually or in combination, cannot induce hyperketonemia in individuals with normal insulin secretory capacity (Kinsell et al., 1951; Schade and Eaton, 1976). Occasionally, however, presumably because of catecholamine inhibition of insulin secretion during a stress response, an individual may exhibit acetonuria in the presence of a normal blood glucose.

Psychological stress can lead to ketoacidosis in diabetic subjects who require insulin (Rosen and Lidz, 1949; Schless and von Laveran-Stiebar, 1964; MacGillivray et al., 1981). Studies have also demonstrated an increase in free fatty acids and ketone bodies during emotional arousal in diabetic patients (Hinkle et al., 1950; Vandenbergh et al., 1966; Vandenbergh et al., 1967). But sudden, short-lived psychological stimuli sufficient to cause marked cardiovascular responses and moderate increases in plasma concentrations of catecholamines and cortisol are unlikely to disturb metabolic control in patients suffering from insulin-dependent diabetes mellitus (Kemmer et al., 1986). It seems that the stressor needs to be either of unusual intensity or of long duration before it has significant metabolic consequences.

Summary

The accumulated experience concerning the influence of stress on the metabolic control of diabetic patients may be summarized as follows. Emotional stress, like physical stress (such as the physical trauma of an accident or operation, or a serious infection such as pneumonia or pyelonephritis), may precipitate a diabetic state, interfere with stable metabolic control of the disorder, or induce uncontrolled diabetic ketoacidosis. Patients may need increased amounts of insulin

(Templeton, 1967) or their diabetes may become "brittle," fluctuating between unacceptably high blood glucose readings, with or without ketoacidosis, and hypoglycemia (Orr et al., 1983; Boehnert and Popkin, 1986; Nathan, 1985). In addition, stress may be associated with higher blood glucose values in patients with non–insulin-dependent diabetes mellitus (Goetsch et al., 1990). However, while earlier workers groped for a solution to the chicken-or-egg dilemma of which came first, the emotional problems or the diabetes (Dunbar et al., 1936 ; Alexander, 1950), there is no basis for concluding that emotional stress causes diabetes mellitus in any individual not predisposed to the condition.

REFERENCES

Alexander F (1950). Psychosomatic Medicine: Its Principles and Application. New York, WW Norton.

Anda R, Williamson D, Jones D, et al. (1993). Depressed affect, hopelessness, and the risk of ischemic heart disease in a cohort of U.S. adults. Epidemiology 4:285–294.

Bairey CN, Kranz DS, Rozanski A (1992). Mental stress as an acute trigger of ischemic left ventricular dysfunction and blood pressure elevation in coronary artery disease. Am J Cardiol 66:28G–31G.

Barefoot JC, Helms MJ, Mark DB, et al. (1996). Depression and long-term mortality risk in patients with coronary artery disease. Am J Cardiol 78:613–617.

Barglow P, Hatcher R, Edidin DV, et al. (1984). Stress and metabolic control in diabetes: psychosomatic evidence and evaluation of methods. Psychosom Med 46:127–144.

Barry J, Selwyn AP, Nabel EG, et al. (1988). Frequency of ST-segment depression produced by mental stress in stable angina pectoris from coronary artery disease. Am J Cardiol 61:989–993.

Benedek T (1948). An approach to the study of the diabetic. Psychosom Med 10:284–287.

Boehnert CE, Popkin MK (1986). Psychological issues in treatment of severely noncompliant diabetics. Psychosomatics 27:11–20.

Bosma H, Peter R, Siegrest J, et al. (1998). Alternative job stress models and the risk of coronary heart disease: the effort–reward imbalance model and the job strain model. Am J Public Health 88:68–74.

Burch G, Phillips J (1962). The role of emotional factors in the etiology and course of diabetes mellitus: a review of recent literature. Am J Med Sci 244:93–109.

Carney RM, Rich MW, Freedland KE, et al. (1988). Major depressive disorder predicts cardiac events in patients with coronary artery disease. Psychosom Med 50:627–633.

Deanfield JE, Shea M, Kensett M, et al. (1984). Silent myocardial ischemia due to mental stress. Lancet 2:1001–1005.

Devereux RB, Pickering TG, Harshfield GA, et al. (1983). Left ventricular hypertrophy in patients with hypertension: importance of blood pressure response to regularly recurring stress. Circulation 68:470–476.

Dunbar HF, Wolfe TP, Rioch JM (1936). Psychiatric aspects of medical problems. Am J Psychiatry 93:649–679.

Eigler N, Sacca L, Sherwin RS (1979). Synergistic interactions of physiological increments of glucagon, epinephrine, and cortisol in the dog: a model for stress-induced hyperglycemia. J Clin Invest 63:114–123.

Engel B (1986). An essay on the circulation as behavior. Behav Brain Sci 9:285–318.

Everson SA, Goldberg DE, Kaplan GA, et al. (1996). Hopelessness and risk of mortality and incidence of myocardial infarction and cancer. Psychosom Med 58:113–121.

Everson SA, Kaplan GA, Goldberg DE, et al. (1997). Hopelessness and the 4-year progression of carotid atherosclerosis. Arterioscler Thromb Vasc Biol 17:1490–1495.

Ford DE, Mead LA, Chang PP, et al. (1998). Depression is a risk factor for coronary artery disease in men: the precursors study. Arch Intern Med 158:1422–1426.

Frasure-Smith N, Lesperance F, Talajic M (1993). Depression following myocardial infarction: inpact on 6-month survival. JAMA 270:1819–1825.

Frasure-Smith N, Lesperance F, Talajic M (1995). Depression and 18-month prognosis after myocardial infarction. Ciculation 91:999–1005.

Freemantle N, Cleland J, Young P, et al. (1999). Beta blockade after myocardial infarction: systematic review and meta regression analysis. Br Med J 318:1730–1737.

Frishman WH, Cheng A (1999). Secondary prevention of myocardial infarction: role of beta-adrenergic blockers and angiotensin-converting enzyme inhibitors. Am Heart J 137(4Pt2):S25–S34.

Gavard JA, Lustman PJ, Clouse RE (1993). Prevalence of depression in adults with diabetes: an epidemiological evaluation. Diabetes Care 16:1167–1178.

Gellert GA, Maxwell RM, Siegel BS (1993). Survival of breast cancer patients receiving adjunctive psychosocial support therapy: a 10-year follow-up study. J Clin Oncol 11:66–69.

Gelernt MD, Hochman JS (1992). Acute myocardial infarction triggered by emotional stress. Am J Cardiol 69:1512–1513.

Gill GV, Lucas S, Kent LA (1996). Prevalence and characteristics of brittle diabetes in Britain. Q J Med 89:839–843.

Gill GV, Walford S, Alberti KGMM (1985). Brittle diabetes: present concepts. Diabetologia 28:579–589.

Goetsch VL, Wiebe DJ, Veltum LG, et al. (1990). Stress and blood glucose in type II diabetes mellitus. Behav Res Ther 28:531–537.

Gold PW, Goodwin FK, Chrousos GP (1988). Clinical and biochemical manifestations of depression. relation to the neurobiology of stress. N Engl J Med 319:348–353.

Goodwin JS, Hunt WC, Key CR, et al. (1987). The effect of marital status on stage, treatment, and survival of cancer patients. JAMA 258:3125–3130.

Greene SM (1989). The relationship between depression and hopelessness: implication for current theories of depression. Br J Psychiatry 154:650–659.

Greene WA (1966). The psychosocial setting of the development of leukemia and lymphoma. Ann NY Acad Sci 125:794–801.

Hachamovitch R, Chang JD, Kuntz RE, et al. (1995). Recurrent reversible cardiogenic shock triggered by emotional distress with no obstructive coronary artery disease. Am Heart J 129:1026–1028.

Haynes SG, Feinleib M, Kannel WB (1980). The relationship of psychosocial factors to coronary artery disease in the Framingham study: 3. Eight year incidence of coronary heart disease. Am J Epidemiol 111:37–58.

Helz JW, Templeton B (1990). Evidence of the role of psychosocial factors in diabetes mellitus: a review. Am J Psychiatry 147:1275–1282.

Hemingway H, Marmot M (1999). Psychosocial factors in the aetiology and prognosis of coronary heart disease: systematic review of prospective cohort studies. Br Med J 318:1460–1467.

Hinkle ~~~~~~ nger GB, Wolf S (1950). Studies on diabetes mellitus: the relation of stress ~~~~~ situations to the concentration of blood glucose in diabetic and non-diabetic humans. J Clin Invest 29:754–769.

Hinkle LE Jr, Whitney LH, Lehman EW, et al. (1968). Occupation, education and coronary heart disease. Science161:238–246.

Hollis JF, Connett JE, Stevens VJ, et al. (1990). Stressful life events, type A behavior, and the prediction of cardiovascular and total mortality over six years. MRFIT Group. J Behav Med 13:263–280.

Jacobson AM (1996). The psychological care of insulin-dependent diabetes mellitus. N Engl J Med 334:1249–1253.

Johnson SB (1980). Psychosocial factors in juvenile diabetes: a review. J Behav Med 3:95–116.

Kamarck T, Jennings JR (1991). Biobehavioral factors in sudden cardiac death. Psychol Bull 109:42–75.

Karasek R, Baker D, Marxer F, et al. (1981). Job decision latitude, job demands, and cardiovascular disease: a prospective study of Swedish men. Am J Public Health 71:694–705.

Karasek RA, Theorell T, Schwartz JE, et al. (1988). Job characteristics in relation to the prevalence of myocardial infarction in the US Health Examination Survey (HES) and the Health and Nutrition Examination Survey (HANES). Am J Public Health 78:910–918.

Kemmer FW, Bisping R, Steingruber HJ, et al. (1986). Psychological stress and metabolic control in patients with type 1 diabetes mellitus. N Engl J Med 314:1078–1084.

Kinsell LW, Margen S, Michaels GD, et al. (1951). Studies in fat metabolism III. The effect of ACTH, of cortisone and of other steroid compounds upon fasting-induced hyperketonemia and ketonuria. J Clin Invest 30:1491–1502.

Kobasa SC, Hilker RR (1982). Executive work perceptions and the quality of working life. J Occup Med 24:25–29.

Krumholz HM, Radford MJ, Wang Y, et al. (1998). National use and effectiveness of beta-blockers for the treatment of elderly patients with acute myocardial infarction: National Cooperative Cardiovascular Project. JAMA 280:623–629.

LaVeau PJ, Rozanski A, Krantz DS, et al. (1989). Transient left ventricular dysfunction during provocative mental stress in patients with coronary artery disease. Am Heart J 118:1–8.

Levy SM, Herberman RB, Lippman M, et al. (1991). Immunological and psychosocial predictors of disease recurrence in patients with early-stage breast cancer. Behav Med 17:67–75.

Linden G (1969). The influence of social class in the survival of cancer patients. Am J Public Health 59:267–274.

Lipworth L, Abelin T, Connelly RR (1970). Socioeconomic factors in the prognosis of cancer patients. J Chron Dis 23:105–115.

Liu K, Cedres LB, Stamler J, et al. (1982). Relationship of education to major risk factors and death from coronary heart disease, cardiovascular diseases, and all causes: findings of three Chicago epidemiologic studies. Circulation 66:1308–1314.

Lustman PJ (1988). Anxiety disorders in adults with diabetes mellitus. Psychiatr Clin North Am 11:419–432.

Lustman PJ, Griffith LS, Clouse RE, et al. (1986). Psychiatric illness in diabetes mellitus: relationship to symptoms and glucose control. J Nerv Ment Dis 174:736–742.

MacGillivray MH, Bruck E, Voorhees ML (1981). Acute diabetic ketoacidosis in children: role of stress hormones. Pediatr Res 15:99–106.

McGarry JD, Foster DW (1977). Hormonal control of ketogenesis: biochemical considerations. Arch Intern Med 137:495–501.

Mirsky IA (1948). Emotional factors in the patient with diabetes mellitus. Bull Menninger Clin 12:187–194.

Mittleman MA, Maclure M, Sherwood JB, et al. (1995). Triggering of myocardial infarction onset by episodes of anger: determinants of myocardial infarction onset study investigators. Circulation 92:1720–1725.

Morris AD, Boyle DIR, McMahon AD, et al. (1997). Adherence to insulin treatment, glycemic control, and ketoacidosis in insulin-dependent diabetes mellitus. Lancet 350:1505–1510.

Myers A, Dewar HA (1975). Circumstances attending 100 sudden deaths from coronary artery disease with coroner's necropsies. Br Heart J 37:1133–1143.

Nathan SW (1985). Psychological aspects of recurrent diabetic ketoacidosis in preadolescent boys. Am J Psychother 39:193–205.

Orr DP, Golden MP, Myers G, et al. (1983). Characteristics of adolescents with poorly controlled diabetes referred to a tertiary care center. Diabetes Care 6:170–175.

Orth-Gomer K, Unden A-L, Edwards M-E (1988). Social isolation and mortality in ischemic heart disease: a 10-year follow-up study of 150 middle-aged men. Acta Med Scand 224:205–215.

Podrid PJ, Fuchs T, Candinas R (1990). Role of the sympathetic nervous system in the genesis of ventricular arrhythmia. Circulation 82(suppl 1):103–110.

Popkin MK, Callies AL, Lentz RD, et al. (1988). Prevalence of major depression, simple phobia and other psychiatric disorders in patients with long-standing type I diabetes mellitus. Arch Gen Psychiatry 45:64–68.

Mittelman MA, Maclure M, Sherwood JB, et al. (1995). Triggering of acute myocardial infarction onset by episodes of anger. Determinants of Myocardial Infarction Onset Study Investigators. Circulation 92:1720–1725.

Ray JJ (1991). If 'A-B' does not predict heart disease, why bother with it? A comment on Ivancevich and Matteson. Br J Med Psychol 64:85–90.

Reynolds P, Kaplan GA (1990). Social connections and risk for cancer: prospective evidence from the Alameda County Study. Behav Med 16:101–110.

Rose G, Marmot MG (1981). Social class and coronary heart disease. Br Heart J 45:13–19.

Rosen H Lidz T (1949). Emotional factors in the precipitation of recurrent diabetic acidosis. Psychosom Med 11:211–215.

Rosenman RH, Brand RJ, Sholtz RI, et al. (1976). Multivariate prediction of coronary heart disease during 8.5 year follow-up in Western Collaborative Group Study. Am J Cardiol 37:903–909.

Rozanski A, Bairey CN, Krantz DS, et al. (1988). Mental stress and the induction of silent myocardial ischemia in patients with coronary artery disease. N Engl J Med 318:1005–1012.

Ruberman W, Weinblatt E, Goldberg JD, et al. (1981). Ventricular premature complexes and sudden death after myocardial infarction. Circulation 64:297–305.

Ruberman W, Weinblatt E, Goldberg JD, et al. (1984). Psychosocial influences on mortality after myocardial infarction. N Engl J Med 311:552–559.

Schade DS, Eaton RP (1976). Modulation of fatty acid metabolism by glucagon in man IV. Effects of a physiological hormone infusion in normal man. Diabetes 25:978–983.

Schiffer F, Hartley LH, Schulman CL, et al. (1980). Evidence for emotionally-induced coronary arterial spasm in patients with angina pectoris. Br Heart J 44:62–66.

Schless GL, von Laveran-Stiebar R (1964). Recurrent episodes of diabetic acidosis precipitated by emotional stress. Diabetes 13:419–420.

Schnall PL, Pieper C, Schwartz JE, et al. (1990). The relationship between "job strain," workplace diastolic blood pressure, and left ventricular mass index. JAMA 263:1929–1935.

Schreurs PJG, Taris TW (1998). Construct validity of the demand–control model: a double cross-validation approach. Work and Stress 12:66–84.

Shekelle RB (1969). Educational status and risk of coronary heart disease. Science 163:97–98.

Skala JA, Freedland KE, Carney RM (1995). Depressive symptoms and functional status in patients with congestive heart failure. Ann Behav Med 17:S120.

Templeton B (1967). Psychotherapeutic intervention in insulin resistance: a case report. Diabetes 16:536.

Thomas CB, Duszynski KR (1974). Closeness to parents and the family constellation in a prospective study of five disease states: suicide, mental illness, malignant tumor, hypertension and coronary heart disease. Johns Hopkins Med J 134:251–270.

Vandenbergh RL, Sussman KE, Titus CC (1966). Effects of hypnotically induced acute emotional stress on carbohydrate and lipid metabolism in patients with diabetes mellitus. Psychosom Med 28:382–390.

Vandenbergh RL, Sussman KE, Vaughan GD (1967). Effects of combined physical–anticipatory stress on carbohydrate-lipid metabolism in patients with diabetes mellitus. Psychosomatics 8:16–19.

Veith RC, Lewis N, Linares OA, et al. (1994). Sympathetic nervous system activity in major depression. Arch Gen Psychiatry 51:411–422.

Wassertheil-Smoller S, Applegate WB, Berge K, et al. (1996). Change in depression as a precursor to cardiac events. Arch Intern Med 156:553–561.

Weinblatt E, Ruberman W, Goldberg JD, et al. (1978). Relation of education to sudden death after myocardial infarction. N Engl J Med 299:60–65.

White K, Kolman ML, Wexler P, et al. (1984). Unstable diabetes and unstable families: a psychosocial evaluation of diabetic children with recurrent ketoacidosis. Pediatrics 73:749–755.

Wilder MH (1976). Differentials in health characteristics by marital status, United States, 1971–1972, Vital and Health Statistics Series 10, No.104, data from the National Heath Survey. Rockville, Md: National Center for Health Statistics.

Yeung AC, Vekshtein VI, Krantz DS, et al. (1991). The effects of atherosclerosis on the vasomotor response of coronary arteries to mental stress. N Engl J Med 325:1551–1556.

Chapter

8

Interplay of Mind and Body in Medical Practice: Pathophysiological Mechanisms

This chapter is about the emotional reaction to disease and to symptoms, and in turn the impact of that reaction on the disease or symptom. The sometimes serious prognostic influence of anxiety or depression on the natural history of a particular disease too often receives scant consideration in clinical discussion. The impact on the natural history of the disorder, however, may be profound. For example, the recognition of depression as a major risk factor in patients with coronary artery disease and the use of catecholamine β-receptor blockers as the mainstay of secondary prevention after myocardial infarction highlight the central role of emotion in the survival of these patients (Chapter 5). Similarly, there is a tendency to view repeated attacks of any kind of pain or allergy syndrome, or a patient's failure to obtain an analgesic effect from regular doses of nonnarcotic analgesics, as progression or exacerbation of the underlying condition, usually without consideration of a potential emotional cause for the clinically unresponsive or relapsing state. The clinical condition may thus provoke an escalation of therapeutic options such as the use of steroids in high doses or of narcotics, both steps where the side effects of the medication carry potentially serious morbidity.

This chapter attempts to explain how these processes may develop and deals with some central features of the integrated pathophysiology of the interplay be-

TABLE 8–1. Mechanisms of Psychophysiological Processes

MECHANISM	CLINICAL EXPRESSION	CHAPTER
Facilitated autonomic responses: symptom anticipation	Any recurrent symptoms, especially pain	8
Anticipation of recovery or improvement	Placebo effects	9
Lowered pain threshold; organ activation syndromes	Irritable bowel syndrome; MVP; esophageal motility disorders; syndrome X	11, 13
	Fibromyalgia	15
Hyperventilation	Dizziness; presyncope panic attacks	14
Immune modulation	Respiratory viruses, herpes viruses; atopic conditions	6, 16
Marked physical deconditioning	MVP: exaggerated autonomic responses	13

tween nervous system and viscera or somatic structures, usually to the detriment of the patient's clinical condition. Table 8-1 lists examples of important psychophysiological mechanisms that are discussed elsewhere in the text. This list tends to emphasize the versatile repertoire of physiological channels for mind–body interactions, in addition to the central mechanisms described here. From examining these mechanisms, one can see that the much emphasized "fight-or flight reaction" of Cannon, which characterizes the acute stress response, does not have a significant role in the great majority of psychosomatic ("stressed") states that we consider in this book.

While the problems just described may represent a blind spot in clinical practice, no less problematic are the somatization syndromes in which the patient's symptom often represents the expression of emotional distress, whether in response to a current stressor or as an expression of much more profound, long-standing, unmet needs or unresolved emotional conflicts (Chapter 2). In societies where health issues are widely publicized, ill-defined or chronic symptoms may be reattributed to new disease entities such as multiple chemical sensitivities, sick-building syndrome, chronic Lyme disease, and candidiasis hypersensitivity. At the same time the symptom intensity of sufferers may be amplified by the media attention given to the disorder (Barsky and Borus, 1999). In addition, many somatization syndromes, involving different systems of the body, have considerable overlap with clinical symptoms and substantial similarities with them in their epidemiology and psychosocial characteristics—although these are seldom sought out (Wessely et al., 1999).

THE INTEGRATED MIND–BODY RESPONSE

Thought content, particularly when it arouses strongly felt emotions, may produce a physiological response in certain organs (Schwartz, 1971; Andrus, 1975). Similarly, stress and anxiety states, if recurrent or sustained, may be associated with visceral responses that produce troublesome symptoms. Despite the importance of the subject to medical practice, however, we lack a clear understanding of the physiology of *functional disorders*. A functional disorder is characterized by physiologically inappropriate functional responses of an organ in the absence of observable pathological changes. Typically, there is a major discrepancy between the severity of the symptoms and degree of disability and the demonstrable tissue abnormality. Functional disorders usually occur under circumstances where the affect is negative, to the extent that it reflects states of anxiety or depression, particularly when this condition is prolonged or recurs frequently (e.g., on a daily basis). As pointed out by Gelder (1996), functional symptoms are a feature of many conditions most frequently associated with adjustment, somatoform, and mood anxiety disorders.

There are, however, still many important unanswered questions in this field. For example: What mechanisms link emotions with exaggerated or inappropriate organ responses? When emotion is expressed consistently through symptoms due, say, to asthma, migraine, abdominal pain, or diarrhea, what process selects the target organ and why does the symptom tend to recur in the same organ? What role does the emotional state play in perpetuating the symptoms and vice versa?

In this chapter we consider psychophysiological mechanisms common to many clinical situations, namely, symptom anticipation and the likely basis of facilitated autonomic responses in psychosomatic disorders.

NEUROSOMATIC INTERACTION: A BIDIRECTIONAL PROCESS

Traditional explanations of how mental processes influence body function tend to relegate the somatic aspects of the psychosomatic equation to secondary status. In almost every case, common sense sees the emotional state as the "driver" and the somatic response as "driven." However, it is important to properly evaluate the bidirectionality of psychophysiological processes in order to better understand their likely mechanism. Thus, I propose here that **somatopsychic** influences may also be responsible for perpetuating a psychosomatic condition. This is especially true in medical disorders where the emotional state develops primarily in response to symptoms produced by the disease. As a result, the presence of symptoms, the extent of suffering, and the success of treatment and rehabilitation programs may all be considerably influenced by the subject's emotional reaction to the disease.

The physiology of psychosomatic disorders may be better understood if we assume that certain pathways of communication between the central nervous system (CNS), particularly the autonomic nervous system, and a specific peripheral site (organ or tissue) are *facilitated* by adaptive processes that take place at all levels of the CNS in response to tissue pathology and/or altered organ function (plasticity; discussed below). While the organ or tissue response may be initiated centrally by thoughts and (usually intense) feelings of anxiety or apprehension, the facilitating processes in the periphery may be expressed as a wider recruitment of afferent neurons associated with a site of pathological change (see below), or exaggerated functional activity due to a lower threshold of stimulation of the afferent neurons innervating the particular organ or tissue.

Two processes that are clearly important in the genesis of psychophysiological states are the mechanism the brain uses to selectively influence the function of an organ or tissue and (in the reverse direction) the way in which the nervous system responds to a pathological visceral-somatic process. Knowledge about these issues helps explain how communication between the brain and a particular body part may be facilitated, as it often seems to be, in psychosomatic disorders. It may also help explain why, in many people, stress-induced symptoms may be stereotypic, that is, may follow a similar pattern on each occasion.

All organs and tissues have their representation in the CNS, which controls the integrated responses aimed at preserving the homeostasis of the *milieu intérieu*. The nervous control of visceral function, in particular, is reflex in character, and the strict interdependence and integration of physiological and biochemical function is very much the hallmark of the normal state. Familiar examples are the direct correlation of a rising pulse rate with the increasing utilization of oxygen by exercising muscle (Mitchell and Blomqvist, 1971) and the reflex bradycardia induced by a sudden rise in blood pressure. Other than these integrated reflexes, most viscera are silent areas in that we cannot directly control their responses. Thus, we need to consider mechanisms that may change this fundamental mechanism of response. In the following section I will try to show how diseases may influence the nervous system to produce changes in a more directed manner—in a particular organ or tissue—independently of normal reflex responses and often also in excess of physiological requirements. The central principle of biofeedback has something important to teach us in this regard.

The Central Principle of Biofeedback Control

The experience of biofeedback indicates that when given some signal *which our special senses can detect*, we are able to influence body function or perceive changes with heightened ability. Basmajian (1963) demonstrated that single motor units (i.e., the cluster of muscle fibers innervated by a single axon) could be trained discretely to contract when needle electrodes were inserted into a muscle. The subject's feedback signal was the transduction of the energy of the motor unit potentials into sound, which could also be seen as a graph on a monitor. In the same year, Hefferline and Perera (1963) used electromyographic feedback to teach subjects to discern a small muscle twitch not otherwise perceptible. With practice, the subjects were able to discriminate changes in muscle activity of the order of 10 nanovolts (nV), an approximately one millionfold enhancement in sensitivity.

The brain is also able to modulate its own activity. For example, Sterman et al. (1974) trained human subjects through biofeedback to increase their sensorimotor rhythm, a 12–14 Hz signal appearing over the sensory motor cortex and usually associated with suppression of movement. He and others (Lubar and Bahler, 1976) used this technique to inhibit seizure activity in epileptic patients. Similarly, biofeedback and conditioning techniques have been used to influence a wide variety of visceral responses, including the modulation of blood pressure (Benson et al., 1969; Shapiro et al., 1970), penile tumescence (Quinn et al., 1970; Rosen et al., 1975), and intestinal (Engel et al., 1974) and urinary tract sphincter control (Cardozo et al., 1978; Burgio et al., 1985). They have also been used to influence pain awareness (Victor et al., 1978).

From here it is a short step to the next question: Can we envisage a natural counterpart of the electronically generated biofeedback signal? This would signal the brain from an organ or other location in the body, much like a needle in the muscle or an electroencephalographic signal. As to the nature of the signal, *any of a variety of pathological processes could serve this function*, including the metabolic or paracrine effects of inflammation or neoplasia. The main difference between classical biofeedback as just described and the processes we are about to consider, however, is that in biofeedback an external signal is delivered to the brain through one of the special senses (usually the eye or ear), whereas afferent impulses from disordered or dysfunctional tissues or organs are generated endogenously and reach the brain through sensory fibers innervating them. Thus, through the presence of either pathology or dysfunction, a previously silent area or process will "reveal" its location to the nervous system, permitting the nervous system in turn to exercise an increased measure of directed (i.e., facilitated) control of the involved tissue or organ.

Plasticity of the Nervous System: The Neurological Response to Peripheral Processes

Plasticity of the CNS, or adaptation of function, is another one of the properties that is central to an understanding of mechanisms involved in the genesis or perpetuation of psychophysiological processes. The CNS used to be viewed as rigidly wired with respect to both structure and function. This concept derived partly from the highly organized anatomical substructure of lobes, nuclei, tracts, and so on, each with its own particular function, and partly from the knowledge that the CNS has the lowest regenerative ability of any organ in the body. As clinical and experimental studies have shown, however, adaptive changes of function do take place in the CNS.

The nervous system shows functional plasticity in its response to different pathological processes. For example, transection of a peripheral nerve in the upper limbs of primates, or of the sensory tract within the spinal cord, leads to a reorganization of topographical maps in the somatosensory cortex. This means that areas of the cortex that formerly responded to stimulation of a particular anatomical locality now become responsive to stimulation of new parts of the body surface (Merzenich et al., 1983). Thus, if the median nerve in primates is sectioned and the cut end sutured to prevent regeneration, a large expanse of cortex is deprived of its normal activating input. When the deprived cortex is examined several months later, it is found to respond to stimuli on parts of the hand innervated by intact radial and ulnar nerves. These two nerves have clearly expanded their receptive fields in the absence of signals from median nerve stimulation.

This placticity of response resulting in reorganization of cortical maps in primates has similarly been demonstrated with digital amputation (Merzenich et al., 1984; Calford and Tweedale, 1988), surgically induced syndactyly, that is, webbed fingers (Allard et al., 1985), and behavioral modification (Jenkins et al., 1990; Recanzone et al., 1992). In the latter studies, training of owl monkeys to detect differences in the frequency of a tactile vibratory stimulus, or a period of trained hand use, resulted in remodeling as well as increased topographic complexity of the corresponding areas of the somatosensory cortex.

Neurological plasticity and inflammation

More subtle adaptive changes of CNS function may also be of considerable functional significance. Studies of the response of the rat nervous system to experimental arthritis induced by the injection of Freund's adjuvant (an agent derived from the bacteria responsible for tuberculosis and used to stimulate immune system activity) have provided insight into the adaptive changes associated with the presence of persistent inflammation. This model has many clinical similarities with rheumatoid arthritis (Pearson and Wood, 1959). In rats, following induction of arthritis, which usually develops within two weeks of beginning injections, joint afferents take on a resting discharge not seen in normal rats. The rats become very sensitive to pressure on the ankle and to small degrees of flexion or extension, stimuli that normally fail to produce a nervous discharge (Guilbaud et al., 1985; Calvino et al., 1987). In the spinal cord, neurons receiving input from inflamed tissues are characterized by high levels of background activity, which follows increased sensitivity to light pressure on the inflamed skin and gentle movement of the affected joint.

At higher levels in the CNS—in the thalamus and somatosensory cortex—a disproportionate number of cells respond to stimulation of the arthritic joint compared to controls (Lamour et al., 1983; Kayser and Guilbaud, 1984). In all experiments, the nervous system was completely normal on microscopic examination. Clearly, then, these are adaptive changes of neural function induced by the peripheral inflammatory process—arthritis. Changes in the response pattern to different stimuli thus reflect long-term alterations in central neuron activity as well as changes in primary afferent responses. The joints' inflammation is now recorded in the CNS through increased neuronal activity and more extensive neurological representation.

The experimental induction of colitis in rats has similarly been shown to produce an increase in background activity of postsynaptic dorsal column cells in the lumbar 6 to sacral 1 spinal cord segments (Al Chaer et al., 1997). This inflammatory state potentiates the responses of the same cells to graded colonic distension but not to cutaneous stimulation, suggesting that similar functional neurological changes occur with inflammed viscera, and not only with somatic structures.

Plasticity in humans

In humans, plasticity of the CNS in response to disuse, unusual use, or injury has been widely documented, especially in subjects suffering from nervous system defects that were congenital or were acquired in early life. Cortical reorganization has been demonstrated by electrophysiological studies in deaf children and congenitally deaf adults (Neville et al., 1983; Wolff and Thacher, 1990). In most of the clinical situations considered in this book, however, the states or disorders are of more recent origin. Even if longstanding, that is, of 10 to 20 years duration, they have developed in adolescence or (usually) in adult life.

Mogilner et al. (1993) used magnetoencephalography to plot the somatotopic organization (the orderly projection of the afferent axons of neurons in the somatosensory system to their target in the thalamus or cortex) of the hand area in normal humans with high spatial precision. Magnetoencephalography is a technique in which magnetic impulses resulting from cortical activity may be detected and localized with considerable accuracy—with millimeter precision—through detectors situated on the scalp. In the study reported above, magnetic impulses were recorded from the scalp in the area of the parietal somatosensory cortex in response to tactile stimulation of the digits of the contralateral hand. Mogilner and colleagues then studied somatosensory cortical changes in two other adults before and after surgical separation of syndactyly. Their observations were the counterpart of those described previously in primates by Merzenich and his group (Allard et al., 1985; Allard et al., 1991). The presurgical maps displayed shrunken and nonsomatotopic hand representations. Within weeks following surgery, cortical reorganization occurred over distances of 3 to 9 mm, correlating with the new functional status of the separated fingers. The extent of the response corresponded to the degree of congenital deformity preoperatively. Thus, while both subjects showed a response, neither attained a fully normal somatosensory representation. With the more severely affected subject, the reorganization resulted in distinct cortical locations for the separated fingers, although the hand representation area was smaller than normal and the organization was nonsomatotopic.

Although this study evaluated only the cortical representation of a congenital anatomical anomaly of the fingers, habitual differences in the use of the fingers may also be reflected in differences of cortical representation. Focal hand dystonia involves a loss of motor control of one or more digits and is associated with the repetitive, synchronous movements of the digits made by musicians over periods of many years. Elbert et al. (1998) showed by magnetic source imaging that there is a smaller distance (fusion) between the representations of the digits in the somatosensory cortex for the affected hand of dystonic musicians than for the hands of nonmusician control subjects. Thus, even differences in habitual use may be reflected in differences in cortical representation.

Adaptive responses in humans: evidence from clinical studies

Swarbrick et al. (1980) conducted an important study that has a bearing on the question of adaptation among patients suffering from the irritable bowel syndrome (IBS). This syndrome is a functional condition of the gastrointestinal tract in which recurrent and often severe bouts of abdominal pain are associated with constipation or loose stools. Other abdominal symptoms such as heartburn, nausea, borborygmus, and distention may also occur to varying degrees. The disorder tends to recur and frequently persists over many years (Chapter 11).

Swarbrick and his colleagues examined the localization of the pain caused by inflation of a balloon at the end of a catheter situated at different levels of the gastrointestinal tract lumen in patients suffering from IBS and in normal controls. In normal subjects, distention from the esophagus to the distal colon induced pain mostly in the midline and close to the site of balloon inflation. In the IBS patients, however, there was a much greater tendency for the pain to be localized to remote sites or lateralized to the side of balloon inflation. In this group, distention of the small gut also produced pain in extra-abdominal sites such as the back, one or both breasts, and retrosternally. Thus the IBS patients apparently had developed a much more extensive representation of pain stimuli derived from the intestinal tract.

The gastrointestinal tract of IBS patients differs from that of normal subjects. There are alterations in intestinal motility, which may be increased or decreased, and a stronger secretory response of the intestinal mucosa to secretion induced by dihydroxy bile acid. Pressure studies of the distal colon indicate that IBS patients have more spasm and a greater sensitivity to increased intraluminal pressure, that is, a lower pain threshold, than normal subjects do. At least some of their abdominal discomfort is thought to be attributable to a lower pain threshold and a much greater awareness of normal physiological bowel activity. Whether or not this is true, there is much evidence that the bowel (not only the colon) in IBS patients is more reactive than in normal subjects with respect to both muscular activity and secretory response. It thus seems likely that, in these patients, the part of the nervous system which receives its afferent input from the gastrointestinal tract is subject to a more active bombardment by signals emanating from the more reactive bowel. This could conceivably have the effect of producing adaptive changes similar to those observed in rats with experimental arthritis, namely, increased neuronal activity and more extensive CNS representation. In human subjects, the stimuli that give rise to pain in several visceral tissues appear to be determined by an increased discharge frequency of primary afferent fibers that also respond to innocuous events such as normal motility changes (Janig and Morrison, 1986).

In a different clinical context, patients who had suffered more than one attack of renal or ureteral colic due to stones were found to have lowered pain thresholds on selective electrical stimulation of the muscles, subcutaneous tissue, and skin at the first lumbar segment on the side of the calculus (Vecchiet et al., 1989). This shows that the induction of pain at a specific dermatome level produces central changes (in the spinal cord) which influence the pain threshold in other tissues innervated at the same level.

Conclusions

To summarize, the foregoing observations suggest that changes in body structure or function may bring about adaptive neurological changes. These occur in response to enhanced and possibly sustained afferent activity resulting from the tissue changes. A distinctive feature of the adaptive neurological changes is a greater recruitment of afferent neurons in the spinal cord, brain stem, and cerebral cortex. Thus, the site of the pathological process, through enhanced afferent neuronal discharge, registers in the CNS as a discrete "address." In effect, this means that this particular locality can now be more easily identified by the nervous system and selected from surrounding tissue for communication. These processes are likely to help facilitate exchange between the CNS and the affected peripheral tissues.

Behavior and the Conditioning of Visceral (Autonomic) Responses

Engel (1993) defines *behavior* as "any response that can be reliably elicited by a stimulus and that can be modified on the basis of experience (i.e., learning)." Similarly, any response that is elicited *in anticipation of a stimulus* is behavior.

From the experimental and clinical evidence presented below it seems that any autonomic response elicited by a stimulus, whether environmentally or endogenously derived, can be learned. Thus, even the innate reflexes are not immutable; *they vary according to the conditions under which they are elicited* and they should be viewed as an integral part of any behavioral response (Engel, 1986).

Most reflexes are behaviors because they are usually not unvarying in their expression; that is, they can be modified by contingent stimuli (stimuli that follow a response and increase or decrease its likelihood of recurring, depending on whether it is rewarding or punishing), and the contingencies can be learned. Therefore, although the responses described below are not attainable through willful intention, innate reflex activity may be modulated, sometimes quite drastically, *through the influence of emotional factors*. A familiar example is the nausea and vomiting on entering hospital, often experienced by patients receiving chemotherapy (Morrow, 1982). This type of learning has been termed "associative conditioning," defined as "a process by which neutral stimuli (e.g., the hospital building) acquire the capacity to elicit responses after repeated pairing with adequate stimuli (the chemotherapeutic agent/s)."

Visceral responses may also be modulated by *operant* (or *instrumental*) *conditioning*, a process by which "organisms learn to emit responses to produce or prevent the occurrence of stimuli that are either rewarding or aversive, respectively" (Engel and Talan, 1991). Unlike classical conditioning, in which the animal is passive or restrained, in operant (or instrumental) conditioning the animal (or human) actively behaves in such a way as to win a reward. Learning is achieved as a result of a specific action. The reward, usually food (the contingent stimulus), acts as the reinforcing stimulus and is awarded in response to the specific action. These principles are central to a great deal of what follows in this chapter.

In an elegant series of studies on monkeys, Engel and his collaborators provided experimental support for the preceding generalizations. They showed that

- Monkeys can be trained to slow down or speed up their heart rates to avoid electric shocks to their tails (Engel and Gottlieb, 1970).
- This was not necessarily mediated by somatomotor responses (Engel et al., 1976) but could be modulated by conditioning procedures independent of musculoskeletal activity. The confirmation that pulse rate, for example, could be modulated independently of muscular activity was important because of the normally sensitive and predictable cardiovascular response to even mild muscular activity (Rowell, 1980).
- When animals self-regulate their heart rates, they also *attenuate the sensitivity of their cardiac baroreflexes* when these reflexes will cause a heart rate change resulting in a tail shock (Engel and Joseph, 1982).

- Animals that slow their heart rates *can override even direct electrical stimulation of the hypothalamus*, which ordinarily produces tachycardia (Joseph and Engel, 1981).
- Through operant reinforcement, animals can modify even those cardiovascular responses that were established earlier through associative conditioning (Ainslie and Engel, 1974).

These studies clearly illustrate how cardiovascular reflexes, though not under direct voluntary control, *may be modulated or even completely overridden in a defined behavioral context*. More broadly, the conditioning principles highlighted by these studies provide an important physiological basis for evaluating the repercussions of disease and for explaining the mechanisms of the exceedingly wide range of psychophysiological processes observed in clinical practice.

DIRECTING THE AUTONOMIC RESPONSE

Individual-Response Specificity

In trying to define factors that determine whether an individual will develop specific symptoms in response to stress, early physiological studies focused on autonomic patterns in response to a stressor. An autonomic response may be specific to the stimulus that elicited it (stimulus-response specificity), for example, the tachycardia that almost always occurs with the cold pressor test, or to the individual responding to a particular stimulus (individual-response specificity) (Engel, 1972). Stimulus-response specificity implies that a given stimulus consistently evokes the same pattern or hierarchy of physiological responses (also referred to as "stereotypy" of response) among most subjects in a group. In the case of individual-response specificity, the responses are idiosyncratic and are therefore of particular interest in psychosomatic medicine. Here too the individual may display stereotypy of response to a variety of different stressful stimuli. This generalization appears to be true for normal controls (Lacey et al., 1953; Engel, 1960), for psychiatric patients with a variety of somatic complaints (Malmo and Shagass, 1949), and for asymptomatic subjects suffering from essential hypertension (Engel and Bickford, 1961).

Lacey et al. (1953) studied response stereotypy in 85 male college students. Each subject was exposed to four consecutive stresses and their autonomic responses as expressed in palmar conductance (reflecting sweat gland activity), heart rate, and heart rate variability were continuously and simultaneously recorded. For a given set of autonomic functions, individuals tended to respond with a pattern of autonomic activation in which maximal activation occurred in the same physiological function, whatever the stress. There was also a strong tendency for the entire pattern of autonomic activation to be reproduced with each new stress. Some individuals responded with a consistent hierarchical pattern of autonomic activation whatever the stress; others showed greater fluctuation from stress to stress but still exhibited one pattern of response more frequently than others; others displayed a completely random pattern of autonomic responses. It would appear from this and other studies that there is a tendency to stereotypy of autonomic response patterns, regardless of the stressor.[1]

For example, in a study by Malmo and Shagass (1949), patients with complaints localized to the head (e.g., headache) or with tightness or tension in the region of the head and neck exhibited greater disturbances in neck muscle potential in response to a standard thermal stress than patients without such complaints. Engel and Bickford (1961) applied five different stress stimuli to 20 female hypertensive patients and 20 age- and sex-matched normotensive subjects. Individual-response specificity, as shown by maximal activation, was found to occur with similar frequencies in the two groups. Of the 20 hypertensive patients, 15 developed marked blood pressure changes, however, as compared to only 5 of the 20 normotensive subjects. The hypertensives usually responded with an elevation of systolic blood pressure while the normotensives never did. These results were interpreted to mean that the hypertensives tend to overreact to environmental stressors with blood pressure elevation and to respond with more consistent individual-response patterns than do normotensives. Similarly, a group of hypertensive patients when challenged with stressful stimuli of all kinds reacted with blood pressure elevation to a greater extent than did the patients with rheumatoid arthritis; the arthritic patients, in contrast, reacted more with tension in the muscles surrounding symptomatic joints than did the hypertensive patients (Moos and Engel, 1962).

To summarize, evidence to support the idea that stereotypy of autonomic response may predict a particular clinical syndrome in those subjects who subsequently develop a defined psychophysiological problem is very weak, other than in perhaps a very small number of subjects. Reevaluation of the stability of response specificity by Marwitz and Stemler (1998) showed that only 15% of sub-

---

[1]Commonly employed experimental stressors include the following:

1. *Mental arithmetic* such as the multiplication of a two-digit number by a one-digit number and the subsequent addition of a two-digit number; for example, "multiply 4 by 67 and then add 39." As soon as the answer is announced another problem is given.

2. *Hyperventilation*, at the rate of one complete respiration per second for 45 seconds.

3. *Letter association*, in which the subject is asked to name words beginning with a particular letter. With every pause, the subject is immediately requested to continue.

4. *Cold pressor*, in which a foot is immersed to the level of the internal malleolus for 60 seconds in water maintained at 4°.

5. *Pain stimulus*, delivered through a heating electrode under controlled conditions. Frequently measured indexes of autonomic activation include heart rate and heart rate variability, blood pressure, respiration rate, palmar galvanic skin resistance, and skeletal muscle potentials.

jects retained some stability of response with time. In addition, these authors suggest that psychological factors such as neuroticism may also have an important influence in the pattern of response and that this factor was not properly evaluated in earlier studies. Furthermore, in the early studies of response stereotypy the influence of underlying disease on the response was also not considered. Thus, in certain diseases such as rheumatoid arthritis, the neurological adaptations to the peripheral inflammatory process, as described in a previous section, may well be important in predisposing to the tendency of muscles pulling across inflamed joints to develop tension in response to stressors, as demonstrated by Moos and Engel (1962).

The Interplay of Emotion and Disease

While a stereotypical autonomic response does not, in the majority of subjects, appear to determine the localization of psychosomatic symptoms, the thesis developed here is that the presence of disease or abnormal organ function does influence the process. To what extent can autonomic activity, subsequent to activation of the limbic system, be directed in a precise neuroanatomical sense? The answer to this question is suggested by observations in a patient severely distressed by attacks of Raynaud's phenomenon, where spasm of the finger arteries was induced, in particular, by exposure to cold (Melmed et al., 1986). Arterial pulsations from the index finger of both hands were recorded with a finger plethysmograph. While in a state of deep relaxation, the patient was encouraged through suggestion to imagine herself putting *only her right hand* into the deep freeze of her refrigerator; as a result, the pulsations diminished and disappeared from the right index finger only (the only finger of her right hand being monitored) (Figure 8-1). At this point the patient was asked to *imagine* that she was withdrawing her right hand from the freezer and plunging it into a bowl of warm water in order to warm her cold fingers. Within seconds, the digital arteries of the right finger had so dilated that the recorded impulse exceeded the limits of the plethysmograph settings. Thus, the typical phases of an attack of Raynaud's phenomenon had been reproduced and completely controlled through guided imagery.

This specific localization of response is supported by clinical experience with a patient in whom unilateral Raynaud's symptoms were evoked while he was reporting a dream in which he had used the affected hand to shoot a number of people (Szajnberg et al., 1987).

The Concealed Logic of Autonomic Responses

One of the most interesting observations to emerge from the various clinical examples described concerns the appropriateness of autonomic responses in specific clinical situations. If, as is claimed here, many psychophysiological

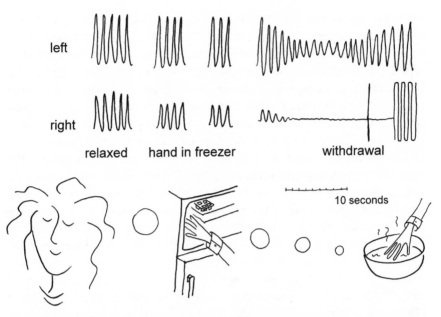

left   relaxed   hand in freezer   withdrawal

right

10 seconds

FIGURE 8.1 Plethysmographic tracing of the right (test) and left (control) index finger pulses of a patient suffering from Raynaud's phenomenon. Under deep relaxation, the patient was first asked to imagine that she put her right hand only into the deep freeze, and then (from the vertical line), that the hand be withdrawn and put into a bowl of warm water. The initial intense vasospasm is followed by pronounced vasodilatation. (Adapted from Melmed et al., 1986, with permission of *Lancet*.)

processes such as symptom anticipation, anxiety-mediated symptom production, and placebo responses (Chapter 9) are sometimes precisely directed, then we have to assume that autonomic responses are well-integrated with the mechanisms controlling cognition and emotion. It would appear, from a consideration of autonomic responses in a physiological context, say, at a fairly basic level of cardiovascular reactivity, that the autonomic system is controlled in a task-driven manner. For example, in numerous studies involving situations that raise the blood pressure, such as emotional arousal (Brod, 1963), isometric exercise, which requires the contraction of muscles against resistance, as in weight lifting (Sannerstedt and Julius, 1972), cold stimulation (Andren and Hansson, 1981), or noise (Andren et al., 1980), it has been demonstrated that the *primary hemodynamic mechanism* (either a *rise in cardiac output*, as with mental arousal and isometric exercise, or an *increase in peripheral resistance*, as with cold stimulation and noise) may be changed without affecting the blood pressure increase.

Thus, Ulrych (1969) observed that the initial blood pressure response while speaking quietly was due to a substantial elevation of cardiac output. When this elevation was inhibited by β-adrenergic blockade the blood pressure response was sustained but was now due to an increase in peripheral resistance. A shift from an increased cardiac output response before β-adrenergic blockade to an increase in peripheral resistance after it was also observed with the blood pressure response during isometric exercise (MacDonald et al., 1966). Similarly, in a study of the blood pressure elevating effects of mental arithmetic, Schmieder et al. (1987) observed that although β-blockade decreases the average blood pressure, it does not decrease the magnitude of the blood pressure response to mental arithmetic. Before β-blockade the blood pressure response was due to a 35% increase in cardiac output and a decrease of 11% in vascular resistance. After blockade the cardiac output increased by only 5%, but instead of decreasing, the vascular resistance increased by 11%. Nifedipine, a calcium channel blocking agent, lowered the average blood pressure to a similar extent without affecting the magnitude of the blood pressure response. Following nifedipine, the elevation in cardiac output due to mental arithmetic increased from 35% before treatment to 42% after treatment. This apparently universal propensity to maintain blood pressure (or the increase in blood pressure) following a wide variety of stimuli, if necessary by switching mechanisms, has been referred to by Julius (1988) as the "blood pressure seeking properties of the central nervous system."

Examples of task-driven control in a more complicated behavioral setting come from experiments performed in the laboratory of B. T. Engel. In these studies, monkeys were taught by operant conditioning to slow their pulse rate. Cholinergic blockade with methylatropine bromide attenuated but did not abolish the ability of monkeys to slow their heart rates at rest while β-blockade with propranolol increased the ability of the animals to slow the heart rate (Gottlieb and Engel, 1979). The authors concluded that expression of the learned control of heart rate does not depend exclusively on either the sympathetic or the parasympathetic branches of the autonomic nervous system. Other studies from the same laboratory, in which monkeys were taught to slow their heart rates while exercising and while under the influence of either atenolol (a β-blocker) or methylatropine (an anticholinergic), similarly demonstrated that the control of heart rate was not confined to a particular effector system (Engel and Talan, 1991). Remarkably, this was true even when the monkeys were performing a set of complex motor acts in which additional metabolic and cardiovascular responses were activated by exercise.

As operant conditioning depends on the reinforcement of a particular action with a reward, execution of the learned response must always be associated with the *anticipation* of gratification. In this respect, the operant conditioning model is of particular relevance to the clinical processes considered in this chapter. Moreover, the versatility of autonomic effector responses observed in these experimental studies parallels the experience of clinical practice in which an autonomic blocking agent is frequently inadequate for the relief of symptoms "driven" by strongly felt emotions such as anxiety, fear, anger, and guilt.

CENTRALLY MEDIATED SYMPTOMATOLOGY

The foregoing discussion has related to factors that primarily *influence the peripheral expression* of psychophysiological processes. Since the subject matter concerns emotions and stress, it may seem strange to use the term "centrally mediated" in the heading above, as it may be conjectured that everything comes from the brain and so must be "central"! However, the preceding section, in an attempt to illustrate the *bidirectionality* of psychophysiological processes, emphasized the interplay of peripheral processes, both organic and functional, with the nervous system. This section presents a number of centrally mediated mechanisms of importance in the initiation and persistence of symptoms.

Mechanisms Driving Symptoms

Somatic representation of anxiety

Most physicians today accept the idea that extreme forms of anxiety may, in a susceptible individual, precipitate an attack of any one of a variety of disorders, such as migraine, asthma, angina pectoris, or even myocardial infarction. However, the conventional clinical wisdom does not see these processes as "directed" in a neuroanatomical sense. Indeed, anxiety and tension for any reason could lead to such an attack without the individual consciously anticipating its occurrence.

The anatomical localization of pain or discomfort as an expression of anxiety is sometimes suggested to the patient by symptoms in a close relative, such as a mother or father. For example, a daughter who has spent months or years nursing a parent suffering from angina pectoris may, when she feels particularly anxious, complain of pain or discomfort in the left chest or arm. Moreover, any left-sided chest or arm symptoms are likely to be interpreted by the same individual as indicating heart disease, which leads to considerable anxiety. The fundamental assumption here is that the patient, even in this situation, is in fact feeling something, not imagining it. If this is true, it must then also be assumed that the state of anxiety, deriving as it does from a concern centered on sensation in a certain part(s) of the body, brings about changes in the nervous system which project the pain, that is, facilitate its referral, specifically in the direction of the anatomical area of concern.

Symptom anticipation and the learned visceral response

The occurrence of a symptom, whether it be headache, palpitations, vertigo, dyspnea, diarrhea, or another, may be an extremely stressful experience even though some individuals undergo the same experience without suffering nearly as much anxiety. The emotional reaction to the symptom or clinical condition,

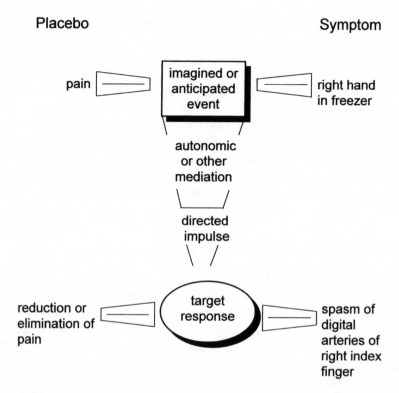

FIGURE 8.2. Schematic presentation of the thesis that symptom anticipation and the placebo effect are two sides of the same coin. On the left the placebo example relates to pain, and on the right the symptom anticipation example is Raynaud's phenomenon

in the form of *anticipatory anxiety*, may play a role both in initiating and in mediating recurrent symptomatology. This implies a process in which abnormal body function is induced or aggravated by anxiety associated with the fear that a particular symptom may recur. The process is also called *symptom anticipation* (Melmed et al., 1990). Whereas the development of anticipatory anxiety is considered of central importance in panic attacks and has been extensively written about in that context (Chapter 12), it has hardly been considered in general medical practice. The anticipation by the patient of symptoms or a worsening of the clinical condition is also called the *nocebo effect* (Benson, 1997). Furthermore, in Chapter 9, we will extend this idea to suggest that the placebo effect, as opposed to the nocebo effect described here, is dependent on the anticipation of improvement or cure activating mechanisms that may work to promote that effect (Figure 8-2).

Anticipatory distress in relation to an expected pain may be manifested early in life. Infants from the age of six months have been observed to show fear in expectation of an immunization injection from a doctor or nurse (Levy, 1960).

A study of the incidence and prevalence of headache fear in migraine sufferers showed that it was a common occurrence which increased in frequency, in a statistically significant manner, with increasing severity of the headache syndrome (Saadah, 1997). Of patients defined as suffering from intractable headache (15 headache days or more per month), 73% had a maximum fear score. Associated with this fear of further migraine attacks was a greater compulsion to take analgesic tablets in anticipation of an attack.

When it first develops in relation to specific symptoms, symptom anticipation tends to link the anxiety felt by the individual to a discrete physical response (which is driven by the anxiety). In this regard it differs from the stress-induced effects described below, in which the stress is derived in the first instance not from the symptom itself, but from any of a wide variety of experiences or life events. Clearly, however, symptom anticipation may develop in relation to any symptom regardless of the primary cause. The process implies a precise neuroanatomical representation linking the experience of anxiety with the organ dysfunction producing the particular symptoms. Accordingly, we now need to consider possible mechanisms that could provide the neurophysiological basis for this type of reaction.

Mechanisms of learning visceral responses

When a stressful experience becomes the trigger for symptom development, the symptom may be considered to be *conditioned* in the classical Pavlovian sense as the patient has no control over its occurrence. In such situations the *conditioned stimulus* may be a specific trigger, either endogenous (such as the memory of a traumatic event) or environmental, and the *unconditioned stimulus*, which is the factor common to all cases, is the anxiety (occult or overt).

Subjects who have experienced a particular event, which they feel sure played a role in the genesis of their symptoms, are likely to believe that symptoms will recur whenever that event happens. For example, although exposure to a cold wind may reflexly induce angina pectoris, a patient's conviction that cold wind causes angina may become at least of equal importance in inducing further attacks under similar circumstances. Similarly, the belief that the severest attacks of rhinitis, bronchitis, or asthma are seasonally related may be the very thing that increases the severity of the attacks during the appropriate season. The element common to all of these situations is the anxiety or apprehension felt at the prospect of an attack. In a lecture on angina pectoris, the cardiologist Samuel A. Levine (1959) clearly described the phenomenon: "Patients may have an attack repeatedly under the same circumstances, such as going to the garage or walking a short distance to the train or shaving in the morning, and have no spells doing much more strenuous things at other times. There is much about all this that makes one think of a conditioned reflex. The number of foot-pounds of work is not the whole story."

The importance of the anticipatory component of a subject's response was demonstrated in the classical study of Luparello et al. (1968). Nebulized physiological saline was given to each of 40 asthmatic subjects, with the information that they were inhaling a substance known to them as a bronchial allergen or irritant. In 19 subjects there was a significant and reproducible increase in airway resistance. Similarly, replacement of the "noxious" agent by a placebo that was presented to the subject as a bronchodilator resulted in rapid relief of the bronchospasm. One of the subjects participating in this study developed both bronchospasm and hay fever when informed that she was inhaling pollen; in another experiment she developed bronchospasm without hay fever when told that the inhalant was dust.

Several case reports in the literature illustrate the phenomenon of symptom anticipation. In a patient reported by Lown (1977), angina pectoris with marked ST segment depression on the electrocardiograph was consistently induced after 44 cycles during a Master two-step test, a form of exercise test. When the counting was faked so that the number 44 was presented earlier in the test (say, at a true count of 31), it had the same physical effect in a reproducible manner. It is clearly impossible to differentiate here between conditioning and anticipation.

The response described more than 100 years ago by MacKenzie (1886), an ear, nose, and throat surgeon to the Baltimore Charity Hospital, who, with the aid of an artificial rose, induced an attack of severe vasomotor rhinitis and asthma in a patient supposedly sensitive to roses, could be ascribed to either symptom anticipation or conditioning. His dramatic description of the episode is worth recounting:

> Decidedly sceptical as to the power of (rose) pollen to produce a paroxysm in her particular case, I practiced the following deception upon her . . . For the purpose of the experiment, I obtained an artificial rose of such exquisite workmanship that it presented a perfect counterfeit of the original . . . When the patient entered my consultation-room, she expressed herself as feeling unusually well . . . Her conjunctivae were normal, the nasal passages free, and there was nothing to indicate the presence of her trouble . . . I produced the artificial rose from behind a screen where it had been secreted, and, sitting before her held it in my hand, at the same time continuing the conversation. In the course of a minute she said she felt that she must sneeze. This sensation was followed almost immediately by a tickling and intense itching in the back of the throat and at the end of the nose. The nasal passages, at the same time, became suddenly obstructed, and the voice assumed a hoarse, nasal tone. In less than two minutes the puncta lachrymalia began to itch violently, the . . . conjunctiva became intensely hyperaemic and photophobia and lachrymation supervened. To these symptoms were added, almost immediately, itching in the auditory meatuses and the secretion of a thin fluid in the previously dry nasal passages. In a few minutes the feeling of oppression in the chest began, with slight embarrassment of respiration. In other words, in the space of five minutes she was suffering from a severe coryza, the counterpart of that which the presence of natural roses invariably produced in her case.

A similar experience was reported by Dekker and Groen (1956), who were able to induce an attack of bronchospasm in a young woman by showing her an artificial presentation of a goldfish in a bowl. When the patient was a child her mother had flushed her pet fish down the toilet. Later in life she developed asthma at the sight of a goldfish. The dispute with her mother, which had led to the fish being unkindly discarded and her distressing childhood memory of that act that killed her pet goldfish, was undoubtedly the event that initially gave the goldfish special significance in this woman's life. However, the experience of developing asthma when seeing a goldfish served to reinforce the association and to imprint this cycle of symptom anticipation in her mind.

The Neurophysiological Basis of Symptom Anticipation

The neuroanatomical basis of emotion is centered mainly in limbic structures, which in turn communicate with the hypothalamus to initiate or influence autonomic activity (Le Doux, 1987). Evidence for this in humans comes from various sources. One important piece of work that illuminates aspects of neurophysiology relevant to the mechanism of symptom anticipation is an early study by Lesse et al. (1955). In this study, human subjects with stereotactically placed electrodes in limbic and subcortical structures had enhanced electrical activity localized to the limbic system (amygdaloid and rostral hippocampal regions) during the *recollection of emotionally significant events*. On the other hand, anger over current events or the recollection of events without special emotional significance to the subject did not elicit this electrical response. The amygdala are regarded as being critically involved in emotional memory (Le Doux 1993), and particularly in the conditioning of fear responses and the development of anxiety states (Le Doux, 1998); this is discussed in more detail in Chapter 12. Since symptom anticipation occurs in relation to symptoms that induce or may have induced anxiety, sometimes of considerable intensity, recollection of the event may lead to activation of limbic structures, as observed in the study cited above.

The activation of neuronal pathways in the anticipation of carrying out a familiar action has been clearly demonstrated in the operant conditioning of monkeys taught to reach out and turn off a heat stimulus applied to the skin. The monkeys were rewarded with orange juice. Recordings from cells of the cerebral cortex showed that, before training, the cells simply signaled the stimulus as expected. After training, however, many of the cells emitted a burst when the monkey received a stimulus that the activity was about to begin. The monkeys responded a second time when the test stimulus was actually presented (Dubner et al., 1981). These findings reproduce those of other studies in which activation of cortical neurons or deeper ganglia occurred in anticipation of motor activity (Schmidt et al., 1974; Tanji and Evarts, 1976; Alexander, 1987).

That this anticipatory activity of the nervous system may produce a defined organ response was well illustrated by Bolme and Novotny (1969) in their studies of classically conditioned, treadmill-induced exercise responses in dogs. After dogs were trained to walk on a treadmill at two different work levels that were signaled by discriminable cues, the animals showed reliable increases in leg blood flow in response to the cues, before the onset of exercise. Furthermore, there was a greater increase in blood flow in response to the cue for the higher work level than for the lesser load.

Task demands for motor readiness may produce an increase in both pulse rate and metabolic activity in anticipation of motor activity (Obrist et al., 1970). A study of anticipatory anxiety in humans used positron emission tomography to measure regional blood flow, a measure of local neuronal activity (Reiman et al., 1989). Healthy volunteers were told that a painful shock would be delivered within a specified two-minute period; they were also told that the severity of the shock was likely to increase with the passage of time. In this state, significant blood flow increases were recorded in bilateral temporal poles, the same regions that were previously implicated by the same authors in a lactate-induced anxiety attack (Chapter 12). The temporopolar cortex, through its anatomical connections with the sensory association areas and the amygdala, has been referred to as a "paralimbic area" (Mesulam and Mufson, 1982; Moran et al., 1987). These authors suggest that it is involved in the evaluation of environmental information, leading to an appropriate response.

This section has described documented neurophysiological processes that underlie anticipatory responses, but there are changes at the cellular level that work to facilitate these integrated responses. These cellular changes should provide a basis for the fundamental characteristic of the defined responses we are considering here, such as those associated with either anxiety states or depression, to be triggered by stimulation of lesser and lesser intensity. The next section describes such changes.

Neural plasticity and the imprinting of affective states

The regional functional reorganization, or plasticity, that occurs in the nervous system in response to peripheral inflammatory processes, congenital defects, and unusual behavioral demands has been discussed. Another important type of plasticity, resulting from the physicochemical changes in the neurons, determines how the neuron will function, as in memory and learning. These cellular and intercellular (synaptic) processes determine the integrated function of nervous tissue. We consider here two processes that are derived from just these kinds of plasticity changes, kindling and long-term potentiation (LTP).

Many features of symptom anticipation are reminiscent of kindling, an experimental process in which *subthreshold* electrical stimulation, especially of the hippocampus, produces increasing effects on electrical activity and behavior. Thus, in experimental animals, a stimulus that initially produces no effects eventually results, after repeated exposure, in major motor convulsions (Delgado and Sevillano, 1961). Goddard et al. (1969), who first used the word "kindling" to describe this process, demonstrated that it depends on intermittent, not continuous, stimulation of hippocampal structures. They also showed that once developed, the ability to respond with a full seizure to subthreshold stimulation was retained and could occur even after a prolonged interval without stimulation.

McEachern and Shaw (1999) suggested that kindling may be viewed as the pathological end of a spectrum of neuron changes in which LTP, believed by many to be the substrate for learning and memory, represents the physiological end. Long-term potentiation is a persistent increase in synaptic strength (as measured by excitatory postsynaptic potentials) that can be rapidly induced by brief neural activity, changes considered necessary for the encoding and retrieval of information (Beggs et al., 1999). A relationship between LTP and neuropathology is suggested in part by the fact that many of the molecular processes involved in LTP induction or maintenance are the same as those activated during excitotoxic events in neurons. Thus, Adamec (1999) demonstrated in studies in the cat that partial kindling of the amygdala produced LTP of efferent transmission from the amygdala to the ventromedial hypothalamus and periaqueductal gray in left and right hemispheres.

Although kindling was first studied in an attempt to understand the electrophysiology of epileptic seizures, this characteristic pattern of responsiveness is now also thought to explain processes other than epilepsy (Weiss and Post, 1998). For example, from a consideration of the natural history of affective disorders in particular, it seems that these may involve a similar mechanism. In many of the anxiety-associated conditions discussed here, the symptoms are typically episodic and attacks may occur with increasing frequency and intensity, much like a kindled response. Furthermore, the attacks may be triggered by anxiety, either in response to an environmental cue or simply out of fear that the symptom itself may recur. After suffering repeated attacks, the intensity of the stimulus that induces further attacks may be fairly small. Post and Kopanda (1975) postulated that a change in limbic activity, as in kindling, could occur after repeated endogenous or psychic stimulation, providing a potential mechanism for some aspects of psychosis as well as depression. In depression, too, while the early episodes may be in response to a significant environmental stressor, if untreated, the tendency to intractability typically increases with increasing bouts of depression (Chapter 16). Later episodes of depression may occur without significant environmental stress, an observation that underlies the therapeutic imperative of vigorous treatment of early bouts of major depression.

Anticipation of death

The idea that the anticipation of death may actually lead to death is a phenomenon reported anecdotally over many hundreds of years (Benson, 1997). Whereas it seems perfectly plausible that, a bout of intense apprehension and anxiety could trigger a lethal ventricular arrhythmia in a subject with preexisting heart disease such as ischemic heart disease, the process is more difficult to understand when it occurs in a supposedly healthy individual. The most substantial claims of this happening emanate from cultures with the embedded belief that this can in fact happen, such as the Australian aborigines and the Maori of New Zealand. Among the aborigenes, it apparently may occur when the shaman hexes a member of the tribe by pointing a bone at him, and among the Maori it is said to result from breaking some taboo. The two possible mechanisms suggested by Benson are norepinephrine-induced myofibrillar degeneration, as described in assault victims who do not have obvious lethal wounds on autopsy (Cebelin and Hirsch, 1980), and the stimulation of an area in the insular cortex that has been shown to lead to ventricular fibrillation in animals (Oppenheimer et al., 1991).

SUMMARY

In analyzing the pathophysiology of psychosomatic processes commonly encountered in clinical practice, we have considered the interplay of elements along two mirror-image paths. The first runs from the diseased or disordered tissue or organ to the CNS and then back again to aggravate symptoms, as an expression of disturbed function. The second arises in the CNS as an expression of emotional distress, passes to the tissue or organ, and then returns to influence neural responses. In both cases the outcome is similar: increased suffering. In either case, there may be plastic changes at different levels of nervous system structure and function that work to promote or sustain the clinical syndrome. The plasticity of nervous system innervation of and responsivity to tissue and organs altered by disease states provides one level of control through enhancing autonomic influence to the diseased area. As observed in the studies described in this chapter, the varying patterns of autonomic activity are integrated into the demands of a broad spectrum of behavioral responses and physiological needs. All aspects of autonomic activity are sensitively modulated by emotional (limbic) input and the superimposition of more intense emotional responses, anxiety in particular, will tend to intensify symptoms.

There seems to be substantial similarity between the operant conditioning model and clinical experience with regard to the expression of autonomic activity as an integral part of learning processes in which fear or suffering is a prominent component of the experience. The key to understanding the occult logic of autonomic responses thus appears to be task-driven, functioning principally in the clinical context that we are most interested in here as the effector of the physical component of anxiety states. Clinical experience, furthermore, strengthens the validity of the comparison introduced in the first paragraphs of this chapter:

there is a behavioral equivalence in the significance of signals that reach the CNS either through the special senses (as with biofeedback) or through afferent activity from the organs and tissues of the body (as with functional or organic disorders), particularly when the signals are coupled with a negative emotional reaction.

The integrated reflexes of cardiovascular and respiratory control with metabolic demands provides another important level of control. However, the studies by Engel and colleagues impressively demonstrate how even apparently immutable cardiovascular reflexes such as the tachycardia of muscular activity may be overridden by fear or anticipation of pain and discomfort. Finally, we have considered processes influencing neuronal function such as kindling and LTP, which may provide the cellular basis for many psychosomatic conditions. Although ending this review with the neuron runs counter to the time-honored practice of building up the picture from the simple to the more complex, a proper understanding of the dynamics of the mind–body interaction that precede it would seem to provide a clearer basis for understanding what probably happens at a cellular level. It is the interplay of the sum total of all these components that determines the impressive unity of mind and body.

REFERENCES

Adamec RE (1999). Evidence that limbic neural plasticity in the right hemisphere mediates partial kindling induced lasting increases in anxiety-behavior: effect of low frequency stimulation (quenching?) on long term potentiation of amygdala efferents and behavior following kindling. Brain Res 839:133–152.

Ainslie GW, Engel BT (1974). Alteration of classically conditioned heart rate by operant reinforcement in monkeys. J Comp Physiol Psychol 87:373–382.

Al Chaer ED, Westlund KN, Willis WD (1997). Sensitization of postsynaptic dorsal column neuronal responses to colon inflammation. Neuroreport 8:3267–3273.

Alexander GE (1987). Selective neuronal discharge in monkey putamen reflects intended direction of planned limb movements. Exp Brain Res 67:623–634.

Allard T, Clark SA, Jenkins WM, et al. (1985). Syndactyly results in the emergence of double-digit receptive fields in somatosensory cortex in adult owl monkeys. Soc Neurosci Abstr 11:965.

Allard T, Clark SA, Jenkins WM, et al. (1991). Reorganization of somatosensory area 3b representations in adult owl monkeys after digital syndactyly. J Neurophys 66:1048–1058.

Andren L, Hansson L (1981). Circulatory effects of stress in essential hypertension. Acta Med Scand Suppl 646:69–72.

Andren L, Hansson L, Bjorkman M, et al. (1980). Noise as a contributory factor in the development of elevated arterial pressure: a study of the mechanisms by which noise may raise blood pressure in man. Acta Med Scand 207:493–498.

Andrus EC (1975). Emotional factors and cardiac function. Biol Psychiatry 10:581–598.

Barsky AJ, Borus JF (1999). Functional somatic syndromes. Ann Intern Med 130:910–921.

Basmajian JV (1963). Control and training of individual motor units. Science 141:440–441.

Beggs JM, Brown TH, Byrne JH, et al. (1999). Learning and memory: basic mechanisms. In: Zigmond MJ, Bloom FE, Landis SC, et al., eds. Academic Press. London, New York, Sydney, Tokyo.

Benson H (1997). The nocebo effect: history and physiology. Prevent Med 26:612–615.

Benson H, Herd JA, Morse WH, et al. (1969). Behavioral induction of arterial hypertension and its reversal. Am J Physiol 217:30–34.

Bolme P, Novotny J (1969). Conditional reflex activation of the sympathetic cholinergic vasodilator nerves in the dog. Acta Physiol Scand 77:58–67.

Brod J (1963). Hemodynamic basis of acute pressor reactions and hypertension. Br Heart J 25:227–245.

Burgio KL, Whitehead WE, Engel BT (1985). Urinary incontenence in the elderly: bladder-sphincter biofeedback and toileting skills training. Ann Intern Med 103:507–515.

Calford MB, Tweedale R (1988). Immediate and chronic changes in responses of somatosensory cortex in adult flying-fox after digit amputation. Nature Lond 332:446–448.

Calvino B, Villanueva L, Le Bars D (1987). Dorsal horn (convergent) neurons in the intact anesthetized arthritic rat. 1. Segmental excitatory influences. Pain 28:81–98.

Cardozo LD, Abrams PD, Stanton SL, et al. (1978). Idiopathic bladder instability treated by biofeedback. Br J Urol 50:521–523.

Cebelin MS, Hirsch CS (1980). Human stress cardiomyopathy: myocardial lesions in victims of homicidal assaults without injuries. Hum Pathol 11:123–132.

Dekker E, Groen J (1956). Reproducible psychogenic attacks of asthma. J Psychosom Res 1:58–67.

Delgado JMR, Sevillano M (1961). Evolution of repeated hippocampal seizures in the cat. Electroencephalog Clin Neurophysiol 13:722–733.

Dubner R, Hoffman DS, Hayes RL (1981). Neuronal activity in medullary dorsal horn of awake monkeys trained in a thermal discrimination task, III. Task-related responses and their functional role. J Neurophysiol 46:444–464.

Elbert T, Candia V, Altenmuller E, et al. (1998). Alteration of digital representations in somatosensory cortex of focal hand dystonia. Neuroreport 9:3571–3575.

Engel BT (1960). Stimulus-response and individual-response specificity. Arch Gen Psychiatry 2:305–313

Engel BT (1972). Response specificity. In: Greenfield NS, Sternbach RA, eds. Handbook of Psychophysiology. New York: Holt Rinehart and Winston, pp 571–576.

Engel BT (1986). An essay on the circulation as behavior. Behav Brain Sci 9:285–318.

Engel BT (1993). Autonomic behavior. Exp Gerontol 28:499–502.

Engel BT, Bickford AF (1961). Response specificity. stimulus-response and individual-response specificity in essential hypertensives. Arch Gen Psychiatry 5:82–93.

Engel BT, Gottlieb SH (1970). Differential operant conditioning of heart rate in the restrained monkey. J Comp Physiol Psychol 73:217–225.

Engel BT, Gottlieb SH, Hayhurst VF (1976). Tonic and phasic relationships between heart rate and somato-motor activity in monkeys. Psychophysiology 13:288–295.

Engel BT, Joseph JA (1982). Attenuation of baroreflexes during operant cardiac conditioning. Psychophysiology 19:609–614.

Engel BT, Nikoomanesh P, Schuster MM (1974). Operant conditioning of rectosphincteric reflexes in the treatment of fecal incontinence. N Engl J Med 290:646–649.

Engel BT, Talan MI (1991). Autonomic blockade does not prevent learned heart rate attenuation during exercise. Physiol Behav 49:373–382.

Engel BT, Talan MI (1991). Cardiovascular responses as behavior. Circulation 83(suppl II):9–13.

Gelder M (1996). Psychiatry and medicine. In: Gelder M, ed. Oxford Textbook of Psychiatry. New York: Oxford University Press, p 348.

Goddard GV, McIntyre DC, Leech CK (1969). A permanent change in brain function resulting from daily electrical stimulation. Exp Neurol 25:295–330.

Gottlieb SH, Engel BT (1979). Autonomic interactions in the control of heart rate in the monkey. Psychophysiology 16:528–536.

Guilbaud G, Iggo A, Tegner R (1985). Sensory receptors in ankle joint capsules of normal and arthritic rats. Exp Brain Res 58:29–40.

Hefferline RF, Perera TB (1963) Proprioceptive discrimination of a covert operant without its observation by the subject. Science 139:834–835.

Janig W, Morrison JFB (1986). Functional properties of spinal visceral afferents supplying abdominal and pelvic organs, with special emphasis on visceral nociception. Prog Brain Res 67:87–114.

Jenkins WM, Merzenich MM, Ochs MT, et al. (1990). Functional reorganization of primary somatosensory cortex in adult owl monkeys after behaviorally controlled tactile stimulation. J Neurophys 63:82–104.

Joseph JA, Engel BT (1981). Instrumental control of cardioacceleration induced by central electrical stimulation. Science 214:341–343.

Julius S (1988). The blood pressure seeking properties of the central nervous system. Editorial Review. J Hypertens 6:177–185.

Kayser V, Guilbaud G (1984). Further evidence for changes in the responsiveness of somatosensory neurons of arthritic rats: a study of the posterior intralaminar region of the thalamus. Brain Res 323:144–147.

Lacey JI, Batemen DE, Vanlehn R (1953). Autonomic response specificity: an experimental study. Psychosom Med 15:8–21.

Lamour Y, Guilbaud G, Willer JC (1983). Altered properties and laminar distribution of neuronal responses to peripheral stimulation in the SmI cortex of the arthritic rat. Brain Res 273:183–187.

Le Doux JE (1987). Emotion. In: Handbook of Physiology. Section 1: The Nervous System. Vol 5, Higher Functions of the Brain. Bethesda, MD: American Physiological Society, pp. 419–439.

Le Doux JE (1993). Emotional memory systems in the brain. Behav Brain Res 58:69–79.

Le Doux JE (1998). Fear and the brain: where have we been, and where are we going? Biol Psychiatry 44:1229–1238.

Lesse H, Heath RG, Mickle WA, et al. (1955). Rhinencephalic activity during thought. J Nerv Ment Dis 122:433–440.

Levine SA (1959). Some notes concerning angina pectoris. [Editorial] JAMA 171:1838–1840.

Levy DM (1960). The infant's earliest memory of inoculation. J Genetic Psychol 96:3–46.

Lown B (1977). Verbal conditioning of angina pectoris during exercise testing. Am J Cardiol 40:630–634.

Lubar JF, Bahler WW (1976). Behavioral management of epileptic seizures following EEG biofeedback training of the sensorimotor rhythm. Biofeedback Self-Regulation 1:77–104.

Luparello T, Lyons HA, Bleeker RR, et al. (1968). Influences of suggestion on airway reactivity in asthmatic subjects. Psychosom Med 30:819–825.

MacDonald HR, Sapru RP, Taylor SH, et al. (1966). Effect of intravenous propranolol on the systemic circulatory response to sustained handgrip. Am J Cardiol 18:333–344.

MacKenzie JN (1886). The production of "rose asthma" by means of an artificial rose. Am J Med Sci 91:45–56.

Malmo RB, Shagass C (1949). Physiological study of symptom mechanisms in psychiatric patients under stress. Psychosom Med 11:25–29.

Marwitz M, Stemmler G (1998). On the status of individual response specificity. Psychophysiology 35:1–15.

McEachern JC, Shaw CA (1999). The plasticity–pathology continuum: defining a role for the LTP phenomenon. J Neurosci Res 58:42–61.

Melmed RN, Roth D, Beer G, et al. (1986). Montaigne's insight: the placebo effect and symptom anticipation are two sides of the same coin. Lancet 2:1448–1449.

Melmed RN, Roth D, Edelstein EL (1990). Symptom anticipation and the learned visceral response: a major neglected determinant of morbidity in functional and organic disorders. Isr J Med Sci. 26:43–46.

Merzenich MM, Kaas JH, Wall JT, et al. (1983). Progression of change following median nerve section in the cortical representation of the hand in areas 3b and 1 in adult owl and squirrel monkeys. Neuroscience 10:639–665.

Merzenich MM, Nelson RJ, Stryker MP, et al. (1984). Somatosensory cortical map changes following digit amputation in adult monkeys. J Comp Neurol 224:591–605.

Mesulam MM, Mufson EJ (1982). Insula of the old world monkey. I. Architectonics in the insulo-orbito-temporal component of the paralimbic brain. J Comp Neurol 212:1–22.

Mitchell JH, Blomqvist G (1971). Maximal oxygen uptake. N Engl J Med 284:1018–1022

Mogilner A, Grossman JA, Ribary U, et al. (1993). Somatosensory cortical plasticity in adult humans revealed by magnetoencephalography. Proc Natl Acad Sci 90:3593–3597.

Moos RH, Engel BT (1962). Psychophysiological reactions in hypertensive and arthritic patients. J Psychosom Res 6:227–241.

Moran MA, Mufson EJ, Mesulam MM (1987). Neural inputs into the temporopolar cortex of the rhesus monkey. J Comp Neurol 256:88–103.

Morrow GR (1982). Prevalence and correlates of anticipatory nausea and vomiting in chemotherapy patients. J Natl Cancer Inst 68:585–588.

Neville HJ, Schmidt A, Kutas M (1983). Altered visual-evoked potentials in congenitally deaf adults. Brain Res 266:127–132.

Obrist PA, Webb RA, Sutterer JR, et al. (1970). The cardiac–somatic relationship: some reformulations. Psychophysiology 6:569–587.

Oppenheimer SM, Wilson JX, Guirouden C, et al. (1991). Insular cortex stimulation produces lethal cardiac arrhythmias: a mechanism of sudden death? Brain Res 550:115–121.

Pearson CM, Wood FD (1959). Studies of polyarthritis and other lesions induced in rats by injection of mycobacterial adjuvant. 1. General clinical and pathological characteristics and some modifying factors. Arthritis Rheum 2:440–459.

Post RM, Kopanda RT (1975). Cocaine, kindling and reverse tolerance. Lancet 1:409–410.

Quinn JT, Harbison JJM, McAllister H (1970). An attempt to shape human penile responses. Behav Res Ther 8:213–216.

Recanzone GH, Merzenich MM, Jenkins WM, et al. (1992). Topographical reorganisation of the hand representation in cortical area 3b of owl monkeys trained in a frequency-discrimination task. J Neurophys 67:1031–1056.

Reiman EM, Fusselman MJ, Fox PT, et al. (1989). Neuroanatomical correlates of anticipatory anxiety. Science 243:1071–1074.

Rosen RC, Shapiro D, Schwartz GE (1975). Voluntary control of penile tumescence. Psychosom Med 37:479–483.

Rowell LB (1980). What signals govern the cardiovascular responses to exercise? Med Sci Sports Exerc 12:307–315.

Saadah HA (1997). Headache fear. J Okla State Med Assoc 90:179–184.

Sannerstedt R, Julius S (1972). Systemic haemodynamics in borderline arterial hypertension: responses to static exercise before and under the influence of propranolol. Cardiovasc Res 6:398–403.

Schmidt EM, Jost RG, Davis KK (1974). Cortical cell discharge patterns in anticipation of a trained movement. Brain Res 75:309–311.

Schmieder RE, Rueddel H, Neus H, et al. (1987). Disparate hemodynamic responses to mental challenge after antihypertensive therapy with beta blockers and calcium entry blockers. Am J Med 82:11–16.

Schwartz GE (1971). Cardiac responses to self induced thoughts. Psychophysiology 8:462–467.

Shapiro D, Tursky, B, Schwartz GE (1970). Control of blood pressure in man by operant conditioning. Circ Res 27(suppl 1):27–41.

Sterman MB, Macdonald LR, Stone RK (1974). Biofeedback training of the sensorimotor electroencephalogram rhythm in man: effects on epilepsy. Epilepsia 15:395–416.

Swarbrick ET, Hegarty JE, Bat L, et al. (1980). Site of pain from the irritable bowel. Lancet 2:443–446.

Szajnberg NM, Zalneraitis E, Zemel L (1987). Unilateral Raynaud's symptoms evoked during dream report. Lancet 2:802.

Tanji J, Evarts EV (1976). Anticipatory activity of motor cortex neurons in relation to direction of intended movement. J Neurophysiol 39:1062–1068.

Ulrych M (1969). Changes of general haemodynamics during stressful mental arithmetic and non-stressing quiet conversation and modification of the latter by beta-adrenergic blockade. Clin Sci 36:453–461.

Vecchiet L, Giamberardino MA, Dragani L, et al. (1989). Pain from renal/ureteral calculosis: evaluation of sensory thresholds in the lumbar area. Pain 36:289–295.

Victor R, Mainardi JA, Shapiro D (1978). Effect of biofeedback and voluntary control procedures on heart rate and perception of pain during the cold pressor test. Psychosom Med 40:216–225.

Weiss SR, Post RM (1998). Kindling: separate vs. shared mechanisms in affective disorders and epilepsy. Neuropsychobiology 38:167–180.

Wessely S, Nimnuan C, Sharpe M (1999). Functional somatic syndromes: one or many? Lancet 354:936–939.

Wolff AB, Thatcher RW (1990). Cortical reorganisation in deaf children. J Clin Exp Neuropsychol 12:209–221.

Chapter

9

Interplay of Mind and Body in Medical Practice: The Placebo Response

Why do doctors begin by practising on the credulity of their patients with so many false promises of a cure, if not to call the powers of the imagination to the aid of their fraudulent concoctions? They know, as one of the masters of their craft has given to them in writing, that there are men on whom the mere sight of medicine is operative.

All this nonsense has come into my head through my recalling a tale told me by an apothecary who served in the household of my late father. He was a simple man and a Swiss—a people not much given to vanity and lying. He had known some years before, a merchant of Toulouse who was sickly and subject to stone, and who often resorted to enemas, which he had made up for him by the physicians in different ways according to the phases of his illness. When they were brought to him none of the usual formalities was omitted; and he often tried them to see if they were too hot. Imagine him then, lying on his stomach, with all the motions gone through except that no application had been made! This ceremonial over, the apothecary would retire, and the patient would be treated just as if he had taken the enema; the effect was the same as if he actually had. And if the doctor found the action in-

> sufficient, he would administer two or three more in precisely the same way. My witness swears that when, to save the expence—for he paid for the enemas as if he had really taken them—the patient's wife tried sometimes to make do with warm water, the result betrayed the fraud; this method was found useless and they had to return to the first.
>
> (de Montaigne, "On the Power of the Imagination," circa 1572)

The placebo effect is one of the most real and yet at the same time one of the most elusive of clinical phenomena. It usually involves some form of treatment or intervention (by word, tablet, injection, or any other maneuver) without direct biological effects that leads to a patient's improvement or recovery more rapidly than could be expected to occur spontaneously, without such intervention. This implies that the patient's belief system, presumably stimulated by the intervention, is activated to drive or potentiate the recovery process. In a review of 15 studies involving 1082 patients with a range of medical, surgical, and emotional disorders, Beecher (1955) found a therapeutic effect of 35% on average. Evaluation of the placebo effect in major surgery produced a comparable figure, 37% (Beecher, 1961). More recent surveys similarly indicate placebo effects of 30% in treatment trials of ulcerative colitis (Ilnyckyj et al., 1997) or the premenstrual syndrome (Freeman and Rickels, 1999) and 47% for depression (Malt et al., 1999).

It follows that the validity of a therapeutic trial is usually questionable if a placebo group is not included in the design, although the control and placebo groups are often considered the same. The addition of a placebo group is intended to help differentiate specific from nonspecific therapeutic effects. There is, nevertheless, an important difference between a "control" and "placebo." The control subject serves as a marker of the rate and extent of natural recovery with time. The placebo effect is the part played in a patient's recovery by the patient's belief in *or anticipation* of recovery, "that aspect of treatment not attributable to specific pharmacologic or physiologic properties" (Benson and Friedman, 1996). Benson and Friedman also emphasize that "the administration of a placebo is not necessary to evoke the placebo response." Common sense would indicate that in any medical intervention there will be some degree of placebo effect derived from the rapport between doctor and patient, the medical setting, and the credibility of the medication including its size, shape, color, and taste (Kleijnen et al., 1994). Thus, in reality, nonspecific factors will unavoidably interact with specific therapeutic factors.

While the gold standard of therapeutic evaluation is the double-blind, placebo-controlled randomized clinical trial, there are circumstances where the use of a placebo group may be unethical. If effective treatment already exists, withholding treatment could potentially endanger the patient or allow irreversible pathological changes to occur, as in withholding treatment for rheumatoid arthritis

(Stein and Pincus, 1999). Examples of clinical situations in which placebo-controlled trials are unethical include treatment of some cancers, many infectious diseases, and myocardial infarction. With chronic diseases in particular, ethical decisions about placebo controls will need to take into account the severity of the disease, the rate at which the disease causes irreversible damage, and the demonstrated capacity of treatment to alter the outcome of the disease. In some cases, the placebo group has fared better than the treatment group, as in a study of drug treatment of cardiac arrhythmias (Echt et al., 1991). Here the treatment group had more fatal episodes of myocardial infarction than did the placebo group.

PLACEBO: NONSPECIFIC OR SPECIFIC PROCESS?

Attempts to describe the biology of the placebo effect are complicated not only by the ill-defined, unphysiological basis for concepts such as "belief system" or "anticipation," but also by the difficulties inherent in the scientific measurement of biological processes that are moving toward normalcy. The true role of most physiological systems has been clearly delineated only after the effects of their absence or dysfunction have been studied. Physicians are educated to understand clinical problems in terms of pathological processes. In contrast, the placebo effect seems to open a rift between the scientifically immeasurable belief system of an individual and the body where its effects are supposed to play out. One could, however, rephrase the question by asking how the energy of anticipation and belief may be captured and harnessed to affect the functioning of cells, tissues, and organs.

In clinical medicine there are two main schools of thought concerning the nature of the placebo response. In the first, placebo is understood to refer to a process that exists in the patient's mind or imagination and does not produce physiological changes. It expresses itself by the degree to which patients may be convinced, or convince themselves, that their condition is better than it appears to be when viewed objectively. In essence, the placebo effect is most easily induced in the most suggestible patients, or it serves as an indication of the subject's distractibility. The result is a generally more satisfied patient, who complains less and needs less medication for the alleviation of symptoms.

The alternative viewpoint, which I hold, is that the placebo effect is a psychophysiological process in which the patient's belief in or anticipation of recovery can influence specific biological parameters to counteract somatic dysfunction or pathology (*specific effects*) or, by relieving patients' anxiety or pessimism, leads to the alleviation of symptoms (*nonspecific effects*). These two mechanisms may result, for example, in the improvement of mood, the reduction or elimination of pain or inflammation, or the reversal of skeletal or smooth muscle spasm.

This second school of thought puts maximal emphasis on the doctor–patient interaction in promoting the placebo effect, particularly the physican's empathic, supportive role in nurturing and reinforcing the patient's own belief in the healing process. Benson and Friedman (1996) describe the essential ingredients of the placebo response as (1) positive beliefs and expectations on the part of the patient; (2) positive beliefs and expectations on the part of the physician or health care professional; and (3) a good relationship between doctor and patient.

The specific mechanisms of the placebo response vary with the circumstances. In the case of angina pectoris, arterial spasm may be inhibited or vessel dilatation mechanisms activated. In arterial occlusive disease of the legs, systemic blood pressure may rise. In patients suffering from pain, mechanisms for inhibiting pain may be activated (Wall, 1993). Potentially, then, the mechanisms mediating the placebo effects may be as varied as those inducing the pathological change. Nonspecific alleviation of symptoms may result simply from routine medical and nursing attention as well as from aspects of the doctor–patient relationship that promote confidence and the relief of anxiety (Kaptchuk, 1998).

There may also be *spurious* placebo effects when a physician's misleading initial evaluation of the patient's condition leads to the mistaken impression of improvement. Inadequate or erroneous baseline evaluation, influenced by a patient's anxiety at the time of the test, unfamiliarity with the diagnostic technique, and the attitude of the testing physician may substantially influence results (Packer, 1990). This means that subsequent evaluative data are compared to an unreliable baseline. This factor would also contribute to the statistical observation of "regression to the mean," in which a seemingly deviant initial value becomes normal with repeated measurement (McDonald et al., 1983).

NONSPECIFIC FACTORS CONTRIBUTING TO A FAVORABLE PLACEBO RESPONSE

Attitude of the Treating Physician

Not surprisingly, a major factor contributing to a patient's anticipation of improvement is the doctor's enthusiasm (Gracely et al., 1985). This was well illustrated by Beecher (1961), who found that the outcome of surgical procedures later demonstrated to be valueless was largely a function of the surgeon's enthusiasm for the operation. For example, "enthusiasts" described ligation of the internal mammary artery for angina pectoris (a totally useless procedure) as providing "complete pain relief" in 38% of 213 patients in four separate series. In some patients the relief lasted for up to one year. "Skeptical" surgeons reported "complete pain relief" in only 10% of the 59 patients in three smaller series (Fish et al., 1958).

The skeptic might communicate his message to the patient by explaining that the proposed operation is unproven, that there is no generally accepted physiological basis for apparent good results, and that there is no way of knowing in advance whether the angina would be improved. The enthusiast, on the other hand, is likely to use phrases such as "exciting new approach," "full of optimism," "your problem seems ideally suited." The enthusiastic practitioner is likely to convey the feeling that it would make no sense at all to refuse the proposed intervention.

The role of optimism on the part of the treating physician is stressed by Basmajian (1978). While evaluating the treatment of back problems, he noted that seeing the electronic gear of the recording devices (inserted electrodes, electromyographic equipment, various electronic devices, and a computer) raised the placebo response in almost 200 patients from the usual 30% for sugar pills to about 50%. This impressive show of equipment must have contributed to the patients' feeling that something worthwhile was being done.

Degree of Patient Distress

In writing about the placebo response, some authors have emphasized that patients experiencing great stress or suffering are likely to be more responsive to the placebo effect than those who suffer less (Beecher, 1956; Wolf, 1959). Clearly, an adequate definition of the "degree of distress" must include an evaluation not only of the severity of pain or impaired function but also of the associated anxiety about its likely implications. Angina pectoris that is chronic and incapacitating, for example, is likely to generate a realistic fear of death and, consequently, considerable apprehension. The favorable clinical responses to the earliest surgical attempts at revascularization of the myocardium, which we know to have been worthless interventions, may be considered placebo responses. The intensity of pain also influences the response to placebos. Patients reporting intense pain are more likely to respond to placebos than those with less pain (Levine et al., 1979).

Relief of Anxiety

Optimism, whatever its source, fosters an antianxiety and antidepression frame of mind. Intuitively, it does not seem possible for great optimism and considerable anxiety about any given subject to coexist in the same individual. In biological terms, sustained activation of autonomic pathways, which may occur in an anxious personality or in an individual under chronic stress, may be expressed in a variety of symptoms and in the exacerbation of a number of common pathological processes. Relief from anxiety will therefore serve to remove an important influence tending to worsen the condition. Thus, any process which eliminates apprehension about a particular physical state or symptom will help promote relief or recovery in many clinical situations (the nonspecific placebo effect) (Turner et al., 1994). These nonspecific aspects of patient management are generally included in any discussion of the placebo effect (Wolf, 1950; Fields, 1987). The question we address here, however, is the following: What processes can reverse or reduce the intensity of the pathological process? The next section presents the clinical evidence for such mechanisms.

COMPLIANCE IN DRUG TAKING

Anticipation of Improvement or Recovery

The anticipation of improvement or recovery is recognized as an important component of the healing process. This attitude clearly embodies an optimistic frame of mind, but what I mean is something more specific, namely, a definite belief that recovery will take place. Implicit in all these cases is the assumption that the patients' compliance in drug taking, particularly when it is of a high order, reflects her or his belief that the drug will help cure or control the disease.

Patterns of behavior concerning compliance in drug taking may be much more fateful for the patient than is generally appreciated. With many diseases, it seems logical to assume that the efficacy of medical treatment depends on the extent to which the patient follows medical advice (Eraker et al., 1984). Though we assume that by taking the medication patients are maximizing their chances of recovery, there are now indications that patients who differ in their adherence to treatment differ in the outcome of their illness even when they are receiving a placebo. This was observed, for example, in drug trials of secondary prevention in patients suffering from ischemic heart disease, that is, trials aimed at preventing a progression of the heart disease to recurrent myocardial infarction or sudden death. In the Coronary Drug Project, a randomized, controlled trial evaluating the efficacy of lipid-lowering drugs on mortality in men who had survived a myocardial infarction (Coronary Drug Project, 1980), the five-year mortality rate for men treated with clofibrate was 20%, compared with 20.9% for men who received placebo. But when these results were assessed by *adherence to treatment*, patients who took at least 80% of their prescribed clofibrate (good adherers) had a significantly lower five-year mortality rate than did poor adherers (15% versus 24.6%). Remarkably similar findings were noted in patients who received placebo (15% mortality for good adherers and 28% for poor adherers).

A similar trend relating treatment adherence to mortality was noted among 2175 participants in the Beta Blocker Heart Attack Trial, a multicenter, randomized, double-blind trial comparing propranolol with placebo in patients surviving an acute myocardial infarction (Horwitz et al., 1990). Overall, patients who did not adhere well to treatment—those who took 75% or less of the pre-scribed medication—were 2.6 times more likely than good adherers to die within a year of follow-up. Poor adherers, whether on propranolol or placebo, had an increased risk of death, which could not be explained by measures of the sever-ity of myocardial infarction, sociodemographic features (race, marital status, ed-ucation), smoking, or psychological characteristics (severe life stress or social isolation). In reviewing 21 original research articles on the influence of medica-tion nonadherence on coronary artery disease outcome, McDermott et al. (1997), found seven studies (including the two just cited) that showed a significant re-lationship between medication adherence and outcome. These authors suggested that adherence behavior may be a marker of better prognosis. It should be noted that none of the studies specifically aimed to test the influence of a compliance-enhancing intervention on outcome.

While the studies discussed above dealt with ischemic heart disease, a similar association of compliance in drug taking with improved outcome has been found in other clinical contexts. Richardson et al. (1990) studied 94 newly diagnosed patients with hematological malignancies for compliance with oral medication and scheduled clinic appointments over a six-month period. Compliance with drug taking was assessed with serial serum drug and metabolite levels; allopuri-nol was used as a surrogate for self-medication with other chemotherapeutic agents. The three variables found to be most related to survival were the disease severity, high compliance with allopurinol (i.e., compliance in taking the pre-scribed drug), and an education program cohort, in that order. It may be argued, however, that high compliance in taking medication simply means better disease control, as no placebo group was used. In a number of well-controlled studies of various diseases where a placebo group was included, compliance with drug tak-ing, whether of placebo or active drug, improved the outcome, just as it did for ischemic heart disease. This has been reported in studies of prophylactic antio-biotic therapy for chemotherapy-induced granulocytopenia (Pizzo et al., 1983), chlorpromazine treatment of schizophrenia (Hogarty and Goldberg, 1973), and disulfiram treatment of alcoholism (Fuller et al., 1983).

This remarkable observation clearly hints at the importance of psychophysio-logical factors in the ultimate outcome of serious disease. Those who complied with the instruction to take their medication, whether active agent or placebo, presumably took the drug in the belief that by so doing they would favorably af-fect the outcome of their disease. It may have been precisely this belief that in some important way influenced the outcome (Chapter 8).

Experimental Studies

The process by which compliance in drug taking affects outcome has been in-vestigated in a direct manner. Black et al. (1963) assessed the influence of suggestion under hypnosis in individuals with positive Mantoux tests. (This test is an intradermal injection of an extract derived from the tuberculosis-producing bacteria *Mycobacterium tuberculosis*, which will produce a red skin reaction if the individual has been, at some stage, infected by the organism. It is not an indication necessarily of active disease.) In a small group of highly hypnotizable subjects, all Mantoux-positive, the suggestion not to react to the Mantoux injection resulted in a considerable reduction in the extent of erythema that would otherwise have developed. Skin biopsies, both before and after hypnosis, were performed under light general anesthesia. Histological evaluation was performed blindly, and sections were evaluated for the presence of edema and infiltration by inflammatory cells. Significantly, microscopic examination showed a reduction in tissue edema at the injection site in all four subjects to whom nonresponse to the injection had been suggested. However, there was no difference in the extent or composition of cellular infiltrate. These biopsies were compared to biopsies taken from the same subjects before the hypnosis and suggestion protocol was begun. This study elegantly demonstrated that the inflammatory response may be inhibited through suggestion, which presumably had a particular influence on the vascular component.

Failure by Locke et al. (1987) to reproduce these findings might be explained by the difference in the degree to which the subjects were prepared before being injected with the antigen. In this latter, unsuccessful study, subjects were injected under hypnosis on the second day of the experiment, following a single session of hypnosis on the preceding day, whereas Black and colleagues' subjects were prepared with repeated hypnosis over about five days. Similarly, in a negative study reported by Beahrs et al. (1970), subjects not normally reactive to two antigens were injected under hypnosis. Attempts to either enhance or diminish the reaction by suggestion failed. Here too there were important differences in protocol compared to that of Black et al., especially with regard to the lack of intensive preparation of the subjects. Another significant point of difference is that whereas those of Black et al. had started by testing positive, subjects in the study of Beahrs et al. were nonreactive to begin with.

In a study by Smith and McDaniel (1983), seven healthy Mantoux-positive subjects were tested monthly in the same arm, for six consecutive months. At the same time, saline was injected into the other arm. On the sixth occasion, however, the Mantoux antigen was injected, without the subject's knowledge, into the arm that had previously received the saline control injections. Each subject showed a striking reduction in the Mantoux reaction, consistent with their expectation of no reaction in that arm, as had occurred with each of the previous five saline injections. Subsequent injection of the Mantoux material into the "correct" arm resulted in a reaction of normal intensity.

In the study by Luparello et al. (1968) described in the previous chapter patients with bronchospasm, when given saline to inhale and told that they were inhaling a bronchodilator, responded with relief of the bronchospasm. The induction and relief of bronchospasm by suggestion in this study indicate that both bronchial constriction and dilatation may occur in response to the patient's expectation.

Conclusions

A patient's anxiety, whether derived from a realistic appraisal of the clinical situation or not, appears to be an important factor in promoting a favorable placebo response. Anxious patients tend to respond to the doctor's enthusiasm with an enhanced expectation of improvement. The more desperate the patient feels, the stronger the anticipation of improvement may be in response to the suggested therapy. To this extent, the placebo response mirrors anticipatory anxiety, in which apprehension associated with the fear of further attacks becomes the "force" promoting the symptom (Chapter 8). In the case of the placebo response, however, the direction is toward relief of whatever process is causing the symptom. It has thus been suggested that mechanistically symptom anticipation and the placebo effect are two sides of the same coin (Melmed 1986). In the former, the patient's apprehensions work to enhance the symptom, whereas in the latter the expectation of relief diminishes the symptom severity. The studies cited showing a relationship between compliance in drug taking and survival data in patients with ischemic heart disease, whether the drug is an active compound or placebo, emphasize just how profoundly a patient's belief system may influence the natural history of a disease.

SPECIFIC PLACEBO EFFECTS

Placebo Response in Angina Pectoris

The history of angina pectoris therapy is replete with claims made about the efficacy of particular interventions, both surgical and medical, that were never documented in properly conducted trials (Benson and McCallie, 1979). Internal mammary artery implantation in the myocardium (Vineberg procedure) of patients with angiographically proven coronary artery disease was found to produce subjective improvement in approximately 60%–80% of cases (Bjork et al., 1968; Balcon et al., 1970; Langston et al., 1972). This intervention, which was initially believed to stimulate revascularization of ischemic myocardium, was in fact worthless. In one study, 58% of 48 patients had increased exercise tolerance after surgery (Langston et al., 1972). As none of the three studies cited above showed a correlation between improvement in exercise tolerance and angiographic evidence of revascularization, it was speculated that the clinical success was due to some other mechanism (Balcon et al., 1970).

In the 1950s, internal mammary artery ligation was performed in patients with coronary artery disease in the mistaken belief that it promoted the growth of collateral vessels proximal to the point of ligation. In a double-blind study undertaken to evaluate the efficacy of the procedure, one of the subjects suffering from severe angina was chosen as a control to undergo the bilateral skin incisions but without ligation of the internal mammary arteries. He of course believed that the full procedure had been performed. Before the sham operation he could manage only 4 minutes of exertion, which produced pain and a striking inversion of T waves; 6 weeks after the operation he managed 10 minutes of exertion, without pain and with a normal ECG (Cobb et al., 1959).

A tendency for objective indexes of improvement to parallel the patients' feelings of well-being following ineffective therapeutic interventions, such as ligation of the internal mammary arteries, has been reflected in increased effort tolerance (Brown and Riseman, 1937; Cobb et al. 1959; Dimond et al., 1960; Bjork et al., 1968), reduced nitroglycerin requirements (LeRoy, 1941; Cobb et al.,1959; Dimond et al., 1960), and improved electrocardiographic results (Cobb et al., 1959). This implies that the patients' sense of anticipation activates mechanisms that work either to inhibit the sympathetically mediated coronary artery spasm or, less likely, to induce vasodilatation directly. The fact that an improvement in angina pectoris is accompanied by decreased electrocardiographic evidence of ischemia indicates that we are not dealing simply with inhibition of pain sensation.

The Placebo Effect in Heart Failure

The course of heart failure might seem so predictable that spontaneous variability would be unlikely to occur to any significant degree. Indeed, so pervasive was this view that many of the drug therapies for heart failure were evaluated without controls. It is now known that 25%–35% of heart failure patients show significant clinical benefits from placebo therapy (Franciosa et al., 1982; Captopril Multicenter Research Group, 1983; Massie et al., 1985). This is true for patients with mild or severe symptoms. The placebo-associated improvement in exercise tolerance, even in patients with severe cardiac failure (functional class 3 or 4), may be as much as 35% (Massie et al., 1985). This classification of the severity of heart failure is based on symptoms and the amount of effort required to provoke them. In functional class 3, patients have marked limitation of physical activity because, although they may feel comfortable at rest, less than ordinary activity leads to symptoms. In class 4, patients are unable to carry out any physical activity without discomfort and usually have symptoms even at rest. In the first two classes the disability is much milder (New York Heart Association, 1964).

Packer (1990) has commented on the difficulties of analyzing drug or placebo effects on left ventricular function and exercise capacity, two cardinal parameters in the assessment of improvement in heart failure patients. The problem of accurately evaluating baseline function in a complex clinical disorder such as heart failure inevitably makes it difficult to assess improvement following some therapeutic intervention. It is especially in this type of situation that an erroneous impression of improvement may give rise to spurious placebo effects.

The problem of assessing the impact of a specific therapeutic measure in heart failure is compounded by the fact that in heart failure patients there is not a good correlation between changes in left ventricular performance, as assessed by non-invasive measures such as echocardiography or radionuclide ventriculography, and the the clinical status or functional capacity (Franciosa et al, 1981; Engler et al., 1982). Indeed, as emphasized by Packer (1987), most vasodilator and inotropic drugs can produce marked hemodynamic and clinical benefits without notable change in the left ventricular ejection fraction. Conversely, the left ventricular ejection fraction may increase significantly despite clinical deterioration due to cardiac failure (McKay et al., 1985).

Hemodynamic changes that mimic a beneficial drug response may be seen in the absence of effective therapy if measurements are performed immediately after catheterization of the right side of the heart, or after ingestion of a normal meal (Packer et al., 1985; Cornyn et al., 1986). It appears that the process of intravascular instrumentation may produce systemic vasoconstriction (possibly due to anxiety), which dissipates in 12 to 24 hours. If baseline measurements are performed during this postcatheterization vasoconstricted state, any subsequent measurement may be interpreted to show improvement. Subsequent catheterization may not provoke similar degrees of systemic vasoconstriction. Consequently, unless hemodynamic measurements are delayed by 12 to 24 hours after catheterization, investigators may report sustained hemodynamic improvement in patients receiving ineffective treatment (Packer, 1990).

Exercise tolerance is the most common parameter used in multicenter trials to evaluate the efficacy of new drugs for the treatment of heart failure. However, the duration of exercise in patients with heart failure is influenced by the motivation of both the patient and the physician. In addition, repeated testing generally results in improved performance because the patient is now more familiar with the test and the physician is more willing to encourage the patient to exercise to exhaustion (Franciosa et al., 1982; Massie et al., 1985). The magnitude of the placebo effect is also influenced by the criteria used for baseline reproducibility before randomization (Pinsky et al., 1989). When only one or two baseline exercise tests are applied, exercise duration during placebo therapy can increase by as much as 90 to 120 seconds, but the increase may be reduced to 10 to 30 seconds if 3 to 10 baseline tests are carried out. Even the use of gas exchange measurements during exercise, however, does not completely eliminate the placebo response (Leier et al., 1987).

Placebo Effects in Severe Limb Ischemia

Ischemia of the legs causing pain at rest, with or without gangrene, is a serious condition. Drugs are usually not of much value in this situation (Coffman, 1979) and if angioplasty, endarterectomy, and fibrinolytic therapy are ineffective or contraindicated, then the patient may require amputation of part of the limb. In a randomized, cross-over, double-blind study of 41 patients suffering from severe leg ischemia associated with pain at rest and gangrene, patients received injections of either the vasodilator drug naftidrofuryl or a placebo, isotonic sodium chloride (Vayssairat et al., 1988). The change in blood flow to the ischemic leg was evaluated by transcutaneous measurement of the partial pressure of oxygen ($TcpO_2$), a technique shown to be useful in the diagnostic and prognostic evaluation of severe lower limb ischemia and in deciding on the level of amputation (Vayssairat et al., 1984; Editorial, 1984). Two important findings emerged from this study. First, both the drug and the placebo raised the $TcpO_2$ significantly ($P < 0.001$ and < 0.01, respectively), and the difference between placebo and drug was not significant. Second, the systolic blood pressure was significantly raised in both groups, by an average of 13 mm Hg in the drug group and 9 mm Hg in the placebo group, not a significant difference. Furthermore, the increase in systolic blood pressure was correlated with the increase in $TcpO_2$ ($P < 0.05$). The authors emphasized the fact that ischemic leg pain at rest depends on local perfusion pressure, which reflects mean arterial blood pressure. Furthermore, acute ischemic pain in the leg may be quickly and reliably relieved by intravenous infusion of a hypertensive drug such as angiotensin (Dahn et al., 1969), which also induces a parallel increase in skin and muscle blood flow (Ahlstrom and Westling, 1971).

Thus, the placebo mechanism appears to be the appropriate physiological one of increase in systolic blood pressure. The vascular perfusion pressure, particularly when the artery is severely stenosed, is critically dependent on the systemic blood pressure. Even a small rise in systolic blood pressure may increase blood flow through ischemic tissue (Westling, 1988). In peripheral vascular disease, as opposed to coronary artery disease, local spasm of the artery seems to play no significant role in the tissue ischemia. It has long been known that contraction of an ischemic muscle is accompanied by a marked rise in blood pressure (Alam and Smirk, 1937). As to the mechanism mediating this effect, experiments in humans have demonstrated that sympathetic discharge to muscle is tightly coupled with muscle cell pH during exercise (Victor et al., 1988). The onset of sympathetic activation coincides with the development of cellular acidification in active muscle, as measured by phosphorus 32 (^{32}P) nuclear magnetic resonance spectroscopic evaluation of phosphorylated metabolites. As ischemic muscle produces lactic acid in increased amounts, this in turn stimulates chemosensitive afferents (Kaufman et al., 1984), signaling to the brain the mismatch between muscle blood flow and metabolism (Rowell et al., 1976; Wyss et al., 1983). It therefore seems logical to conclude that in patients who experience ischemic muscle pain, first on exertion and then at rest, this mechanism would stimulate sympathetic activity leading to a rise in blood pressure. In the patients described above, expectation of relief following the placebo injection may have led to increased sympathetic activation and increased blood pressure, thus eliminating the pain.

PLACEBO-MEDIATED PAIN RELIEF

It seems likely that the experience of pain can be influenced by the anticipation of either its occurrence or its disappearance. The central role of the affective component in pain received important impetus from the gate control theory (Melzack and Wall, 1965), which postulates that central control mechanisms inhibit or facilitate the input of pain signals from the periphery to the spinal cord. In their relay through the spinal cord, pain messages are modulated by descending impulses from the brain, which in turn reflect cognitive, attentional, and emotional factors.

The subjectivity of pain makes it difficult to investigate clinically, and the great importance of emotional factors in influencing pain intensity tends to reinforce the widespread but mistaken view that pain is simply a psychological construct. The problem is further complicated by the frequent observation that there are two aspects to the pain experience, its sensory quality and the suffering or distress associated with it (Chapman and Gavrin, 1999). Narcotic analgesia, for example, may in some cases be due more to a reduction in suffering than to changes in intensity of the sensory experience (Beecher, 1959). Similar observations have been made about analgesia induced by prefrontal leukotomy, hypnosis, diazepam, and placebo. Thus, the patient feels the pain but is less distressed by it. In general, any measure that reduces anxiety should enhance the efficacy of a pain-relieving intervention.

Experimental studies, mostly in animals but also in humans, have helped to delineate a number of systems which, once activated, serve to inhibit the sensation of pain. These include the release of endogenous opioid peptides (Khachaturian et al., 1985) as well as a number of brain stem centers and pathways that, when stimulated, are associated with the induction of an analgesic state (Reynolds, 1969; Mayer and Liebeskind, 1974). Structures involved in the descending inhibitory systems include the periaqueductal gray (Behbehani and Fields, 1979; Beitz, 1982), locus ceruleus, and parabrachial area (Willis and Westlund, 1997). It seems likely, therefore, that placebo-mediated relief of pain involves the active mediation of these systems in some circumstances.

The explorer David Livingstone's account of being mauled by a lion in Africa vividly illustrates how at times of considerable stress the experience of pain may be suppressed completely:

> It causes a kind of dreaminess, in which there is no sense of pain or feeling of terror. It was like what patients under chloroform describe who see all the operation but feel not the knife . . . This peculiar state is probably produced in all animals killed by the carnivores; and, if so, is a merciful provision by our benevolent creator for lessening the pain of death.[1]

REFERENCES

Ahlstrom H, Westling H (1971). Prolonged measurement of ^{133}xenon disappearance from subcutaneous tissue of the foot. Scand J Clin Lab Med 28:401–407.

Alam M, Smirk FH (1937). Observations in man upon a blood pressure raising reflex arising from the voluntary muscles. J Physiol 89:272–383.

Balcon R, Leaver D, Ross D, et al. (1970). Clinical evaluation of internal mammary-artery implantation. Lancet 1:440–443.

Basmajian JV (1978). Cyclobenzaprine hydrochloride effect on skeletal muscle spasm in the lumbar region and neck: two double-blind controlled clinical and laboratory studies. Arch Phys Med Rehabil 59:58–63.

Beahrs JO, Harris DR, Hilgard ER (1970). Failure to alter skin inflammation by hypnotic suggestion in five subjects with normal skin reactivity. Psychosom Med 32:627–631.

Beecher HK (1955). Powerful placebo. JAMA 159:1602–1606.

Beecher HK (1956). Evidence for increased effectiveness of placebos with increased stress. Am J Physiol 187:163–169.

Beecher HK (1959). Measurement of Subjective Responses: Quantitative Effects of Drugs. New York: Oxford University Press.

Beecher HK (1961). Surgery as placebo. JAMA 176:1102–1107.

Behbehani MM, Fields HL (1979). Evidence that an excitatory connection between the periaqueductal grey and nucleus raphe magnus mediates stimulation produced analgesia. Brain Res 170:85–93.

Beitz AJ (1982). The organization of afferent projections to the midbrain periaqueductal gray of the rat. Neuroscience 7:133–159.

Benson H, Friedman R (1996). Harnessing the power of the placebo and renaming it "remembered wellness." Annu Rev Med 47:193–199.

Benson H, McCallie DP (1979). Angina pectoris and the placebo effect. N Engl J Med 300:1424–1429.

Bjork L, Cullhed I, Hallen A, et al. (1968). Results of internal mammary artery implantation in patients with angina pectoris.Scand J Thorac Cardiovasc Surg 2:1–9.

Black S, Humphrey JH, Niven JSF (1963). Inhibition of Mantoux reaction by direct suggestion under hypnosis. Br Med J 2:1649–1652.

Boivie J, Meyerson BA (1982). A correlative anatomical and clinical study of pain suppression by deep brain stimulation. Pain 13:113–126.

Brown MG, Riseman JEF (1937). The comparative value of purine derivatives in the treatment of angina pectoris. JAMA 109:256–258.

---

[1]From *Missionary Travels*, quoted in Chatwin (1988), p. 243.

Captopril Multicenter Research Group (1983). A placebo-controlled trial of captopril in refractory chronic congestive heart failure. J Am Coll Cardiol 2:755–763.

Chapman CR, Gavrin J (1999). Suffering: the contributions of persistent pain. Lancet 353:2233–2237.

Chatwin B (1988). The Songlines. New York: Penguin Books, p 243.

Cobb LA, Thomas GI, Dillard DH, et al. (1959). An evaluation of internal mammary artery ligation by a double-blind technique. N Engl J Med 260:1115–1118.

Coffman JD (1979). Vasodilator drugs for peripheral vascular disease. N Engl J Med 300:713–717.

Cornyn JW, Massie BM, Unverferth DV, et al. (1986). Hemodynamic changes after meals and placebo treatment in chronic congestive heart failure. Am J Cardiol 57:238–241.

Coronary Drug Project (1980). Influence of adherence to treatment and response of cholesterol on mortality in the coronary drug project. N Engl J Med 303:1038–1041.

Dahn I, Hallbook T, Larsen OA, et al. (1969). Treatment of acute ischemia pain in the leg by induced hypertension. Acta Chir Scand 135:391–394.

De Montaigne M (1958). Essays. On the Power of the Imagination. New York: Penguin Books.

Dimond EG, Kittle CF, Crockett JE (1960). Comparison of internal mammary artery ligation and sham operation for angina pectoris. Am J Cardiol 5:483–486.

Echt DS, Liebson PR, Mitchell LB, et al. (1991). Mortality and morbidity in patients receiving encainide, flecainide, or placebo. N Engl J Med 324:781–788.

Editorial (1984). Transcutaneous oxygen measurement in skin ischemia. Lancet 2:329.

Engler R, Ray R, Higgins CB, et al. (1982). Clinical assessment and follow-up of functional capacity in patients with chronic congestive cardiomyopathy. Am J Cardiol 49:1832–1837.

Eraker SA, Kirscht JP, Becker MH (1984). Understanding and improving patient compliance. Ann Intern Med 100:258–268.

Fields H (1987). Pain. New York: McGraw-Hill Book Company.

Fish RG, Crymes TP, Lovell MG (1958). Internal-mammary-artery ligation for angina pectoris; its failure to produce relief. N Engl J Med 259:418–420.

Franciosa JA, Park M, Levine TB (1981). Lack of correlation between exercise capacity and indexes of resting left ventricular performance in heart failure. Am J Cardiol 47:33–39.

Franciosa JA, Weber KT, Levine TB, et al. (1982). Hydralazine in the long-term treatment of chronic heart failure: lack of difference from placebo. Am Heart J 104:587–594.

Freeman EW, Rickels K (1999). Characteristics of placebo responses in medical treatment of premenstrual syndrome. Am J Psychiatry 156:1403–1408.

Fuller R, Roth H, Long S (1983). Compliance with disulfuram treatment of alcoholism. J Chronic Dis 36:161–170.

Gracely RH, Dubner R, Deeter WR, et al. (1985). Clinicians' expectations influence placebo analgesia. Lancet i:43.

Hogarty GE, Goldberg SC (1973). Collaborative Study Group: drug and sociotherapy in the aftercare of the schizophrenic patient: one year relapse rates. Arch Gen Psychiatry 28:54–64.

Horwitz RI, Viscoli CM, Berkman L, et al. (1990). Treatment adherence and risk of death after a myocardial infarction. Lancet 336:542–545.

Ilnyckyj A, Shanahan F, Anton PA, et al. (1997). Quantification of the placebo response in ulcerative colitis. Gastroenterology 112:1854–1858.

Kaptchuk TJ (1998). Powerful placebo: the dark side of the randomized controlled trial. Lancet 351:1722–1725.

Kaufman MP, Rybicki KJ, Waldrop TG, et al. (1984). Effect of ischemia on responses of group III and IV afferents to contraction. J Appl Physiol 57:644–650.

Khachaturian H, Lewis ME, Schafer MK-H, et al. (1985, March). Anatomy of the CNS opioid systems. Trends Neurosci: 111–119.

Kleijnen J, De Craen AJM, Everdingen J, et al. (1994). Placebo effect in double-blind clinical trails: a review of interactions with medications. Lancet 344:1347–1349.

Langston MF Jr, Kerth WJ, Selzer A, et al. (1972). Evaluation of internal mammary artery implantation. Am J Cardiol 29:788–792.

Leier CV, Binkley PF, Randolph PH, et al. (1987). Chronic indoramin therapy in congestive heart failure: a double-blind, randomized, parallel placebo-controlled trial. J Am Coll Cardiol 9:426–432.

LeRoy GV (1941). The effectiveness of xanthine drugs in the treatment of angina pectoris. 1. Aminophylline. JAMA 116:921–925.

Levine JD, Gordon NC, Bornstein JC, et al. (1979). Role of pain in placebo analgesia. Proc Nat Acad Sci USA 76:3528–3531.

Locke SE, Ransil BJ, Covino NA, et al. (1987). Failure of hypnotic suggestion to alter immune response to delayed-type hypersensitivity antigens. Ann NY Acad Sci 496:745–749.

Luparello T, Lyons HA, Bleeker RR, et al. (1968). Influences of suggestion on airway reactivity in asthmatic subjects. Psychosom Med 30:819–825.

Malt UF, Robak OH, Madsbu H-P, et al. (1999). The Norwegian naturalistic treatment study of depression in general practice (NORDEP). 1: Randomized double blind study. Br Med J 318:1180–1184.

Massie B, Bourassa M, DiBianco R, et al. (1985). Long-term oral administration of amrinone for congestive heart failure: lack of efficacy in a multicenter controlled trial. Circulation 71:963–971.

Mayer DJ, Liebeskind JC (1974). Pain reduction by focal electrical stimulation of the brain: an anatomical and behavioral analysis. Brain Res 68:73–93.

McDermott MM, Schmitt B, Wallner E (1997). Impact of medication nonadherence on coronary heart disease outcomes: a critical review. Arch Intern Med 157:1921–1929.

McDonald CJ, Mazzuca SA, McCabe GP (1983). How much of the placebo "effect" is really statistical regression? Stat Med 2:417–427.

McKay CR, Nana M, Kawanishi DT, et al. (1985). Importance of internal controls, statistical methods and side effects in short term trials of vasodilators: a study of hydralazine kinetics in patients with aortic regurgitation. Circulation 72:865–872.

Melmed RN, Roth, Beer G, et al. (1986). Montaigne's insight: placebo effect and symptom anticipation are two sides of the same coin. Lancet II:1448–1449.

Melzack R, Wall PD (1965). Pain mechanisms: a new theory. Science 150:971–979.

New York Heart Association (1964). Criteria Committee, Disorders of the Heart and Blood Vessels. Nomenclature and Criteria for Diagnosis, 6th ed. Boston: Little Brown, p 114.

Packer M (1987). How should we judge the efficacy of drug therapy in patients with chronic congestive heart failure? The insights of six blind men [editorial]. J Am Coll Cardiol 9:433–438.

Packer M (1990). The placebo effect in heart failure. Am Heart J 120:1579–1582.

Packer M, Medina N, Yushak M (1985). Hemodynamic changes mimicking a vasodilator drug response in the absence of drug therapy after right heart catheterization in patients with chronic heart failure. Circulation 71:761–766.

Pinsky DJ, Ahern D, Wilson PB, et al. (1989). How many exercise tests are needed to minimize the placebo effect during repeated exercise in patients with chronic heart failure? Circulation 80(suppl II):426. Abstract.

Pizzo PA, Robichaud KJ, Edwards BK, et al. (1983). Oral antibiotic prophylaxis in patients with cancer: a double-blind randomized placebo controlled trial. J Pediatr 102:125–133.

Reynolds DV (1969). Surgery in the rat during electrical analgesia produced by focal brain stimulation. Science 164:444–445.

Richardson JL, Shelton DR, Krailo M, et al. (1990). The effect of compliance with treatment on survival among patients with hematological malignancies. J Clin Oncol 8:356–364.

Rowell LB, Hermansen L, Blackmon JR (1976). Human cardiovascular and respiratory responses to graded muscle ischemia. J Appl Physiol 41:693–701.

Smith GR, McDaniel SM (1983). Psychologically mediated effect on the delayed hypersensitivity reaction to tuberculin in humans. Psychosom Med 45:65–70.

Stein CM, Pincus T (1999). Placebo-controlled studies in rheumatoid arthritis: ethical issues. Lancet 353:400–403.

Turner JA, Deyo RA, Loeser JD, et al. (1994). The importance of placebo effects in pain treatment and research. JAMA 271:1609–1614.

Vayssairat M, Baudot N, Sainte-Beuve C (1988). Why does placebo improve severe limb ischemia [letter]? Lancet 1:356.

Vayssairat M, Mathieu JF, Priollet P, et al. (1984). Mesure transcutanée de la pression partielle d'oxygène: une nouvelle méthode d'exploration fonctionnelle en pathologie vasculaire. Press Med 13:1683–1686.

Victor RG, Bertocci LA, Pryor SL, et al. (1988). Sympathetic nerve discharge is coupled to muscle cell pH during exercise in humans. J Clin Invest 82:1301–1305.

Wall PD (1993). Pain and the placebo response. In: Experimental and Theoretical Studies of Consciousness. Chichester: Wiley (Ciba Foundation Symposium 174), pp 187–216.

Westling H (1988). Correspondence. Lancet I:1057.

Willis WD, Westlund KN (1997). Neuroanatomy of the pain system and of the pathways that modulate pain. J Clin Neurophysiol 14:2–31.

Wolf S (1950). Effects of suggestion and conditioning on the action of chemical agents in human subjects: the pharmacology of placebos. J Clin Invest 29:100–109.

Wolf S (1959). The pharmacology of placebos. Pharmacol Rev 11:689–704.

Wyss CR, Ardell JL, Scher AM, et al. (1983). Cardiovascular responses to graded reductions in hindlimb perfusion in exercising dogs. Am J Physiol 245:H481–486.

CHRONIC OR RECURRENT PAIN SYNDROMES

> The pain did not grow less, but Ivan Ilych made efforts to force himself to think that he was better. And he could do this so long as nothing agitated him. But as soon as he had any unpleasantness with his wife, any lack of success in his official work, or held bad cards at bridge, he was at once acutely sensible of his disease . . . now every mischance upset him and plunged him into despair. He would say to himself: "There now, just as I was beginning to get better and the medicine had begun to take effect, comes this accursed misfortune, or unpleasantness . . ."
>
> (Tolstoy, *The Death of Ivan Ilych*, 1886)

Chronic or recurrent pain syndromes are often among the most complex of clinical problems to diagnose and effectively manage. The clinical aspects of this group of disorders span a number of fields of practice. Thus, if patients suffering from either recurrent or intractable pain are not managed in a comprehensive manner, failure is guaranteed. A comprehensive approach to diagnosis and management usually offers the only chance of success and requires that the following issues be considered:

1. To what extent is the pain due to an underlying pathological process that requires specific treatment? Our concern is always to exclude an underlying neoplastic, inflammatory, or metabolic process and to manage pain appropriately.

2. What is the emotional status of the individual with pain? Regardless of the cause, it is wise to assume that every chronic or recurrent pain syndrome has a concomitant significant emotional content. The reasons are clear and usually well defined. Thus, suffering caused by pain, if unremitting, may often result in depression; or there may be anxiety that the pain and attendant suffering will recur (symptom anticipation), or the patient may fear both the suffering and what the pain may mean, that is, that it represents a sinister, life-threatening disease. When present, fear will work to intensify the anxiety and/or depression and vice versa. In all cases, the emotional state will promote further attacks or intensify pain already present and this in turn will aggravate the patient's mood changes.

3. Pain may be the physical expression of an affective state such as depression or anxiety, or of unexpressed, intensely felt emotion such as anger or guilt. Speaking about "feeling pain" as a reaction to some life experience has as much validity in common parlance as does feeling "anxious" or "depressed." Whether pain may also be considered the equivalent of an affective condition such as depression is still debated, but on pragmatic grounds alone there is substantial good clinical sense in sometimes regarding it as such.

This chapter first elaborates on various central issues connected to the complex interplay between chronic or recurrent pain syndromes and emotion. We then try to understand the physiological basis of chronic pain, especially musculoskeletal pain, which, because of its frequent occurrence in the clinic in one form or another, is well researched. The difficulty we encounter here in demonstrating a clearly defined pain mechanism tends to be representative of many chronic pain syndromes that do not occur on the basis of identifiable pathology. Finally, two major pain syndromes are presented in some detail. The first, lower backache, is one of the most frequently encountered debilitating pain disorders of the labor force in the industrialized world. Although it has substantial economic consequences and a frequently recognized major psychosocial component, it has remained in many cases a difficult problem to effectively manage. The second, migraine, is also very common. It is a pain syndrome with distinctive clinical features and has, as opposed to the lower back pain syndrome, a specific drug treatment; nevertheless, it may similarly be extremely resistant to medical management. These pain syndromes, with their distinctive differences in clinical expression and pathogenesis, encompass many aspects of the interplay of chronic or recurrent pain and emotion.

DEFINING PAIN

In discussing a scientific subject, the normal procedure is to define it at the outset. When the subject is pain, however, this is not easily done because we do not know enough about it to offer a comprehensive definition (Melzack and Wall, 1988). The International Association for the Study of Pain (1994) defines *pain* as "an unpleasant sensory and emotional experience associated with actual or potential tissue damage, or described in terms of such damage." Although this definition would probably suffice for most acute pain situations, it does not cover adequately the severe pain resulting from muscular spasm in the walls of hollow muscular systems such as the uterus (childbirth and menstruation), biliary tract (gallstones), ureter (calculus), or gastrointestinal tract (gastroenteritis), to give one set of examples. In nearly all of these situations the "actual or potential tissue damage," if present, may have little to do with the muscular spasm producing the pain. For example, ureteric or biliary colic is produced by the ureter or gall bladder or common bile duct contracting—sometimes violently—to eject intraluminal content such as a stone or sand. The severe pain of natural childbirth is another common example.

The difficulty of producing an adequate definition increases when pain is experienced in chronic pain syndromes. Some chronic sufferers may be diagnosed as having conversion disorder, or Briquet's syndrome, (Merskey, 1982). In such cases patients are experiencing pain as the expression of a psychological conflict or need and are not intentionally malingering. Both the DSM-IV and the ICD-10 call this condition "somatoform pain disorder," a distinct variant of conversion disorder. In attempting to define pain in this context, it is instructive to consider these questions: When the patient complains of pain, what feelings underlie the pain? Could the physical experience of pain be a representation of a state of emotion?

I believe that the answer to the last question is yes—there are at least some occasions when psychological distress such as anxiety, anger, or guilt is experienced as physical discomfort and perceived by the patient as pain, whether it be headache, lower backache, irritable bowel syndrome, or temporomandibular joint pain. Facilitated neural pathways may have been established by previous injury (prolapsed intervertebral disc, degenerative changes of the vertebrae), learned behavior, or perhaps inherited predisposition. Thus, while the experience of pain may have originally developed from peripherally induced processes, it becomes a psychological problem in that peripheral stimulation is no longer required to provoke it. Because of what the pain represents in these instances, "it comes to occupy a key position of the total psychic economy" (Blumer and Heilbronn, 1982).

A growing body of literature on the most common chronic pain problems in clinical practice point to the role of psychological factors in mediating symptoms. Among depressed patients, the complaint of pain has a high reported frequency (Von Knorring, 1975; Ward et al., 1979). Conversely, chronic pain is often associated with depressive illness (Walters, 1961; Sternbach, 1974; Black, 1975; Kramlinger et al., 1983) and suicidal behavior (Dorpat et al., 1968). In a study of 150 chronic nonmalignant pain patients consecutively referred to a Danish multidisciplinary pain center, Becker et al. (1997) found that 58% of the patients suffered from a depressive or anxiety disorder. Compared to the normal non-patient population, quality of life and psychological well-being of the group of chronic pain patients were severely reduced. Furthermore, they used the health services five times more often than the normal population in the year before referral. The common association between chronic pain and depression in clinical practice, and the considerable overlap of symptoms, suggests that chronic somatic pain syndromes may mask depression (Lesse, 1968; Forrest and Wolkind, 1974) or represent a somatic equivalent of depression (Blumer and Heilbronn, 1982). It should be remembered, however, that both symptom complexes are common and that a physical basis for the pain cannot be identified in many chronic pain patients. The coincidence of these two conditions does not necessarily imply a causal linkage but may in some instances point to a common constitutional predisposition to both the affective state and the pain syndrome (Merikangas, 1995).

Personality Characteristics of Patients Suffering from Chronic Pain of Obscure Origin

In an attempt to define more clearly the personal and emotional characteristics of patients suffering from chronic pain of obscure origin (i.e., in whom a neoplastic, inflammatory, or metabolic cause had been excluded), Blumer and Heilbronn (1982) presented a comprehensive description of the clinical features of 900 such patients. Their principal aim was to determine whether it was possible to characterize certain people as "pain prone" according to personal characteristics, a notion that has since found very little utility or acceptance in clinical practice. More important, however, is the educational value to the physician when encountering a chronic pain problem. Their analysis of the demographics and attitudes of chronic pain patients may help to facilitate accurate diagnosis, avoid unnecessary costly and sometimes dangerous examinations and interventions, and in general more effectively guide the patient toward an appropriate path of management.

In the Blumer and Heilbronn (1982) study, the mean age of onset was 39 years and most of the patients were women. Pain had lasted for an average of 6.5 years by the time of evaluation. The average education level was grade 12 and the disorder was most prevalent among the lower middle class (67%). The main clinical features of these patients suffering from pain of obscure origin were the following:

- Most sufferers complained of a continuous pain, which was present on going to sleep at night and on waking in the morning.
- Despite repeated negative examinations, they displayed a hypochondriacal preoccupation with the painful body parts.
- Every patient in the group had undergone at least one surgical procedure because of pain and most of them insisted that the problem required a surgical solution.
- Despite years of disabling pain and dependence on others, most patients tried to project an image of solidity, denying difficulties in interpersonal relationships, describing their family relationships in idealized terms, and viewing themselves as independent types.
- In contrast to the typical loss of initiative and enthusiasm for work following the onset of the pain, there was usually a history of excessive work performance and relentless activity before its onset. The extreme lassitude after onset was associated with decreased ability to enjoy social life, leisure time, and sexual relations (anhedonia). Patients maintained their appetite but tended to develop insomnia. About one-third strongly denied feeling depressed while admitting to feeling despair over the pain.
- Patients were often unable to recognize or verbalize their feelings. They tended to give an impression of stoicism by avoiding comment with emotional content, and they typically showed a lack of imagination and fantasy.

There are marked similarities in personality characteristics between this group of patients and those suffering from the chronic fatigue syndrome (CFS) (Abbey, 1993; Ware, 1993; Clauw and Chrousos, 1997). Often CFS patients show symptoms of extreme inability to function and lassitude after onset of the illness, although until then they had been exceptionally active in their personal and professional lives. They also tend to aggressively deny the possibility of an emotional basis for their disorder and try hard to convince the physician of its organic basis. Similarly, they tend to deny depression, presenting their emotional state rather as "despair." If they admit to feeling depressed, they may rationalize it as a reaction to their clinical state. This particular constellation of personality characteristics compounds the difficulty of correctly managing the problem, as the doctor is often persuaded by the patient's insistence that there must be some underlying disease process to explain the symptoms, leading to excessive investigations as well as inappropriate surgical interventions in the case of the chronic pain patient. The most unfortunate consequence is that the doctor's attempts to direct the patient to some form of psychological intervention often meet with the patient's refusal to cooperate, leading to prolonged incapacity and suffering.

Many with chronic pain conditions report diminished symptoms as their age increases. This is true for low back pain syndromes as well as headache and temporomandibular disorders, although not for arthritis-related diseases (Dworkin et al., 1990; Dworkin, 1991). In those with lower back pain, for instance, the decrease in symptomatology and disability from back pain contrasts with the general worsening of spinal degenerative changes with increasing age. This apparent paradox highlights the role of psychological and behavioral factors.

Cognitive Aspects of Pain

The experience of pain may conveniently be considered to have three important components (Weisenberg, 1989):

1. *Sensory-discriminative*, those aspects of the neurophysiology of pain considered above.
2. *Cognitive-evaluative*, relating to the implication of the pain—patients' perception of what the pain means and what resources they feel they have to deal with the pain.
3. *Motivational-affective*, relating to the predominant emotion associated with the pain, which is the suffering associated with it and possibly also its metaphorical meaning.

It is clear that the second and third points are related, in that cognitive-evaluative restructuring can substantially alter the motivational-affective response to pain, even if the sensory-discriminative component remains the same. The understanding that cognition plays a central role in the pain experience led to an emphasis on cognitive aspects in the treatment of pain. The Gate Control Theory of Pain as formulated by Melzack and Wall (1965), by suggesting the important influence of higher cerebral function in up- or downregulating pain awareness, played a major role in integrating physiologically our present-day ideas of the importance of cognitive factors in pain perception.

This recognition is related to the development of the field of cognitive and behavioral therapy, which is based on the idea that belief systems exert an influence on cognitive evaluation or appraisal, and that emotion is conditioned by this cognitive process. Patients are taught how to monitor negative, automatic thoughts, to recognize the connections among cognition, affect, and behavior, and to recognize irrational beliefs that lead them to distort experience (Ellis and Grieger, 1977; Beck, 1991: Weisenberg, 1999). Cognitive evaluation influences the way individuals react to and cope with stress. Thus, their responses reflect their perception of the event, its importance to their well-being, and their coping resources. Cognitive appraisal is a dynamic process that may change with scrutiny and reconsideration, leading to an altered perception of an event or experience and a consequent change in emotions. The use of cognitive therapy in managing chronic or recurrent pain problems has proved particularly successful. Cognitive–behavioral therapies directed at chronic pain aim to modify irrational perceptions and thoughts centered on the pain symptoms as well as to enhance active (as opposed to) passive coping behaviors (Turk and Flor, 1984; Fordyce et al., 1985; Keefe and Gill, 1986; Tan and Leucht, 1997).

WHAT CAUSES CHRONIC PAIN?

The origins of chronic or recurrent pain may be difficult to determine and are likely to differ according to the location of the pain. A brief history of ideas about the origin of musculoskeletal pain is instructive, however, as a representative example for showing how our understanding of the problem has evolved. The focus of ideas about the generation of the pain syndromes typically moves from concrete, limited perceptions about local changes, such as spasm in the painful muscles, to a more holistic appreciation of the subtle interplay and importance of sleep physiology and mood changes on the heightened sensitivity of the muscles, to physiological activity.

For instance, many of the relatively common muscular pain syndromes that encompass a large number of patients complaining of chronic pain, such as muscle tension headaches, chronic lower back pain, temporomandibular disorders, and myofascial pain or fibromyalgia, were popularly assumed to derive from abnormal muscle activity. This idea was fueled by early electromyographic (EMG) recordings of painful muscles, when several workers reported abnormal activity indicative of spasm or spastic contractures. It soon became clear, however, that most patients with chronic muscle pain show no histological or biochemical signs of pathological processes. Thus, after conducting clinical, biochemical, EMG, and muscle biopsy evaluations, Mills and Edwards (1983) were unable to establish a tissue diagnosis in 72 of 109 (66%) patients presenting with muscle pain. It is this group of patients that we are most interested in here. Of the 37 patients in whom muscular pain was an expression of a disease state, 16 (15%) had an enzyme defect, 8 (7%) a noninfective inflammatory (collagen) disorder such as polymyositis, 7 (6%) a neurogenic disorder, and 6 (5%) an endocrine or metabolic disorder. After exhaustive testing most patients remained undiagnosed, though the disability caused by their chronic pain was often great.

The potential mechanism of musculoskeletal pain induction has been the subject of numerous investigations. One of the earliest hypotheses was that of Travell et al. (1942), who suggested that pain and dysfunction are reciprocally linked to set up a "vicious cycle" in which one reinforces the other. This idea, initially proposed for pain and spasm in the muscles of the shoulder girdle, where it is most probably valid, was then generalized to other muscular pain syndromes such as temporomandibular joint syndromes (Cobb et al., 1975; Michler et al., 1987; Blasberg and Chalmers, 1989; Parker, 1990) and fibromyalgia (Bengtsson and Bengtsson, 1988; Yunus, 1988). Yet extensive research aimed at establishing hyperactivity as an etiological factor in chronic muscle pain conditions has failed to support the hypothesis (Nouwen and Bush, 1984; Chapman, 1986; Ahern et al., 1988; Henriksson and Bengtsson, 1991). In temporomandibular pain, for example, resting EMG activity is no higher on the painful side of the mandible than on the nonpainful side (Majewski and Gale, 1984; Dolan and Keefe, 1988). Similarly, when EMG activity in patients suffering from "muscle tension headaches" was compared to that in age- and sex-matched controls, there was no evidence of elevated EMG activity in the frontalis, neck (Martin and Mathews, 1978; Sutton and Belar, 1982), or temporalis (Majewski and Gale, 1984) muscles in the affected patients. On the basis of these findings and of other data, Lund et al. (1991) proposed a model of pain adaptation in order to describe more accurately the relationship between chronic musculoskeletal pain and motor activity. They pointed out that the ability to contract muscles forcefully in chronic pain syndromes is reduced rather than increased, and that the only situation in which EMG activity appears to be higher than normal in the presence of chronic pain is when the muscle acts as an antagonist. They interpreted the latter observation as an adaptive response that serves to limit the range and velocity of motion, thus helping to reduce pain and minimizing damage when present. However, the real source of the pain in these conditions is mostly unclear.

In an EMG study of female fibromyalgia patients and age-matched controls, the patients reported significant pain in the biceps brachii, trapezius, and tibialis anterior, but there was no difference in the mean level of resting EMG activity between the two patient groups (Zidar et al., 1990). Of considerable interest in this regard is the work of Moldofsky and his colleagues (Moldofsky et al., 1975; Anch et al., 1991) on the role of sleep disturbances in the genesis of fibromyalgia (Chapter 15). The term "unrefreshing (nonrestorative) sleep" was introduced by Moldofsky et al. (1975), who observed that an anomalous alpha rhythm (7.5–11.0 Hz) on electroencephalographic (EEG) recordings during non–rapid eye movement (NREM) sleep was associated with unrefreshing sleep and an overnight increase in muscle tenderness. Similarly, Anch et al. (1991) reported that fibromyalgia patients had more alpha rhythm in their EEGs during sleep, were more vigilant during sleep, and had more fatigue, sleepiness, and pain than healthy controls. Other authors have also observed an association between disturbed sleep and muscular pain. Saskin et al. (1986) reported anomalous alpha EEG rhythm during sleep, as well as diffuse myalgia, fatigue, and emotional distress, in patients after an emotionally distressing but not physically injurious industrial or motor accident. Also, Kolar et al. (1989) and Jacobsen and Danneskiold-Samsoe (1989) reported a correlation between poor sleep quality and muscle tenderness. As pointed out by Moldofsky (1993), many of the clinical features of fibromyalgia and CFS may be induced by total and partial or selective sleep deprivation (see Chapter 15).

What has not seriously been considered up to now is that in most of the musculoskeletal syndromes, pain may be an expression of a reduced pain threshold analogous to visceral syndromes such as the irritable bowel syndrome, esophageal motility disorder, and chest pain with normal coronary arteries (Chapter 11). In all these situations pain results from physiological activation of the viscera or muscles in question. Thus, activity that may fall within a physiological range causes pain because of the attendant emotional state reducing the pain threshold.

ADULT LOW BACK PAIN

No other painful condition better illustrates the clinical complexity of chronic pain than the low back pain syndrome. It is a condition with substantial economic consequences in all industrialized countries in that the maximum prevalence peaks in the male work force at around the age of 40 years, some 20–40 years before the development of significant degenerative changes of the spinal vertebrae. It is precisely this striking discrepancy between peak occurrence of the clinical syndrome and spinal degenerative changes that offers the key to a proper understanding of the problem. That is, an interplay among social, psychological, and physical factors has to be considered to arrive at an accurate evaluation of any patient suffering from this condition (Andersson, 1999).

Lumbar spine problems affect up to 80% of people at some time during their lives and up to 25% of working men in any given year (Kelsey and White, 1980). In the United States, back problems are the most common cause of disability in adults under the age of 45 (National Center for Health Statistics, 1973; Kelsey and White, 1980; Spengler et al., 1986). Since the age group with maximal incidence of low back problems overlaps the age group of the principal work force, the economic and industrial consequences are substantial. Within the United States and Sweden, low back pain accounts for approximately 25% of all sick-leave absenteeism from work. This represents about 20 million worker-days per year in the United States and a remarkable 25 million in Sweden (Nachemson, 1992). Back pain in the United States is the most frequent cause of activity limitation in people younger than 45 years of age, the second most frequent cause of visits to the physician, the third most frequent cause of surgical procedures, and the fifth ranking cause of admission to hospitals (Taylor et al., 1994; Hart et al., 1995). This high prevalence makes major demands on health care resources, in addition to leading to early retirement and demands for compensation payment (Andersson, 1981; Nachemson, 1992; Frymoyer, 1992). In Sweden the estimated annual cost of this problem is about $10 billion and in the United States between $20 billion and $50 billion (Frymoyer, 1992; Snook and Webster, 1987). In the United Kingdom 7% of the adult population present each year to their general practitioner with low back pain at a cost to the National Health Service in excess of the equivalent of $750 million (United Kingdom Department of Health, 1994).

Despite the scale of these statistics, a relatively small number of people with back pain actually consume most of the resources. About 85% of those who stay away from work because of acute back pain recover without further consequences within six weeks (Frymoyer, 1992). Although in one year up to 50% of adults of working age reported limitation of their activities because of back pain (Bigos and Andary, 1992), only about 2%–10% of the sufferers developed chronic problems. This small percentage spent 80% of the resources consumed in the management of lower back pain (Spengler et al., 1986). Stated more specifically, in the United States and Canada, low back injuries account for 15%–25% of injuries covered by workers compensation and 30%–40% of the payments made under that program (Spengler et al., 1986). It is thus important to have a clear understanding of the natural history of low back pain in relation to degenerative conditions of the spine and of the common clinical syndromes in order to be better able to assess patients complaining of back pain.

Natural History of Degenerative Spinal Changes

The changes most commonly observed in the spine are degenerative. These include disc degeneration, various degrees of herniation of the intervertebral discs, and osteoarthrosis of the apophyseal joints as well as osteoporosis, spondylolisthesis, and fractures and dislocations of vertebrae. Advances in imaging techniques such as computed tomography (CT) and magnetic resonance imaging (MRI) permit much more sensitive evaluation of spinal integrity in all age groups than can be achieved with standard x-rays. Evidence of degenerative spinal changes can be detected as early as childhood and adolescence (Ghabrial and Tarrant, 1989; Banerian et al., 1990; Tertti et al., 1991), but the incidence of degenerative spinal changes naturally increases with age. By the age of 50, autopsy evidence of degenerative disc disease is found in 85%–95% of cases (Miller et al., 1988).

Experimental and clinical evidence indicates that degeneration results from the mechanical effects of weight bearing in the erect posture, with consequent axial loading of the spinal column over time (Ellenberger, 1994). Furthermore, the degenerative process considered here is likely to be promoted by any defect or intervention that alters the normal mechanics of posture, such as congenital neural arch defects (spondylolisthesis or spondylolysis) and previous back surgery. Thus, over a 10-year period, patients who have had one spinal operation are 10 times more likely than unoperated patients to require spinal surgery (Bruske-Hohlfeld et al., 1990).

Origins of Pain in Spinal Disorders

Though not the first to suggest that lumbar disc herniation with spinal root compression causes the radicular pain of sciatica, Mixter and Barr (1934) presented a systematic description of the clinical conditions that may result from this process. It took some years, however, before this view was challenged and modified by the observation that acute peripheral compression neuropathies are usually painless (Howe et al., 1977). Experimentally, acute compression of the root or nerve did not produce more than a few seconds of repetitive firing, in contrast to minimal acute compression of a normal dorsal root ganglion, which caused long periods of repetitive firing (5–25 minutes). In addition, chronic injury of dorsal roots in the cat, or of the sural nerve in the rabbit, markedly increased mechanical sensitivity and altered the reponse to acute compression, which now produced several minutes of repetitive firing. Howe and his coauthors thus suggested that radicular pain resulted from compression of either the dorsal root ganglion or chronically injured nerves.

In a review of pain mechanisms in the lower back, Rydevik et al. (1984) pointed out that mechanical nerve fiber deformity may compromise nerve root microcirculation, leading to intraneural edema and demyelination. These factors are likely to be important in the genesis of pain from nerve root compression. Jinkins et al. (1989) noted that in addition to the syndromes of neurogenic spinal radiculopathy accompanying posterior disc extrusion, anterior and central disc extrusions also may be associated with a definite clinical syndrome of local pain as well as pain referred to the thigh or buttock. The syndrome of anterior extrusion is commonly manifested in the midlumbar spine, whereas posterior extrusion syndromes tended to involve the lower lumbar levels.

Clinical Presentation

The most common presentation of the low back pain syndrome is local pain and muscular spasm in the lower back or pain which also radiates to the leg, buttock, hip, or groin and which is sensitive to position or movement. Limitation of spinal movement, muscle asymmetry, and loss of lumbar lordosis due to spasm are typical features. Clinical evaluation may reveal altered tendon reflexes, motor or sensory deficits, and (rarely) autonomic or sphincter disturbances. Typically, with degenerative disease of the spine, symptoms are intermittent. This is especially true of pain. Persistent or progressive radicular pain or painless motor or sensory deficits referable to the lumbosacral segments should arouse suspicion of other processes, such as tumor.

The main diagnostic procedures in those patients needing investigation are spinal CT and MRI. The latter is considered the procedure of choice for evaluating the spine (Ellenberger, 1994). But the value of diagnostic procedures in the assessment of patients with low back pain syndrome remains questionable in the great majority of cases. This is because investigation often fails to show abnormality, and when it does it may be difficult to relate the finding uneqivocally to the patient's symptoms. A systematic review of publications on the relationship between symptoms of back pain and findings on plain radiography indicates that false positives range from 40% for degeneration to 50% for spondylosis and spondylolisthesis (Van Tulder et al., 1997). Still, for the majority of patients, the origin of back pain remains unknown despite the considerable technical advances in imaging techniques (Holt, 1968; Modic and Ross, 1991).

The greater likelihood of finding abnormalities with techniques like MRI means that misleading false positives are likely to occur more frequently than with plain radiographs (Roland and van Tulder, 1998). That this concern is well founded was borne out by an MRI study of the vertebral column in 98 *asymptomatic* subjects which revealed that only 36% of the subjects had normal discs at all levels, 52% had at least a bulge at one level, 27% had a protrusion, and one subject had an extrusion (Jensen et al., 1994). An abnormality at more than one intervertebral disc was found in 38% of the patients. The prevalence of bulges, but not of protrusions, increased with age. The most common nonintervertebral disc abnormalities were Schmorl's nodules (herniation of the disc into the vertebral body endplate), found in 19% of the subjects; annular defects (disruption of the outer fibrous ring of the disc), seen in 14%; and facet arthropathy (degenerative disease of the posterior articular processes of the vertebrae), seen in 8%. The findings were similar in men and women.

Predicting Low Back Pain Problems: Is It Possible?

Because problems involving back pain tend to recur, it is important to identify people with these problems, especially among industrial workers (Chaffin and Parks, 1973; Svensson and Andersson, 1983; Biering-Sorenson and Thomsen, 1986). Over the years all strategies that focused simply on the mechanical aspects of spinal disorders failed to reveal any reliable predictor of disability due to spinal disorder. In the earliest studies of this problem, it was assumed that back symptoms would be correlated with spinal disorders, and accordingly preemployment roentgenographic screening was recommended (Bohart, 1929; Cushway and Maier, 1929). It was only approximately 30–50 years later, following case-control and cohort studies involving collectively more than 28,000 sets of lumbosacral spinal x-ray films, that x-rays were declared useless as predictors of future back problems (Diveley and Oglevie, 1956; Fullenlove and Williams, 1957; LaRocca and MacNab, 1970; Magora and Schwartz, 1976). Furthermore, neither physical examination (unless a surgical scar is noted) nor preemployment history is reliable in eliciting information about previous back trouble (Rowe, 1971; Biering-Sorenson, 1984). To date, the most dependable predictor of future back trouble is a previous history of this complaint, although job dissatisfaction has also been observed to play a role (Bigos et al., 1992).

One predictor is psychosocial factors, which are consistently present in high frequency in populations with persistent disability—longer than one year—from lower back pain (Burton et al., 1995). Thomas et al. (1999) undertook a prospective study in primary care of 180 patients to quantify those variables most often associated with persistence of back pain. All the patients had consulted their general practitioner because of back pain in the 18 months before the study. Persistence of symptoms was associated with "premorbid" factors such as high levels of psychological distress, poor self-rated health, low levels of physical activity, smoking, and dissatisfaction with employment. A cross-sectional epidemiological study showed that lower back disability was associated with many other health complaints and illness behaviors (Frymoyer et al., 1985). This greater tendency to somatization in chronic lower back sufferers as compared to controls has also been noted by others (Coste et al., 1992; Thomas et al., 1999), as has a higher incidence of psychiatric diagnoses such as depression, generalized anxiety disorder, and substance abuse (Polatin et al., 1993). Regardless of the instrument, however, psychological tests tend to give variable results in the assessment of subjects with low back pain, and they would appear to have little value as prognostic tools (Frymoyer, 1992).

While the discussion so far has focused principally on biological and psychological factors that may operate in cases of recurrent or persistent disability, some consideration should be given as well to the influence of social policies and economic factors on clinical behavior. In general, the frequency and duration of compensation claims are influenced by the level of compensation benefits. Thus, Loeser et al. (1995) estimated that in the United States, where benefit levels differ from state to state, a 10% increase in a compensation benefit was associated with a 1%–11% increase in the frequency and duration of claims. Among patients with back pain, the level of functioning and severity of symptoms after treatment are worse in those who retain an attorney, initiate litigation, or become involved in workers compensation proceedings than in those who do not, even after adjustment for clinical findings (Treif and Stein, 1985; Atlas et al., 2000). Similar trends have been demonstrated for whiplash injury of the spine where elimination of compensation for pain and suffering (so called no-fault insurance, where claimants are compensated for their medical needs following an accident but not for pain and suffering) is associated with a decreased incidence and improved prognosis (Cassidy et al., 2000). How are we to understand the significance of these findings? Deyo (2000) summarized the phenomenon as follows:

> The vast majority of claimants undoubtedly have real symptoms, but how these symptoms are labeled, evaluated, and treated may have important effects on their perceived severity and duration. The mere act of assigning a diagnostic label may

increase illness-related behavior (Haynes et al., 1978), and many physicians believe that excessive testing leads to the conviction that one has a disease, as well as to anxiety and overreaction (Colledge, 1993). Patients may choose to file insurance claims not only because of the severity of their symptoms or disability, but because of an inability to cope with symptoms, anxiety about their implications, and a conscious or unconscious desire for retribution.

Thus, we are beginning to understand much better the substantial influence of social policy decisions and economic factors on illness behavior.

The Pervasive Difficulty in Managing Chronic Lower Back Pain

Educational programs have been set up in the United States to help cope with the widespread problem of lower back pain in the work force (Forssell, 1981; Mattmiller, 1980). These "back schools" were developed by physical therapists to provide information on back anatomy and physiology, the mechanism of pain, pain management, good posture, safe techniques of lifting and handling, and muscle strengthening and stretching. The training is given in small groups. Generally, these programs have reduced back pain and number of sick days, but no program has reduced injury rates. Lahad et al. (1994) concluded that although there is some support for the observation that exercise prevents lower back pain, justification for other prevention strategies is insufficient.

This doubt regarding the efficacy of preventive interventions to reduce the incidence of lower back pain in worker populations at risk is reinforced by the failure of a well-conducted program aimed at preventing back pain to achieve its objective. Daltroy et al. (1997) undertook a randomized, controlled trial of an educational program to prevent low back injuries in about 4000 postal workers. The subjects were followed for more than 5.5 years. Comparison of the intervention and control groups showed that the education program did not reduce the rate of low back injury, the median cost per injury, the time off from work per injury, the rate of related musculoskeletal injuries, or the rate of repeated injury after return to work. Clearly, given the scope and duration of this study this was an unencouraging outcome, and one at variance with the impact of educational programs in other clinical conditions (Chapter 18). These educational programs may have failed because they should have led to increased practice of safe lifting and handling techniques, a behavioral change that did not take place. Moreover, this preventive program was directed specifically at easing the physical strain inherent in a particular type of work (postal work), and it did not address psychosocial issues.

It seems important to stress in conclusion that the outcome of this study in no way negates the value of educating individual back sufferers on the safest way to deal with physical strain that may result from various demands in their day-to-day lives. There is clearly a difference between the management program of a patient suffering from disabling back pain and the outcome of such education in a group of asymptomatic workers participating in a prospective clinical study. It seems clear, however, from the substantial data reviewed here, that in the chronically disabled education should be coupled to the greatest possible extent with comprehensive psychosocial evaluation and appropriate intervention.

THE SPECTRUM OF HEADACHES

In evaluating a patient complaining of headache, one must decide whether the headache is primary or secondary. Primary headaches, while often recurrent, are not associated with underlying pathology, as opposed to secondary headaches, which are (National Headache Foundation, 1997). The common primary types of headaches have long been viewed in clinical practice as representing discrete pathophysiological entities. This attitude was influenced by the distinctive clinical expression of classical migraine headaches compared to the typical tension headache, as well as by the assumption that they differ in pathogenesis. The typical aura and symptoms of migraine, including the pain, were considered to have a vascular basis. Tension headaches, on the other hand, were considered to emanate from tension in the upper cervical and extracranial musculature (Pozniak-Patewicz, 1976). The different therapeutic armamentarium for each of these conditions reinforced the idea that they are different entities. For many years ergot alkaloids were the drugs of choice for migraine, whereas simple analgesics or nonsteroidal anti-inflammatory agents were used for tension headache. Today, that delineation is considered less relevant as migraine may respond well to generic analgesics, and sumatriptan, shown to be most effective in terminating an attack of migraine (Perrin et al., 1989), may be effective in severe tension headache (Cady et al., 1997).

In 1962, the Ad Hoc Committee on Classification of Headache provided definitions for the common headaches. Migraine was defined as "recurring attacks of headache, widely varied in intensity, frequency and duration. The attacks are commonly unilateral in onset, are usually associated with anorexia and sometimes with nausea and vomiting; in some are preceded by, or associated with, conspicuous sensory, motor, and mood disturbances; and often familial." Tension headache was defined as "ache or sensations of tightness, pressure, or constriction, widely varied in intensity, frequency and duration; long lasting and commonly suboccipital; associated with sustained contraction of skeletal muscle; usually as part of the individual's reaction during life-stress." Finally, combined headaches were defined as "combinations of vascular headache of the migraine type and muscle contraction headache prominently coexisting in an attack."

Although these definitions were widely accepted for more than 20 years, clinical experience increasingly indicates that migraine and tension headaches may represent different points on a continuum of responses. This perception is reflected in the revised classification of headaches of the International Headache Society (1988), where "migraine without aura" and "chronic tension headache" are coupled in the same category. Nevertheless, there is a clear distinction in the typical presentation of each headache type. The diagnostic criteria for tension headache as opposed to classical migraine are that they may be bilateral, non-pulsating, mild to moderate, and are not aggravated by movement. In addition, in distinction to classical migraine there is only mild nausea, if any, or photophobia and phonophobia (Ferrari, 1998).

The Clinical Continuum of Migraine and Tension Headaches

Electromyographic recordings in headache sufferers indicate that migraine cannot be distinguished from tension headache on the basis of tension measurements in the extracranial and upper cervical muscles (Bakal and Kaganov, 1977). The fact that migraine sufferers may experience more muscular tension than tension headache patients, both during and between attacks of headache, would appear to exclude extracranial muscle tension as the main cause of tension headaches. It seems likely that the muscle spasm is secondary to the presence of headache, occurring as a facilitated response to the localization of pain to the same somatic segments. That such facilitated pathways indeed exist was indicated by the work of Malmo and Shagass (1949) on response specificity (Chapter 8). These authors showed that in headache sufferers, nonspecific stressors were associated with increased tension in the extracranial muscles rather than with an increase in blood pressure or other stress response.

Attempts to distinguish between these common headache types were further complicated by the fact that the syndromes overlap (Saper, 1986). Classical migraine sufferers may have attacks without an aura and may also suffer from tension headaches. Individuals who usually suffer from tension headaches may have the occasional migraine attack, with or without an aura. In addition, recognized accompaniments of migraine, such as unilateral throbbing pain, nausea, and photophobia, may also be associated with tension headaches. The prevalence of these overlapping syndromes has been the subject of numerous reports (Waters, 1973; Bakal and Kaganov, 1979; Thompson et al., 1980).

Intermittent migraine may evolve into a pattern of daily headaches in some patients, a condition termed "transformed migraine" by Mathew et al. (1982). In a study of 515 patients (mean age 41 years, 3:1 female-to-male gender ratio) suffering from daily headaches, 80% of patients reported experiencing the first migraine attack before the age of 26 (Saper, 1983). In this group the character of the headache had changed over the years from the typical migraine pain to a low-grade, dull feeling of tightness or throbbing, much more consistent with the clinical picture of tension headaches. All of these patients still experienced typical attacks of migraine from time to time. Some authors describe this condition as the "mixed headache syndrome" (Diamond and Freitag, 1988).

One possible explanation for this transformation from intermittent migraine attacks to a tension headache–like clinical picture is that with the involvement of the limbic system, the neurological mechanisms mediating the headache are triggered with increasing ease by a process analogous to "kindling." (Chapter 8) This process may also operate in anxiety states and depression, so that lower levels of stress or anxiety would be sufficient to trigger a headache.

Headache Prevalence and Gender

National prevalence estimates in the United States indicate that migraine headache is the most frequently reported chronic condition of the nervous system or sense organs in noninstitutionalized populations (Collins, 1988). The National Health Interview Study of 1983–1985 projected an annual incidence of 7.7 million cases of migraine headache, with a female-to-male gender ratio of 2.66:1 (47.9 females and 18.0 males per 1000 population). The estimated cost to U.S. employers per year from missed workdays and impaired function resulting from migraine attacks has been calculated to be about $13 billion, with the greatest morbidity falling, as with lower back pain problems, on the 30 to 49 year olds (Hu et al., 1999). Gender differences among migraine sufferers are well documented, both clinically (Blau, 1987) and epidemiologically (Waters, 1970). A survey in the United States demonstrated striking ethnic differences in the prevalence of migraine, although the female preponderance was preserved in all ethnic groups (Stewart et al., 1996). The prevalence in those of Caucasian, African, and Asian origin was, respectively, 20.4%, 16.2%, and 9.2% for women and 8.6%, 7.2%, and 4.2% for men.

The higher prevalence of clinically significant headache (severe enough to induce the patient to consult a physician) among females is cause for speculation. While it is not known whether or to what extent this gender difference is attributable to biological differences, socialization processes in childhood, or role differences between males and females in society, it does seem that the pain associated with headache in general is greater and the average duration of each attack is longer in women than it is in men (Celentano et al., 1990). Thus, although females were twice as likely as males to report recent disability caused by a headache attack, the great majority of headache sufferers in the United States (Celentano et al. 1990), Great Britain (Green, 1977), and Sweden (Ekbom et al., 1978) do not consult physicians because of the problem.

Female hormones appear to influence the frequency of migraine attacks. Oral contraceptives can initiate migraine attacks or increase their frequency (Bickerstaff, 1975). The tendency toward premenstrual and menstrual-related headache attacks among migraine patients is reportedly as high as 60% (De Wit, 1950; MacGregor et al., 1990), and pregnancy has been reported to alleviate migraine in 60%–70% of cases (Somerville, 1972). Waters and O'Connor (1971) found that headaches were more frequent during the first three days of menstruation than later.

Integrating Clinical Observations and Experimental Studies of Migraine

In considering the pathophysiology of the most common headache syndromes, there are a number of good reasons for focusing our attention on migraine: it is common, it has been extensively studied, in its most classical forms it has distinctive neurological changes associated with the development of the character- istic headache, it merges clinically into the syndrome of tension headaches, there are often stress or affective elements associated with its occurrence, and it is fre- quently amenable to specific pharmacotherapy as well as techniques of behav- ioral therapy. It thus fits comfortably into that category of disorder of principal interest to us in which defined physiological responses and the resulting clinical symptoms may be triggered or significantly influenced by psychological processes. Furthermore, the large-scale prospective epidemiological study (with 14,407 participants) conducted by Merikangas et al. (1997) established a signif- icant relationship between migraine and severe nonspecific headache and stroke, particularly among young women. This study provides another dramatic exam- ple of psychophysiological events such as stress acting as a trigger for a process that may lead to a lethal or, more usually here, severely crippling outcome. The other, more familiar example is the influence of stress on ischemic heart disease, discussed in detail in Chapter 7.

Theories of the pathogenesis of migraine have engaged some of the best minds in neurology and pharmacology over the last century. However, while there is still no consensus regarding the primary event that leads to an attack of migraine, we are in a better position, through technological advances in brain imaging tech- niques in particular, to document pathophysiological events associated with the classical attack (Lance and Goadsby, 1998; Edvinsson, 1999). The following dis- cussion attempts to describe the interrelationship of mechanisms thought to be important in an attack of migraine, namely, neurological symptoms, changes in cerebral blood flow, and pain.

The primary event appears to involve brain stem and limbic structures

Proof of involvement of brain stem nuclei has come from Weiller et al. (1995) who used positron emission tomography (PET) in studying a group of nine pa- tients within six hours after the onset of symptoms of unilateral acute migraine attacks. During the attacks, increased blood flow was observed in the cerebral hemispheres, in cingulate, auditory, and visual association cortices, and in the brain stem. However, only the brain stem activation persisted after the injection of sumatriptan, which induced complete relief from headache as well as from phono- and photophobia. While accurate localization of the brain stem activity was not possible, Weiller et al. noted that the foci of maximum vascular increase coincided with the anatomical location of the dorsal raphe nucleus and the locus coeruleus, centers involved in the modulation of both pain and autonomic activity. They further point out that as these brain stem nuclei are involved in decreasing pain ("antinociception") and extra- and intracerebral vascular control, it is tempting to see these brain stem centers as being part of a primary mechanism in the genesis of migraine.

Several clinical observations point to the involvement of the limbic system, also richly connected to the same brain stem structures, in the earliest phases of a classical migraine attack starting with the fact that stress is considered the most important trigger (Blau, 1992). In an analysis of the factors associated with the initiation of migraine attacks in 60 sufferers (41 females and 19 males), Blau (1985) found that 50% of the patients regarded the migraine as being associated with a stressful experience. Even when the onset of migraine was attributed to a physical factor, in most cases there was a stressful component. The list of causes included childbirth, vaginal hemorrhage, traffic accident, head injury, and prolonged lack of sleep. However, a trigger cannot be found in every case.

In classical migraine, the typical aura is frequently preceded by a craving for sweet foods, which if eaten quickly and in quantity may abort the attack. Furthermore, diabetes may alleviate migraine (Blau and Pike, 1970), whereas insulin-induced hypoglycemia in diabetic migraine sufferers can provoke an attack (Martins and Blau, 1989), as can starvation or fasting. The hypothalamus is particularly sensitive to blood glucose levels and, together with the sympathetic–adrenal axis, it is the principal mediator of glucose counterregulation. Similarly, fluid retention and yawning as forerunners of a migraine attack could well reflect hypothalamic and hypothalamic–midbrain influences.

The primary neurophysiological event leads to cortical activity

The aura preceding a migraine attack, when it occurs, may be manifested as scintillating scotomata (indicating involvement of the occipital cortex), numbness ascending from the fingertips to the shoulder (involvement of the sensory cortex), or aphasia (frontal cortex). Furthermore, it does not respect vascular boundaries. Fisher (1971) pointed out that the numbness ascending from the fingertips to the shoulder would have to be explained by a selective sequential spasm of small vessels of the middle cerebral artery, supplying specifically the sensory cortex. Because the motor cortex almost invariably escapes (motor paralysis is very rare as a migraine aura), one would have to assume that the anterior branches of the same vessel are seldom involved—a highly improbable sequence of selective vascular participation.

Thus, the presence of an aura suggests that the cerebral cortex sometimes directly undergoes metabolic change in a migraine attack, and that changes in trigeminovascular activity causing the pain follow it. The trigeminal system provides the only known pain-sensitive innervation of the cranial vasculature by virtue of the convergence of trigeminal and upper cervical pain inputs (Edvinsson, 1999). Spreading depression of neural activity in the cortex, a process so far observed only in the laboratory, has characteristics resembling the progression of a classical migraine attack, as discussed above. The analogy between the similar progression rate of the migraine scotoma during the aura and *cortical spreading depression* was first suggested by Leao and Morrison (1945). However, the process is still regarded today as a potential model of migraine-associated changes in the cortex (Read and Parsons, 1999).

Cortical spreading depression

Spreading depression has been induced in most gray matter regions studied (with the exception of the spinal cord) in a wide variety of mammals, fish, amphibians, reptiles, and birds through the buildup of potassium in the extracellular space. The cessation of neuronal activity at the time of maximal depression is due to massive depolarization (Sugaya et al., 1975), leading to a sustained release of excitatory and inhibitory neurotransmitters. In experimental studies, the transient induction of spreading depression is characterized by depression of evoked and spontaneous electroencephalographic (EEG) activity, which spreads at a rate of 2–5 mm/min across the cortical surface (Leao, 1944). Spreading depression is characteristically a transient process. Although spreading depression has not been demonstrated in humans, considerable circumstantial evidence supports the occurrence of a similar process during attacks of classical migraine.

Classical migraine attacks show a number of striking similarities to spreading depression in their signs, symptoms, and the distinctive pattern of regional cerebral blood flow (rCBF) reduction during an attack. During a typical attack of classical migraine, only the posterior half of the hemicortex is affected (Olesen et al., 1981). Most regional blood flow studies in migraine without aura have produced normal results, unlike those with aura (Olesen et al., 1990). In a very well-documented positron emission tomography study, fortuitously performed while a subject developed an attack of atypical visual aura followed by migraine headache, repeated blood flow studies were performed at closer intervals than had been previously done (Woods et al., 1994). Flow reduction started bilaterally in the visual association areas, not in the primary visual cortex, and spread slowly forward on both sides in a fashion strongly resembling spreading depression.

The vascular response is secondary to the cortical changes and causes the pain

The cortical arterioles are responsive to local neuronal activity and tend to dilate when the adjacent cortex is active. It is mainly this part of the system that was studied in the regional blood flow experiments just described. Despite conflicting data on the two-phase response of cortical vessels during the evolution of an attack—oligemia (presumably vasoconstriction) followed by hyperemia (Olesen et al., 1981)—the fact that infarcts may still be considered rare (given the substantial number of migraine attacks) would tend to support this sequence of events.

A less visible but possibly more important factor in the genesis of migraine pain is the blood supply of the meninges and the venous sinuses of the dura. The brain tissue itself has no pain fibers and the pain probably derives from dilatation of meningeal blood vessels in response to the cortical changes (Blau and Dexter, 1981). Moskowitz and colleagues (1993; Moskowitz et al., 1987) proposed that neurogenic inflammatory neuropeptides such as substance P and calcitonin gene-related peptide (CGRP), released from primary sensory nerve terminals innervating the dural blood vessels, may produce a local inflammatory response called neurogenic inflammation. Neurogenic inflammation may lower the nociceptive threshold required to stimulate meningeal sensory fibers (Johnson et al., 1998). Goadsby et al. (1990) found a marked increase of CGRP but not of neuropeptide Y, vasoactive intestinal polypeptide, or substance P in the external jugular venous blood during migraine headache. Following sumatriptan administration, CGRP returned to control levels with successful relief of the headache (Goadsby and Edvinsson, 1993). One mechanism of action of the serotonin agonists such as sumatriptan or naratriptan is that they inhibit the release of substance P and CGRP from trigeminal sensory afferent neurons surrounding the meninges (Durham and Russo, 1999).

Fozard (1995) proposed that migraine arises as a result of nitric oxide (NO) release activating the release of substance P and CGRP from trigeminal sensory efferents. The tendency of nitroglycerin to induce severe headache in patients with a past history of migraine implicates NO in the process. Here the headache occurs typically approximately five hours after nitroglycerin infusion, suggesting that NO initiates a cascade of events leading to the headache attack. Significantly, Fullerton et al. (1999) showed that sumatriptan substantially improved niroglycerin-induced headaches (administered by infusion) in 9 of 10 healthy male volunteers. Nonmigraine patients may complain of a headache following nitroglycerin close to the time of exposure.

The efficacy of sumatriptan, a receptor agonist similar to $5\text{-}HT_{1D}$ (5-hydroxytryptamine, serotonin) in acute migraine attacks, coupled with the fact that it neither penetrates into the CNS nor exerts a specific antinociceptor action, strengthens the notion that the main antimigraine activity of the drug derives from its vascular effects (Peroutka and McCarthy, 1989; Saxena and Ferrari, 1989) and perhaps from a direct action on trigeminal neurons as well (Goadsby and Hoskin, 1998; Durham and Russo, 1999). As the direct effect on the trigeminal neurons is to inhibit the secretion of the inflammatory mediators, this observation does not seem to challenge the idea that the pain and other migraine-associated symptoms are mediated by the vascular changes.

The ability of the most potent antimigraine drugs to reduce blood flow through intracranial arteriovenous fistuli and to constrict the main cerebral arteries provides additional support for the vascular theory (Feniuk et al., 1987; den Boer et al., 1991). In a study of seven migraine patients during an attack, Heyck (1969) showed that the jugular venous oxygen saturation was elevated on the affected side and could be normalized by treatment with dihydroergotamine. It was suggested by the author that the increase in the oxygen saturation of the venous blood might be due to abnormal dilatation of arteriovenous anastamoses during the migraine attack.

Pain from meningeal structures may provoke extracranial muscle spasm. Extracranial muscles may be painful in all phases of migraine, and the pain may persist after the migraine has gone. Extracranial muscle pain, especially from the neck, may also trigger migraine attacks (Blau, 1992). These findings point to the involvement (via the brain stem) of nociceptive fibers of the trigeminal and upper cervical nerves.

Headache and Emotional State: How Are They Related?

To what extent does headache reflect emotional state? This is not an easy question to answer. The standardized questionnaires used to determine the role of emotional factors are not simple to apply, and the interviewers' experience in using them varies. Selection and diagnostic criteria may also introduce variables that affect the outcome of the study. Some patients may conceal or not recognize the true emotional content of a particular situation, or they may tend to minimize its role. The most dependable answers generally come from surveys based on random population samples or studies using suitably matched controls.

Overall, the evidence from such studies points to higher levels of psychological distress among subjects with migraine, particularly females, than in those without migraine. Although controlled studies have not demonstrated consistent psychological profiles in headache sufferers (Adams et al., 1980), there are strong indications that many migraine patients have psychological symptoms even during headache-free periods (Zeitlin and Oddy, 1984; Hooker and Raskin, 1986). Crisp et al. (1977) examined the psychological status of individuals in a random sample of 722 residents in an English market town. The lifetime prevalence of migraine was 25% in women and 10% in men. Women who suffered from migraine reported significantly greater levels of anxiety, somatic symptoms, depression, and hysteria than women without migraine, but no such differences were found for men. In a nested case-control study of classical migraine and personality, Brandt et al. (1990) found that psychological distress scores of migraine sufferers were significantly higher than those of age- and gender-matched controls. In a nested case-control study, new cases of a disease are identified during a follow-up study of a cohort and are then compared with controls drawn from the same cohort (Abramson, 1988).

Although no particular personality type serves as a predictor of headache, it is worth noting that in evaluating the "locus of control" (see Chapter 4) in headache sufferers, Shulman (1989) asserted that "while most people fall somewhere in the middle [i.e., between internal and external locus of control], headache patients tend to group toward the high internal end of the continuum; they tend to take responsibility on themselves for meeting and coping with the problems that life brings . . . such a person is responsible, conscientious, ambitious and perfectionistic. Such a person will be anxious to control outcome," feelings that may be predicted to lead to stress.

Studies of the association between migraine and depression in both clinical and community studies have provided consistent evidence of comorbidity between these disorders, regardless of the index disorder for which the patient sought treatment in the clinical setting (Merikangas and Stevens, 1997). Ziegler et al. (1978) studied 711 community residents and found that those with histories of "disabling" or severe headaches had higher depression and anxiety scores than did participants with "mild" or no headaches. The pattern was similar for men and women. In a study of 515 migraine sufferers whose headaches had evolved into a pattern of chronic daily headaches, Saper (1986) found that 86% could be diagnosed as suffering from depression and 50% met the criteria for a sleep disturbance. Thus, at least in the case of patients suffering from frequent or debilitating headaches, anxiety and depression appear to be more prevalent than in nonsufferers (Diamond, 1964; Mongini et al., 1997; Guidetti et al., 1998; Mitsikostas and Thomas, 1999).

Managing Migraine

Management of migraine sufferers consists of the following four strategies.

1. *Prevention of attacks by avoidance of triggers:* These triggers may be identifiable ingested substances such as chocolate, cheese, or wine. Similarly, analgesic overuse—whether aspirin, acetaminophen, or nonsteroidal anti-inflammatory compounds (NSAIDs), or ergotamine and serotonin agonists such as sumatriptan (Evers et al., 1999)—when used too intensively, may lead to persistent or frequently recurrent attacks of headache, the so-called analgesic rebound headaches. This latter state is particularly suggested in patients with refractory daily or nearly daily headaches where in approximately 75% the attacks have transformed from episodic episodes in treated patients (Manzoni et al.,

1991). Not infrequently patients consume analgesics in anticipation of headaches. The fear of pain drives them to take the medication before the headache develops (Mathew, 1997a). These patients should be weaned off the medication gradually, with the expectation of spontaneous improvement.

2. *Treatment of the acute attack:* The selective agonists of the serotonin receptor (5-HT$_{1B/D}$) such as sumatriptan and zolmitriptan usually provide the most certain pharmacological means of aborting an attack of migraine (Doenicke et al., 1988). However, the problem of nausea and delayed gastric emptying during an attack as well as the uncertain absorption characteristics of sumatriptan limit the efficacy of these medications. In some instances antiemetics such as metoclopramide are administered with the drug, though the development of preparations suited to intranasal administration have also proven efficacious (Ryan et al., 1997; Tfelt-Hansen, 1998) and more convenient than subcutaneous injection.

The cost of drugs like sumatriptan is still, however, substantially more than the older remedies such as ergotamine derivatives or analgesics such as aspirin, acetaminophen, or NSAIDs, and it is likely to be more than many sufferers of limited economic capability can afford on a regular basis. For this reason, more readily available and cheaper analgesics are usually recommended as a first step, as they are often shown to be as effective, particularly when taken at the start of an attack. In a placebo-controlled study of 156 adults suffering from migraine attacks, the effectiveness of the NSAID diclofenac potassium was compared to sumatriptan. Diclofenac potassium was shown to be faster acting and just as efficacious as sumatriptan in eliminating pain over an eight-hour study period and more efficacious than placebo or sumatriptan in reducing nausea (Diclofenac-K/Sumatriptan Migraine Study Group, 1999). Similarly, ergotamine may be favored in migraine sufferers who have infrequent or long duration headaches and who can be depended on to comply with dosing restrictions in order to avoid peripheral or coronary vasospasm, in particular, as a potential side effect (Tfelt-Hansen et al., 2000).

In view of the common comorbidity of migraine and depression, and the fact that the selective serotonin reuptake inhibitors (SSRIs) and triptans both work to increase serotonin effects on the nervous system, the potential for drug interactions resulting from their combined use is considerable. However, in a survey of fluoxetine use in Canada, of 22 adverse events reported, 6 showed "varying degrees of evidence of a drug interaction between fluoxetine and sumatriptan" (Joffe and Sokolov, 1997). These may include coronary events or, more commonly, malaise, nausea, vomiting, vertigo, tingling, and nasal discomfort (Mathew, 1997b). Thus it appears that while the danger of combined use is not great considering the very widespread use of both classes of drugs, the potential for a significant interaction should be remembered. For patients with migraine and manic depressive disorder or epilepsy, divalproex sodium is the drug of choice (Silberstein, 1998).

3. *Long-term prophylactic therapy:* In spite of the substantial advances made in the specific pharmacotherapy of migraine, it is generally acknowledged that there still remains a very significant group of chronic migraine sufferers. Drugs like sumatriptan with a specific mode of action have had a favorable effect in significantly reducing utilization of health care resources and improving workplace productivity as well as quality of life and patient satisfaction (Lofland et al., 1999), but they have not eliminated the problem of chronic or recurrent attacks. In the long-term management of this more intractable group of patients, the varied list of drugs testifies to the real difficulties encountered in effectively preventing recurrent migraine attacks. Most frequently used for this purpose are β-blockers such as propranolol, metoprolol, and atenolol, but NSAIDs, calcium antagonists, valproate, SSRIs, and amitriptyline, among others, are also used (Tfelt-Hansen, 1997). As with all chronic or recurrent pain syndromes and particularly when migraine attacks are severe and incapacitating it is wise to assume that emotional factors have a role in promoting the attacks.

4. *Response of benign headache disorders to behavioral treatment or psychotherapy:* The conventional management strategies of recurrent or chronic pain problems have relied heavily on the use of drugs and surgery. Because the importance of psychological and behavioral factors in the genesis of chronic pain is now widely accepted, few reputable pain control clinics today function without the active participation of a psychologist as a constant member of the management team (Barber, 1996). As will be discussed in Chapter 18, the question of diagnostic labels is not critical in this context; indeed a psychological label may deter the patient from further cooperation.

The use of nonpharmacological treatments like those suggested in Chapters 18 and 19 may be advocated early on because of the likelihood that these interventions, when successful, will substantially reduce the intensity and frequency of the headache attacks (Young et al., 1997). The mostly only partial efficacy of the drugs used in the interval treatment of migraine (listed above) parallels the sometimes similar difficulty in controlling the pain of the irritable bowel syndrome, another intermittent pain syndrome with a substantial psychosomatic component (Chapter 11). It should be clear that the anxiety state perpetuating the pain syndrome may derive simply from apprehension about the prospect of another attack of pain, or it may be symptomatic of other stressful events in the patient's life of a recent or more distant experience.

The two principal approaches in the behavioral treatment of headache are some form of muscular relaxation and biofeedback training. In the latter, the focus is on learning to relax the muscular tension emanating usually from a forehead site. Comprehensive reviews of the efficacy of these treatments demonstrate their superiority to a control period of headache monitoring (i.e., simply doing nothing) while on a waiting list for inclusion in a treatment program (Andrasik and Blanchard, 1987). In addition, specific combinations of cognitive therapy (Holroyd et al., 1977; Holroyd and Andrasik, 1978), including group discussions on the subject of headache, were shown to be effective, and superior to amitryptilline, in chronic tension headache sufferers (Holroyd et al., 1991).

A detailed review of the gamut of psychotherapeutic techniques indicates that while the common varieties of headaches may be effectively treated with any of the various interventions indicated above, such as biofeedback, relaxation techniques, or cognitive therapy, individuals vary in their responses and may be more favorably disposed to one technique than another (Blanchard, 1992). The combination of biofeedback and cognitive behavioral therapy has been shown to significantly improve the outcome in a group of 38 patients with migraine without aura (Kropp et al., 1997). In general, behavioral treatments appear to be as effective as medication. The good response of headache syndromes to psychological forms of treatment supports the view that headache, particularly as a frequent, recurrent, or chronic problem, may be largely a psychophysiological problem

A broad-based workshop sponsored by the National Institutes of Health (NIH) evaluated the clinical efficacy of behavioral and relaxation therapy for chronic pain and insomnia and concluded that "a number of well-defined behavioral and relaxation techniques now exist and are effective in the treatment of chronic pain and insomnia. The panel found strong evidence for the use of relaxation techniques in reducing chronic pain in a variety of medical conditions as well as strong evidence for the use of hypnosis in alleviating pain associated with cancer. The evidence was moderate for the effectiveness of cognitive-behavioral techniques [CBT] and biofeedback in relieving chronic pain" (NIH, 1996). Medical conditions with a certain organic basis are amenable to the same approaches. In a series of eight well-designed studies reviewed by the panel, CBT proved superior to placebo and to routine care for alleviating low back pain, rheumatoid arthritis, and osteoarthritis-associated pain but inferior to hypnosis for oral mucositis and to EMG biofeedback for tension headache. Similarly, for migraine headaches, biofeedback was better than relaxation therapy and better than no treatment. Multimodal treatment programs have a consistently positive effect on several categories of regional pain, such as back and neck pain, dental or facial pain, joint pain, and migraine headaches. The report emphasized that while the efficacy of different techniques can be rated according to the published scientific evidence, the data are insufficient to conclude that one technique is definitely superior to any other for any given condition or any given patient.

SUMMARY

The syndromes of chronic back pain and migraine are common forms of recurrent pain associated with considerable morbidity. Chronic back pain is often of uncertain pathogenesis and frequently occurs without a clear relationship to co-existent vertebral pathology. Paradoxically, the prevalence of symptomatic back pain decreases strikingly as the severity of vertebral and spinal pathology (degenerative changes and osteoporosis in particular) increases with increasing age. Psychosocial factors appear to be of considerable importance in the pathogenesis of the condition, and there is a significant association between intractability of the back pain and psychiatric diagnoses as well as the prospect of deriving economic benefits from "pain and suffering" through insurance and workers compensation schemes.

Migraine by contrast has a highly defined clinical presentation in its classical form, indicating an involvement of cells of the cerebral cortex as well as the trigeminovascular (nociceptive) axis. Rather than being a totally discrete entity, most evidence favors a continuum of responses between the very common tension headache at one end of the clinical spectrum and migraine with aura at the other end. The pattern of expression of the headache—whether classical migraine or migraine without aura or tension headache syndrome—may well be influenced by constitutional/genetic factors. While a number of analgesics and vasospastic drugs are efficacious in treating the pain, the triptan series of serotonin receptor agonists are highly effective in aborting an attack of migraine and also the pain of tension headache. In spite of the specificity of these drugs in combating the pain of migraine, there is considerable tendency to recurrence of the attacks. There is a significant comorbidity of headache, particularly migraine, with affective states such as depression, and emotional stress is recognized as a significant trigger for migraine (headache) attacks.

The very substantial differences in pathophysiology of lower back pain and migraine highlight the considerable diversity of physical response to, as well as the central importance of psychological stress in diverse syndromes of recurrent or chronic pain. The experience of lower back pain management teaches, among other things, that educating a population at risk to behavioral changes that may serve to diminish the chance of back strain, as was described for postal workers, is a formidable objective not easily achieved. It would appear from clinical experience that real motivation for behavior change arises usually, when it occurs at all out of the discomfort of pain or disability. From lower back pain patients and others with musculoskeletal disorders, we have come to learn how social and economic considerations may significantly influence illness behavior. In addition, the experience of migraine teaches us the very important lesson that even the availability of a specific therapeutic agent does not circumvent the necessity of having to deal with the underlying psychological stressors in an appropriate manner, when they are present, in order to effectively manage the problem.

REFERENCES

Abbey SE (1993). Somatization, illness attribution and the sociocultural psychiatry of chronic fatigue syndrome. In: Kleinman A, Strans SE (Eds,) Chronic Fatigue Syndrome. Chichester: Wiley (Ciba Foundation Symposium 173), pp 238–261.

172   MIND, BODY, AND MEDICINE

Abramson JH (1988). Making Sense of Data. New York: Oxford University Press, p 275.

Ad Hoc Committee on the Classification of Headaches (1962). Arch Neurol 6:173–176.

Adams HE, Feuerstein M, Fowler JL (1980). Migraine headache: review of parameters, etiology and intervention. Psychol Bull 87:217–237.

Ahern DK, Follick MJ, Council JR, et al. (1988). Comparison of lumbar paravertebral EMG patterns in chronic lower back pain patients and non-patient controls. Pain 34:153–160.

Anch AM, Lue FA, MacLean AW, et al. (1991). Sleep physiology and psychological aspects of fibrositis [fibromyalgia] syndrome. Can J Psychol 45:179–184.

Andersson GBJ (1981). Epidemiological aspects on low-back pain in industry. Spine 6:53–60.

Andersson GBJ (1999). Epidemiological features of chronic low-back pain. Lancet 354:581–585.

Andrasik F, Blanchard EB (1987). Task force report on the biofeedback treatment of tension headache. In: Hatch JP, Rugh JD, Fisher JG, eds. Biofeedback Studies in Clinical Efficacy. New York: Plenum, pp 281–321.

Anthony M, Hinterberger H, Lance JW (1967). Plasma serotonin in migraine and stress. Arch Neurol 16:544–552.

Atlas SJ, Chang Y, Kammann, et al. (2000). Long-term disability and return to work among patients who have a herniated lumbar disc: the effect of disability compensation. J Bone Joint Surg Am 82:4–15.

Bakal DA, Kaganov JA (1977). Muscle contraction and migraine headache: psychophysiologic comparison. Headache 17:208–215.

Bakal DA, Kaganov JA (1979). Symptom characteristics of chronic and nonchronic headache sufferers. Headache 19:285–289.

Banerian KG, Wang AM, Samberg LC, et al. (1990). Association of vertebral end plate fracture with pediatric lumbar intervertebral disc herniation: value of CT and MR imaging. Radiology 177:763–765.

Barber J (1996). Psychological evaluation of the patient with pain. In: Barber J, ed. Hypnosis and Suggestion in the Treatment of Pain, New York: WW Norton and Co, pp 50–66.

Beck AT (1991). Cognitive therapy: a 30 year retrospective. Am Psychol 46:368–375.

Becker N, Bondegaard TA, Olsen AK, et al. (1997). Pain epidemiology and health related quality of life in chronic non-malignant pain patients referred to a Danish multidisciplinary pain center. Pain 73:393–400.

Bengtsson A, Bengtsson M (1988). Regional sympathetic blockade in primary fibromyalgia. Pain 33:161–167.

Bickerstaff ER (1975). Neurological complications of oral contraceptives. Oxford: Clarendon Press, pp 81–86.

Biering-Sorenson F (1984). A one year prospective study of low back trouble in a general population: the prognostic value of low back history and physical measurement. Dan Med Bull 31:362–375.

Biering-Sorenson F, Thomsen C (1986). Medical, social and occupational history as risk indicators for low-back trouble in a general population. Spine 11:720–725.

Bigos SJ, Andary MT (1992). The practitioner's guide to the industrial back problem: 1. Helping the patient with symptoms and pathology. Semin Spine Surg 4:42–54.

Bigos SJ, Battie MC, Spengler DM, et al. (1992). A longitudinal, prospective study of industrial back injury reporting. Clin Orthop 279:21–34.

Black RG (1975). The chronic pain syndrome. Surg Clin N Am 55:999–1011.

Blanchard EB (1992). Psychological treatment of benign headache disorders. J Consult Clin Psychol 60:537–551

Blasberg B, Chalmers A (1989). Temporomandibular pain and dysfunction syndrome associated with generalized musculo-skeletal pain: a retrospective study. J Rheumatol Suppl 16:87–90.

Blau JN (1985). Pathogenesis of migraine: initiation. J R Coll Physicians Lond 19:166–168.

Blau JN (1987). Migraine: Clinical, Therapeutic, Conceptual and Research Aspects. London: Chapman and Hall.

Blau JN (1992). Migraine: theories of pathogenesis. Lancet 1:1202–1207.

Blau JM, Dexter SL (1981). The site of pain origin during migraine attacks. Cephalalgia 1:143–147.

Blau JN, Pike DA (1970). Effect of diabetes on migraine. Lancet 2:241–243.

Blumer D, Heilbronn M (1982). Chronic pain as a variant of depressive disease: the pain-prone disorder. J Nerv Ment Dis 170:381–406.

Bohart WH (1929). Anatomic variations and anomalies of the spine: relation to prognosis and length of disabilitity. Illinois Med J 55:356–.

Brandt J, Celentano D, Linet M, et al. (1990). Personality and emotional disorder in a community sample of migraine headache sufferers. Am J Psychiatry 147:303–308.

Bruske-Hohlfeld I, Merritt JL, Onofrio BM, et al. (1990). Incidence of lumbar disc surgery: a population-based study in Olmsted County, Minnesota, 1950–1979. Spine 15:31–35.

Burton KA, Tillotson KM, Main CJ, et al. (1995). Psychosocial predictors of outcome in acute and subchronic low back trouble. Spine 20:722–728.

Cady RK, Gutterman D, Saiers JA, et al. (1997). Responsiveness of non-IHS migraine and tension-type headaches to sumatriptan. Caphalalgia 17:588–590.

Cassidy JD, Carroll LJ, Cote P, et al. (2000). Effect of eliminating compensation for pain and suffering on the outcome of insurance claims for whiplash injury. N Engl J Med 342:1179–1186.

Celentano DD, Linet MS, Stewart WF (1990). Gender differences in the experience of headache. Soc Sci Med 30:1289–1295.

Chaffin DB, Parks KS (1973). A longitudinal study of low-back pain as associated with occupational weight lifting factors. Am Ind Hyg Assoc J 34:513–525.

Chapman SL (1986). A review and clinical perspective on the use of EMG and thermal biofeedback for chronic headaches. Pain 27:1–43.

Clauw DJ, Chrousos GP (1997). Chronic pain and fatigue syndromes: overlapping clinical and neuroendocrine features and potential pathogenic mechanisms. Neuroimmunomodulation 4:134–153.

Cobb CR, De Vries HA, Urban RT, et al. (1975). Electrical activity in muscle pain. Am J Phys Med 54:80–87.

Colledge A (1993). A model for the prevention of iatrogenic disease associated with work-related low back pain. J Occup Rehab 3:223–232.

Collins JG (1988). National Center for Health Statistics, Prevalence of Selected Chronic Conditions, United States, 1983–85. Advance Data from Vital and Health Statistics. No.155. DHHS Publ. No. (PHS) 88-1250. Hyattsville, Md: Public Health Service.

Coste J, Paolaggi JB, Spira A (1992). Classification of nonspecific low back pain. 1. Psychological involvement in low back pain. Spine 17:1028–1037.

Crisp AH, Kalucy RS, McGuinnies B, et al. (1977). Some clinical, social and psychological characteristics of migraine subjects in the general population. Postgrad Med Bull 53:691–697.

Cushway BC, Maier RJ (1929). Routine examination of the spine for industrial employees. JAMA 93:801–.

Daltroy LH, Iversen MD, Larson MG, et al. (1997). A controlled trial of an educational program to prevent lower back injury. N Engl J Med 337:322–328.

De Wit JC (1950). Allergy to oestrone in cases of migraine. Acta Endocrinol 5:173–.

Den Boer MO, Villalon CM, Heiligers JP, et al. (1991). Role of 5HT1-like receptors in the reduction of porcine cranial arteriovenous anastomotic shunting by sumatriptan. Br J Pharmacol 102:323–330.

Deyo RA (2000). Pain and public policy [editorial]. N Engl J Med 342:1211–1213.

Diamond S (1964). Depressive headaches. Headache 4:255–259.

Diamond S, Freitag FG (1988). Mixed headache syndrome: a review. Clin J Pain 4:67–74.

Diclofenac-K/Sumatriptan Migraine Study Group: Acute treatment of migraine attacks: efficacy and safety of a nonsteroidal anti-inflammatory drug, diclofenac-potassium, in comparison to oral sumatriptan and placebo. Cephalagia 19:232–240.

Diveley RL, Oglevie RR (1956). Pre-employment examination of the low back. JAMA 160:856–.

Doenicke A, Brand J, Perrin VL (1988). Possible benefit of GR43175, a novel 5HT1-like receptor agonist, for the acute treatment of severe migraine. Lancet 1:1309–1311.

Dolan EA, Keefe FJ (1988). Muscle activity in myofascial pain-dysfunction syndrome patients: a structured clinical evaluation. J Craniomandib Disord Facial Oral Pain 2:101–105.

Dorpat DL, Anderson WF, Ripley HS (1968). The relationship of physical illness to suicide. In: Resnick HLP, ed. Suicidal Behaviors: Diagnosis and Management. Boston, Little Brown, pp 209–219.

Durham PL, Russo AF (1999). Regulation of calcitonin gene-related peptide secretion by a serotinergic antimigraine drug. J Neurosci 19:3423–3429.

Dworkin SF (1991). Illness behavior and dysfunction: review of concepts and application to pain. Can J Physiol Pharmacol 69:662–671.

Dworkin SF, Huggins KH, LeResche L, et al. (1990). Epidemiology of signs and symptoms in temporomandibular disorders: clinical signs in cases and controls. J Am Dent Assoc 120:273–281.

Edvinsson L, ed. (1999). Migraine and Headache Pathophysiology. London: Martin Dunitz, pp 175.

Ekbom K, Ahlborg B, Schele R (1978). Prevalence of migraine and cluster headache in Swedish men of 18. Headache 18:9–19.

Ellenberger C (1994). MR imaging of the low back syndrome. Neurology 44:594–600.

Ellis A, Grieger R (1977). Handbook of Rational–Emotive Therapy, Vol 1. New York: Springer Publishing Company.

Evers S, Gralow I, Bauer B, et al. (1999). Sumatriptan and ergotamine overuse and drug-induced headache: a clinicoepidemiological study. Clin Neuropharmacol 22:201–206.

Feniuk W, Humphrey PPA, Perren MJ (1987). Selective vasoconstrictor action of GR43175 on arteriovenous anastamoses (AVAs) in the anaesthetized cat. Br J Pharmacol 92:756P.

Ferrari MD (1998). Migraine. Lancet 351:1043–1051.

Fisher CM (1971). Cerebral ischemia—less familiar types. Clin Neurosurg 18:267–335.

Fordyce WE, Roberts AH, Sternbach RA (1985). The behavioral management of chronic pain: a response to critics. Pain 22:113–125.

Forrest AJ, Wolkind SN (1974). Masked depression in men with lower back pain. Rheumatol Rehabil 13:148–153.

Forssell MZ (1981). The back school. Spine 6:104–106.

Fozard JR (1995). The 5-hydroxyamine–nitric oxide connection: the key link in the initiation of migraine? Arch Int Pharmacodyn Ther 329:111–119.

Frymoyer JW (1992). Predicting disability from low back pain. Clin Orthop 279:101–109.

Frymoyer JW, Rosen JC, Clements J, et al. (1985). Psychological factors in low-back-pain disability. Clin Orthop 195:178–184.

Fullenlove TM, Williams AJ (1957). Comparative roentgen findings in symptomatic and asymptomatic backs. Radiology 68:572–.

Fullerton T, Komorowski-Swiatek D, Forrest A, et al. (1999). The pharmacodynamics of sumatriptan in nitroglycerin-induced headache. J Clin Pharmacol 39:17–29.

Ghabrial VA, Tarrant MJ (1989). Adolescent lumbar disc prolapse. Acta Orthop Scand 60:174–176.

Goadsby PJ, Edvinsson L (1993). The trigeminovascular system and migraine: studies characterizing cerebrovascular and neuropeptide changes seen in humans and cats. Ann Neurol 33:48–56.

Goadsby PJ, Edvinsson L, Ekman R (1990). Vasoactive peptide release in the extracerebral circulation of human during migraine headache. Ann Neurol 28:183–197.

Goadsby PJ, Hoskin KL (1998). Serotonin inhibits trigeminal nucleus activity evoked by craniovascular stimulation through a $5HT_{1B/1D}$ receptor: a central action in migraine? Ann Neurol 43:711–718.

Green JE (1977). A survey of migraine in England, 1975–76. Headache 17:67–68.

Guidetti V, Galli F, Fabrizi P, et al. (1998). Headache and psychiatric comorbidity: clinical aspects and outcome in an 8-year follow-up study. Cephalalgia 18:455–462.

Hart LG, Deyo RA, Cherkin DC (1995). Physician office visits for low back pain. Spine 20:11–19.

Haynes RB, Sackett DL, Taylor DW, et al. (1978). Increased absenteeism from work after detection and labeling of hypertensive patients. N Engl J Med 299:741–744.

Henriksson KG, Bengtsson A (1991). Fibromyalgia—a clinical entity? Can J Physiol Pharmacol 69:672–677.

Heyck H (1969). Pathogenesis of migraine. Res Clin Stud Headache 2:1–28.

Holroyd KA, Andrasik F (1978). Coping and the self-control of chronic tension headaches. J Consult Clin Psychol 5:1036–1045.

Holroyd KA, Andrasik F, Westbrook T (1977). Cognitive control of tension headache. Cognit Ther Res 1:121–133.

Holroyd KA, Nash JM, Pingel JD, et al. (1991). A comparison of pharmacological (amitryptilline HCl) and nonpharmacological (cognitive-behavioral) therapies for chronic tension headaches. J Consult Clin Psychol 59:387–393.

Holt EP Jr (1968). The question of lumbar discography. J Bone Joint Surg Am 50:720–726.

Hooker WD, Raskin NH (1986). Neuropsychologic alterations in classic and common migraine. Arch Neurol 43:709–712.

Howe JF, Loeser JD, Calvin WH (1977). Mechanosensitivity of dorsal root ganglia and chronically injured axons: a physiological basis for the radicular pain of nerve root compression. Pain 3:25–41.

Hu XH, Markson LE, Lipton RB, et al. (1999). Burden of migraine in the United States: disability and economic costs. Arch Intern Med 26:813–818.

International Association for the Study of Pain (1994). Classification of Chronic Pain. Second edition. Eds. Merskey H, Bogduk N. IASP Press, Seattle.

International Headache Society (1988). Headache Classification Committee. Classification and diagnostic criteria for headache disorders, cranial neuralgias and facial pain. Cephalalgia 8(suppl 7):1–96.

Jacobsen S, Danneskiold-Samsoe B (1989). Inter-relations between clinical parameters and muscle function in patients with primary fibromyalgia. Clin Exp Rheumatol 7:493–498.

Jensen MC, Brant-Zawadzki MN, Obuchowski N, et al. (1994). Magnetic resonance imaging of the lumbar spine in people without back pain. N Engl J Med 331:69–73.

Jinkins JR, Whittemore AR, Bradley WG (1989). The anatomic basis of vertebrogenic pain and the autonomic syndrome associated with lumbar disc extrusion. Am J Roentgenol 152:1277–1289.

Joffe RT, Sokolov ST (1997). Co-administration of fluoxetine and sumatriptan: the Canadian experience. Acta Psychiatr Scand 95:551–552.

Johnson KW, Phebus LA, Cohen ML (1998). Serotonin in migraine: theories, animal models and emerging therapies. Prog Drug Res 51:219–244.

Keefe FL, Gill KM (1986). Behavioral concepts in the analysis of chronic pain syndromes. J Consult Clin Psychol 54:776–783.

Kelsey JL, White AA (1980). Epidemiology and impact of low back pain. Spine 5:133–142.

Kolar E, Hartz A, Roumm A, et al. (1989). Factors associated with severity of symptoms in patients with chronic unexplained muscular aching. Ann Rheum Dis 48:317–321.

Kramlinger KG, Swanson DW, Maruta T (1983). Are patients with chronic pain depressed? Am J Psychiatry 140:747–749.

Kropp P, Gerber WD, Keinath-Specht A, et al. (1997). Behavioral treatment in migraine. Cognitive-behavioral therapy and blood-volume-pulse biofeedback: a cross-over study with a two-year follow-up. Funct Neurol 12:17–24.

Lahad A, Malter AD, Berg AO, et al. (1994). The effectiveness of four interventions for the prevention of low back pain. JAMA 272:1286–1291.

Lance JW, Goadsby PJ. Mechanism and Management of Headache. 1998, Sixth edition. Butterworth Heinemann, Oxford, Boston.

LaRocca H, MacNab I (1970). Value of pre-employment radiographic assessment of the lumbar spine. IMS Ind Med Surg 39:253–258.

Leao AAP (1944). Spreading depression of activity in the cerebral cortex. J Neurophysiol 7:359–390.

Leao AAP, Morrison RS (1945). Propagation of spreading cortical depression. J Neurophysiol 8:33–45.

Lesse S (1968). The multivariant masks of depression. Am J Psychiatry 124(suppl):35–40.

Loeser JD, Henderlite SE, Conrad DA (1995). Incentive effects of workers' compensation benefits: a literature synthesis. Med Care Res Rev 52:34–59.

Lofland JH, Johnson NE, Batenhorst AS, et al. (1999). Changes in resource use and outcomes for patients with migraine treated with sumatriptan: a managed care perspective. Arch Intern Med 159:857–863.

Lund JP, Donga R, Widmer CG, et al. (1991). The pain-adaptation model: a discussion of the relationship between chronic musculoskeletal pain and motor activity. Can J Physiol Pharmacol 69:683–694.

MacGregor EA, Chia HMY, Vohrah C, et al. (1990). Migraine and menstruation: a pilot study. Cephalalgia 10:305–310.

Magora A, Schwartz A (1976). Relation between the low back syndrome and x-ray findings. 1. Degenerative osteoarthritis. Scand J Rehab Med 8:115–123.

Majewski RF, Gale EN (1984). Electromyographic activity of anterior temporal area pain patients and non-pain patients. J Dent Res 63:1228–1231.

Malmo RB, Shagass C (1949). Physiological study of symptom mechanisms in psychiatric patients under stress. Psychosom Med 11:25–29.

Manzoni GC, Sandrini G, Zanferrari C, et al. (1991). Clinical features of daily chronic headache and its different subtypes. Cephalalgia 11(suppl 11):292–293.

Martin PR, Mathews AM (1978). Tension headaches: psychophysiological investigation and treatment. J Psychosom Res 22:389–399.

Martins I, Blau JN (1989). Headaches in insulin dependent diabetic patients. Headache 29:660–663.

Mathew NT (1997a). Transformed migraine, analgesic rebound, and other chronic daily headaches. Neurol Clin 15:167–186.

Mathew NT (1997b). Serotonin 1_D (5-HT_{1D}) agonists and other agents in acute migraine. Neurol Clin 15:61–83.

Mathew NT, Stubits E, Nigam M (1982). Transformation of episodic migraine into daily headaches: analysis of factors. Headache 22:66–68.

Mattmiller AW (1980). The California Back School. Physiotherapy 66:118–121.

Melzack R, Wall PD (1965). Pain and mechanisms: a new theory. Science 150:971–979.

Melzack R, Wall PD (1988). The Challenge of Pain, 2nd ed. New York: Penguin Books.

Merikangas KR (1995). Association between psychopathology and headache syndromes. Curr Opin Neurol 8:248–251.

Merikangas KR, Fenton BT, Cheng SH, et al. (1997). Association between migraine and stroke in a large-scale epidemiological study of the United States. Arch Neurol 54:362–368.

Merikangas KR, Stevens DE (1997). Comorbidity of migraine and psychiatric disorders. Neurol Clin 15:115–123.

Merskey H (1982). Management of chronic pain. Can Med Assoc J 127:677–678.

Michler L, Bakke M, Moller E (1987). Graphic assessment of natural mandibular movement. J Craniomandibular Disord Facial Oral Pain 2:97–114.

Miller JA, Schmatz C, Schultz AB (1988). Lumbar disc degeneration: correlation with age, sex, and spine level in 600 autopsy specimens. Spine 13:173–178.

Mills KR, Edwards RH (1983). Investigative strategies for muscle pain. J Neurol Sci 58:73–88.

Mitsikostas DD, Thomas AM (1999). Comorbidity of headache and depressive disorders. Cephalalgia 19:211–217.

Mixter WJ, Barr JS (1934). Rupture of intervertebral disc with involvement of the spinal canal. N Engl J Med 211:210–215.

Modic MT, Ross JS (1991). Magnetic resonance imaging in the evaluation of low back pain. Orthop Clin North Am 22:283–301.

Moldofsky H (1993). Fibromyalgia, sleep disorder and chronic fatigue syndrome. In: Chronic Fatigue Syndrome. Chichester: Wiley (Ciba Foundation Symposium 173), pp 262–279.

Moldofsky H, Scarisbrick P, England R, et al. (1975). Musculoskeletal symptoms and non-REM sleep disturbance in patients with "fibrositis syndrome" and healthy subjects. Psychosom Med 37:341–351.

Mongini F, Defilippi N, Negro C (1997). Chronic daily headache: a clinical and psychological profile before and after treatment. Headache 37:83–87.

Moskowitz MA (1993). Neurogenic inflammation in the pathophysiology and treatment of migraine. Neurology 43:S16–20.

Moskowitz MA, Saito K, Moskowitz MA (1987). Neurogenically mediated leakage of plasma protein occurs from blood vessels in dura mater but not brain. J Neurosci 7:4129–4136.

Nachemson AL (1992). Newest knowledge of lower back pain: a critical look. Clin Orthoped Relat Res 278:8–20.

National Center for Health Statistics (1973). Limitation of Activity Due to Chronic Conditions. United States, Series 10: number 80.

National Headache Foundation (1997). Standards of care for treating headache in primary care practice. Cleveland Clin J Med 64:373–383.

NIH Technology Assessment Panel on Integration of Behavioral and Relaxation Approaches into the Treatment of Chronic Pain and Insomnia (1996). JAMA 276:313–318.

Nouwen A, Bush C (1984). The relationship between paraspinal EMG and chronic lower back pain. Pain 20:109–123.

Olesen J (1985). Migraine and regional cerebral blood flow. Trends Neurosci 8:318–321.

Olesen J, Edvinsson L (1991). Migraine: a research field matured for the basic neurosciences. Trends Neurosci 14:3–5.

Olesen J, Friberg L, Olsen TS, et al. (1990). Timing and topography of cerebral blood flow, aura, and headache during migraine attacks. Ann Neurol 28:791–798.

Olesen J, Larsen B, Lauritzen M (1981). Focal hyperemia followed by spreading oligemia and impaired activation of rCBF in classical migraine. Ann Neurol 9:344–352.

Olsen TS (1993). Spreading oligemia in the migraine aura—most likely an artifact due to scattered radiation. Cephalalgia 13:86–88.

Parker MW (1990). A dynamic model of etiology in temperomandibular disorders. J Am Dent Assoc 120:283–290.

Peroutka SJ, McCarthy BG (1989). Sumatriptan (GR43175) interacts selectively with 5-HT_{1B} and 5-HT_{1D} binding sites. Eur J Pharmacol 163:133–136.

Perrin VL, Farkkila M, Goasguen J, et al. (1989). Overview of clinical studies with intravenous and oral GR43175 in acute migraine. Cephalalgia 9 (suppl 9):63–72.

Polatin PB, Kinney RK, Gatchel RJ, et al. (1993). Psychiatric illness and chronic back pain. The mind and the spine: which goes first? Spine 18:66–71.

Pozniak-Patewicz E (1976). "Cephalgic" spasm of the head and neck muscles. Headache 15:261–266.

Read SJ, Parsons AA (1999). Cortical spreading depression and migraine. In: Edvinsson L, ed. Migraine and Headache Pathophysiology. London: Martin Dunitz, p 175.

Roland M, Van Tulder M (1998). Should radiologists change the way they report plain radiography of the spine? Lancet 352:229–230.

Rowe ML (1971). Low back pain disability in industry: updated position. J Occup Med 13:476–478.

Ryan R, Elkind A, Baker CC, et al. (1997). Sumatriptan nasal spray for the acute treatment of migraine: results of two clinical studies. Neurology 49:1225–1230.

Rydevik B, Brown MD, Lundborg G (1984). Pathoanatomy and pathophysiology of nerve root compression. Spine 9:7–15.

Saper JR (1986). Changing perspectives on chronic headache. Clin J Pain 2:19–28.

Saskin P, Moldofsky H, Lue FA (1986). Sleep and posttraumatic rheumatic pain modulation disorder (fibrositis syndrome). Psychosom Med 48:319–323.

Saxena PR, Ferrari MD (1989). 5-HT1-like receptor agonists and the physiology of migraine. Trends Pharmacol Sci 10:200–204.

Shulman BH (1989). Psychological factors affecting migraine. Clin J Pain 5:23–28.

Silberstein SD (1998). Comprehensive management of headache and depression. Cephalalgia 18 (suppl 21):50–55.

Snook SH, Webster BS (1987) The cost of disability. Clin Orthoped 221:77–81.

Somerville BW (1972). A study of migraine in pregnancy. Neurology 22:824–828.

Spengler DM, Bigos SJ, Martin NA, et al. (1986). Back injuries in industry: a retrospective study. 1. Overview and cost analysis. Spine 11:241–245.

Sternbach RA (1974). Pain and depression. In: Kiev A, ed. Somatic Manifestations of Depressive Disorders. Amsterdam: Excerpta Medica, pp 107–119.

Stewart WF, Lipton RB, Liberman J (1996). Variation in migraine prevalence by race. Neurology 47:52–59.

Sugaya E, Takato M, Noda Y (1975). Neuronal and glial activity during spreading depression in cerebral cortex of cat. J Neurophysiol 38:822–841.

Sutton EP, Belar CD (1982). Tension headache patients versus controls: a study of EMG parameters. Headache 22:133–136.

Svensson H-O, Andersson GB (1983). Low back pain in 40- to 47-year old men: work history and work environmental factors. Spine 8:272–276.

Tan SY, Leucht CA (1997). Cognitive-behavioral therapy for clinical pain control: a 15-year update and its relationship to hypnosis. Int J Clin Exp Hypn 45:396–416.

Taylor VM, Deyo RA, Cherkin DC, et al. (1994). Low-back pain hospitalization: recent United States trends and regional variations. Spine 19:1207–1213.

Tertti MO, Salminen JJ, Paajanen HE, et al. (1991). Low-back pain and disc degeneration in children: a case-control MR imaging study. Radiology 180:503–507.

Tfelt-Hansen P (1997). Prophylactic pharmacotherapy of migraine: some practical guidelines. Neurol Clin 15:153–165.

Tfelt-Hansen P (1998). Efficacy and adverse events of subcutaneous, oral, and intranasal sumatryptan used for migraine treatment: a systematic review based on number needed to treat. Cephalalgia 18:532–538.

Tfelt-Hansen P, Saxena PR, Dahlof C, et al. (2000). Ergotamine in the acute treatment of migraine: a review and European consensus. Brain 123:9–18.

Thomas E, Silman AJ, Croft PR, et al. (1999). Predicting who develops chronic low back pain in primary care: a prospective study. Br Med J 318:1662–1667.

Thompson JK, Haber JD, Figueroa JL, et al. (1980). A replication and generalization of the "psychobiological" model of headache. Headache 20:199–203.

Tolstoy L. The Death of Ivan Ilych and Other Stories. New York: Signet Classic, 1960, pp 123–124.

Travell J, Rinzler S, Herman M (1942). Pain and disability of the shoulder and arm: treatment by intramuscular infiltration procaine hydrochloride. JAMA 120:417–422.

Treif P, Stein N (1985). Pending litigation and rehabilitation outcome of chronic back pain. Arch Phys Med Rehabil 66:95–99.

Turk DC, Flor H (1984). Etiological theories and treatments for chronic back pain II. Psychological models and interventions. Pain 19:209–233.

United Kingdom Department of Health, Clinical Standards Advisory Group (1994). Epidemiology Review: The Epidemiology and Cost of Back Pain. London: HMSO.

Van Korff M, Dworkin SF, LeResche L (1990). Graded chronic pain status: an epidemiological evaluation. Pain 40:279–291.

Van Tulder MW, Assendelft WJJ, Koes BW, et al. (1997). Spinal radiographic findings and non-specific low back pain. Spine 22:427–434.

Von Knorring L (1975). The experience of pain in depressed patients: a clinical and experimental study. Neuropsychobiology 1:155–165.

Walters A (1961). Psychogenic regional pain alias hysterical pain. Brain 84:1–18.

Ward NG, Bloom VL, Friedel RO (1979). The effectiveness of tricyclic antidepressants in the treatment of coexisting pain and depression. Pain 7:331–341.

Ware NC (1993). Society, mind and body in chronic fatigue syndrome: an anthropological view. In: Chronic Fatigue Syndrome. Chichester: Wiley (Ciba Foundation Symposium 173), pp 62–82.

Waters WE (1970). Community studies of the prevalence of headache. Headache 9:178–186.

Waters WE (1973). The epidemiological enigma of migraine. Int J Epidemiol 2:189–194.

Waters WE, O'Connor PJ (1971). Epidemiology of headache and migraine in women. J Neurol Neurosurg Psychiatry 34:148–153.

Weiller C, May A, Limmroth V, et al. (1995). Brain stem activation in spontaneous human migraine attacks. Nat Med 1:658–660.

Weisenberg M (1989). Cognitive aspects of pain. In: Wall PD, Melzack R, eds. Textbook of Pain, 2nd ed. Edinburgh: Churchill Livingstone, pp 231–241.

Weisenberg M (1999). Cognitive aspects of pain. In: Wall PD, Melzack R, eds. Textbook of Pain, 4th ed. Edinburgh: Churchill Livingstone, pp 231–241.

Woods RP, Iacobini M, Mazziotta JC (1994). Brief report: bilateral spreading cerebral hypoperfusion during spontaneous migraine headaches. N Engl J Med 331:1689–1692.

Young WB, Silberstein SD, Dayno JM (1997). Migraine treatment. Semin Neurol 17:325–333.

Yunus MB (1988). Diagnosis, etiology and management of fibromyalgia syndrome: an update. Compr Ther 14:8–20.

Zeitlin C, Oddy M (1984). Cognitive impairment in patients with severe migraine. Br J Clin Psychol 23:27–35.

Zidar J, Backman E, Bengtsson A, et al. (1990). Quantitative EMG and muscle tension in painful muscles in fibromyalgia. Pain 40:249–254.

Ziegler DK, Rhodes RJ, Hassanein RS (1978). Association of psychological measurements of anxiety and depression with headache history in a non-clinic population. Res Clin Stud Headache 6:123–135.

Chapter
11

VISCERAL PAIN SYNDROMES

We are now able to recognize relatively common pain syndromes in which the pain results from physiological activation of a particular organ. It would appear that under certain circumstances the pain threshold is reduced in the tissue or organ involved, so that stimuli within the physiological range may produce pain. Evidence of hyperresponsivity to stimulation—that is, a similar stimulus in any other individual does not cause pain—has been obtained through appropriate functional testing, as discussed in this chapter. Common to these pain syndromes is the pronounced occurrence of some affective disturbance, anxiety states in particular. In essence, the clinical pain syndrome seems to represent the somatic counterpart of the affective condition. As with panic disorder, however, the physical symptoms usually receive the treating physician's attention, and, much to the patient's detriment, the affective state is often considered by both doctor and patient to be secondary to the distressing symptoms and perhaps attendant disability.

The syndromes we consider here involve the gastrointestinal tract (irritable bowel syndrome and esophageal motility disorders), the heart (chest pain with normal coronary arteries, syndrome X), and skeletal muscles (fibromyalgia). The main thesis of this chapter is that these clinical syndromes, rather than being discrete, seemingly unrelated, clinical entities are in fact different visceral and somatic expressions of a similar underlying clinical state. This chapter deals with pain syndromes affecting the heart and gastrointestinal tract. Fibromyalgia is discussed in Chapter 15.

THE GASTROINTESTINAL TRACT

There are two main syndromes of gastrointestinal hyperreactivity in which pain is a prominent clinical symptom, the irritable bowel syndrome (IBS) and esophageal motility disorders. There is some evidence that the bouts of pain coincide with episodes of intestinal contraction (Kumar and Wingate, 1985), although Richter et al. (1987) found that chest pain persisted despite normalization of elevated esophageal pressures in patients with "nutcracker esophagus." Nutcracker esophagus and corkscrew esophagus are alternative names for the condition of diffuse esophageal spasm. The condition is a motor disorder of the esophagus characterized by multiple spontaneous contractions or contractions associated with swollowing which are of simultaneous onset. The nutcracker form is usually characterized by means of manometry as large-amplitude peristaltic waves that presumably reflect heightened excitatory activity. Uncoordinated simultaneous contractions may give the esophageal lumen a corkscrew appearance on barium swollow. All forms may be associated with chest pain. It was also noted by Peters et al. (1988) that half the patients examined with suspected esophageal motility dysfunction had motility changes during ambulatory monitoring, following the onset of chest pain often by as long as several minutes.

Studies have shown that IBS patients have both an enhanced perception of physiological bowel motility (Kellow et al., 1991) and a lower pain threshold to a balloon inflated in the rectum—in other words, that painful discomfort is induced by a smaller volume of distention as compared to controls (Ritchie, 1973; Whitehead et al., 1980). Similar observations have been made in IBS patients in whom a balloon dilated in the esophagus elicited pain at pressures significantly lower than those of control subjects (Constantini et al., 1993). This suggests that although IBS has been considered a colonic disorder, evidence of dysfunction may be found throughout the gastrointestinal tract (Whorwell et al., 1981; Kellow et al., 1990). The same tendency had been found in patients with chest pain whose coronary arteries were normal (see below) but who were not considered to be suffering from IBS (Barish et al., 1986; Richter et al., 1986). Patients in the latter group have also been shown to be sensitive to a balloon dilated in their esophagus and although the esophagus is usually assumed to be the source of the chest pain, esophageal sensitivity may with equal validity be regarded as an associated finding. Similarly, an abnormal perception of visceral pain has been demonstrated in response to a balloon inflated in the stomach in a group of patients suffering from chronic dyspepsia of undetermined cause (Leman at al., 1991).

Despite these reports, other studies using experimental colonic or rectal distension have not consistently shown lower discomfort or pain thresholds in patients with IBS compared with controls (Whitehead et al., 1990; Prior et al., 1993). Using a different technique, however, Munakata et al. (1997) demonstrated that repetitive balloon stimulation of the esophagus and rectum results in increasing pain sensation with consecutive distensions of the same balloon volume, a kind of "windup" effect. Thus, for example, in studies of repetitive rectal stimulation, regardless of baseline sensitivity, all patients with IBS developed rectal hyperalgesia as manifested by two of the three following criteria: lowered thresholds for pain and discomfort, more extensive referral of the pain, and lower abdominal discomfort outlasting the experimental stimulation. Swarbrick et al. (1980) had previously shown that inflating a balloon at different sites along the length of the colon resulted in pain that radiated more extensively in IBS patients compared to controls, including extra-abdominal sites such as the chest (see also Chapter 8).

The pain threshold may be modulated by mechanisms acting at different levels along the pathways from the wall of the gut to the brain. It has been shown experimentally in rats that repetitive noxious stimulation of the viscera evokes increases in the excitability of viscerosomatic neurons in the spinal cord (Roza et al., 1998). Stimuli applied simultaneously at different points in the gut amplify the intensity of the perception, as does sympathetic arousal, whereas somatic stimuli or distraction attenuate it (Accarino et al., 1994; Coffin et al., 1994; Iovino et al., 1995). Silverman et al. (1997) used positron emission tomography to study the central responses of normal subjects and patients with IBS following balloon dilatation in the rectum. In the healthy volunteers noxious rectal stimulation stimulated brain activity in the region of the anterior cingulate gyrus, a region associated with perception of the emotional qualities of the pain experience. In the IBS patients there was enhanced activity instead in the dorsolateral prefrontal cortex, in expectation of the visceral stimulus. This finding has been interpreted to reflect the hypervigilance to visceral events that is characteristic of patients with IBS (Cervero and Laird, 1999).

It may be concluded from these studies that in patients with IBS there is altered responsivity of the gastrointestinal tract that is sometimes associated with the full-blown clinical picture of abdominal pain and altered gastrointestinal function, while others express their clinical condition in more restricted terms, as in patients suffering from chest pain without gastrointestinal disturbance. It seems too that regardless of the clinical syndrome, the hyperresponsivity demonstrated by luminal distension studies may just as readily be a concomitant of the emotional (anxiety) state as a specific cause for the pain in question—a state that has been described as abnormal visceral nociception (Cannon and Benjamin, 1993).

The condition may be viewed primarily as the clinical expression of a lowered pain threshold. Thus, even bowel activity that is considered to fall within the normal physiological range may give rise to pain in this group of patients.

Irritable Bowel Syndrome: The Prototypic Functional Disorder

The clinical picture

Irritable bowel syndrome is the most frequently encountered noninflammatory diagnosis in gastroenterological practice (Drossman et al., 1977; Ferguson et al., 1977; Harvey et al., 1983). In a study of 3111 patients attending 36 general practitioners in the United Kingdom, 255 patients were found to have a gastrointestinal problem, and 30% of these patients were diagnosed as suffering from IBS with an additional 14% categorized as functional bowel disorder, a separate subgroup (Thompson et al., 2000).

Clinically, IBS presents as abdominal pain, altered bowel habit, and dyspepsia, all of which may be present to varying degrees. Most characteristic are recurrent bouts of abdominal pain, sometimes quite severe, associated with the passage of small, hard (goatlike) feces called scybala. These patients often complain of constipation, though bouts of alternating constipation and diarrhea are also common. A typical finding on physical examination is an easily palpable and sensitive sigmoid colon. Symptoms are not restricted to the lower bowel: dyspepsia, nausea, vomiting, and dysphagia have been recorded in 85%–100% of IBS sufferers (Svedlund et al., 1985; Whorwell et al., 1986). As all these symptoms may be experienced in the nonpatient population (see below), an international team of experts put together criteria for the diagnosis of IBS, the so-called Rome criteria (Thompson et al., 1999), which define IBS as

> characterized by *continuous or recurrent abdominal pain or discomfort*, relieved by defecation or associated with altered stool frequency or consistency, together with either or both of the following features:
> *Altered pattern of defecation* for at least 25% of the time, i.e., two or more of the following:
>> Altered stool frequency (>3/day or <3/week)
>> Altered stool form (lumpy, hard, loose, watery)
>> Altered stool passage (straining, fecal urgency, feeling of incomplete emptying)
>> Passage of mucus
> *Abdominal bloating* or a feeling of abdominal distension.

These symptoms, of course, are nonspecific and could indicate more defined pathology, particularly of the colon. In most cases IBS is diagnosed by exclusion, after physical examination and routine tests such as stool examination, barium enema, colonoscopy, and abdominal ultrasound produce normal results. Manning et al. (1978) administered a questionnaire listing 15 symptoms thought to be typical of IBS to 109 unselected patients referred to gastroenterology or surgical clinics with abdominal pain, a change in bowel habit, or both. A review of the case records 17–26 months later established a diagnosis of IBS in 32 patients and of organic disease in 33. Symptoms most suggestive of IBS were distention, relief of pain with bowel movement, and looser and more frequent bowel movement at the time of pain onset. The passage of mucus and a sensation of incomplete evacuation were also common in these patients. Other reviewers have emphasized mucus (hence the synonym mucus colitis), flatus, scybala, and relief of pain after defecation (Thompson et al., 1989; Drossman et al., 1990). Painless diarrhea, as the sole manifestation of IBS, is much less common (Chaudhary and Truelove, 1962; Cann and Read, 1985).

Natural history and differential diagnosis

Knowledge of the natural history of IBS is important, both for accurate clinical diagnosis and for evaluating the likely efficacy of any therapeutic intervention. Owens et al. (1995) studied 112 patients who were followed for 1 to 32 years after a diagnosis of IBS had been made. All had presented with abdominal pain and half of them were also suffering from diarrhea. Organic gastrointestinal disease was subsequently diagnosed in only 10 patients, a median of 15 years after diagnosis of IBS, and the survival of patients with IBS did not differ from the normal life span (27 deaths; median survival of >30 years after initial diagnosis). Significantly, a positive physician–patient interaction defined a priori using objective criteria in the written record was associated with fewer return visits for IBS.

In a study by Holmes and Slater (1982), when 77 IBS patients were reexamined six to eight years after the initial diagnosis, 57% retained their diagnosis, 5% had a different gastrointestinal diagnosis, and 38% were symptom-free. In a study of 50 IBS patients who were followed for 12–31 months without treatment, 52% remained the same or got worse, most of them exhibiting intermittent symptoms and only short symptom-free periods (Waller and Misiewicz, 1969). On reevaluation the rest were improved (36%) or asymptomatic (12%). As these studies show, symptoms in IBS may be very persistent, but also intermittent and phasic.

Because the diagnosis is largely based on exclusion, there is often concern, particularly on the part of the patient, that an important condition (usually cancer) has been missed (Thomson et al., 2000). If the diagnosis of IBS is made according to the Rome criteria rather than simply according to the presence or absence of unexplained abdominal pain, and after the exclusion of other disease, then the diagnosis usually holds up very well. Hamm et al. (1999) studied 1452 patients with IBS. All patients' symptoms meet the Rome criteria for IBS for at least 6 months before study entry. If the previous evaluation had been done more than two years before, patients underwent colonoscopy or radiography at study entry. Lactose malabsorption was diagnosed in 22% of patients, a prevalence comparable with the general U.S. population, and there was a very low incidence of thyroid dysfunction (6%, of whom half were hypo- and half hyperthyroid). Positive ova and parasite infestation were noted in 2% and colonic pathology in 2%.

In a certain percentage of patients, the changes that characterize a particular disease may be missed or simply not yet be evident on investigation. But it should be stressed that the severity of the symptoms and the degree of disability they cause must be considered in relation to the objective findings. Thus, for example, in a person complaining of recurrent bouts of distressing lower abdominal pain and alternating constipation and diarrhea, whose colon looks normal on both barium enema and colonoscopy, the symptoms will not be explained by an occult carcinoma of the colon. In general, diagnosis presents less of a dilemma in a patient with a long history, say between 2 and 20 years, of recurrent abdominal pain and bowel irregularity, and in whom repeated investigations including colonoscopy and barium studies are normal. In patients troubled by varying degrees of abdominal pain, flatulence, borborygmi, and loose stools or diarrhea, disaccharide intolerance (especially lactose intolerance) must be excluded. This too is a condition that may be present for many years before being diagnosed. It is also important to exclude rarer toxic and metabolic causes of recurrent bouts of abdominal pain, such as acute intermittent porphyria and lead poisoning, which may cause suffering over an extended period before they are diagnosed. Porphyria is a particularly important diagnosis to consider in this context, as these patients, like those with IBS, are often labeled neurotic, tense, or unstable.

Surveys of apparently healthy populations for the presence of gastrointestinal symptoms, both in Britain (Thompson and Heaton, 1980) and in the United States (Drossman et al., 1982; Greenbaum et al., 1983), have shown that up to 30% of subjects have symptoms of some kind. The symptoms of constipation, diarrhea, and abdominal discomfort are reported by 9%–22% of the population (Drossman et al., 1993), although only approximately 9% of affected individuals were motivated to consult a doctor (Talley et al., 1995). In the British study (Thompson and Heaton, 1980), 21% had abdominal pain more than six times a year; in 14% it was relieved by defecation. An additional 6% had constipation (straining at stool on more than 25% of occasions), typically with scybalous stools and less frequent bowel movements. In a telephone survey in the United States of the bowel habits in the preceding three months of 10,018 eligible individuals 18 years of age or older, 4.6% suffered from functional constipation (an entity distinguished from IBS in this survey) as opposed to about 3% for IBS sufferers (Stewart et al., 1999). Diarrhea (painless, runny stools on more than 25% of occasions) was reported by only 4% of the population. Other studies have indicated that only a small proportion of symptomatic subjects (around 10%) are referred to outpatient clinics for their symptoms and that most of those referred are women (Fielding, 1977; Hillman et al., 1984).

Stress and intestinal activity

The landmark studies of William Beaumont, a U.S. Army surgeon, published in 1883, represent the first account of the effect of emotion on gastrointestinal (gastric) function. The studies were made on the now famous stomach of Alexis St. Martin, who had been wounded in the abdomen by the accidental discharge of a musket. St. Martin was treated by Beaumont, who subsequently employed him as an experimental subject. The stomach lumen was observed directly through a window in the abdominal wall, which had resulted from the trauma. Beaumont observed: "[with] fear, anger, or whatever depresses or disturbs the nervous system—the villous coat . . . loses its healthy appearance; the secretions become vitiated, greatly diminished, or entirely suppressed." This was followed by Cannon (1902) reporting decreased colonic activity in cats in the presence of a growling dog. Almy et al. (1949) recorded motility and vascular changes in the region of the rectosigmoid junction in humans in response to a variety of physical and emotional stimuli, including stress. Their subjects, medical students, were led to believe for a short period that the examining doctor had fortuitously observed a carcinoma! Studies of colostomy patients revealed decreased colonic activity with feelings of depression and increased motility with anger and resentment (Grace et al., 1951). In functional studies of normal subjects, where the stress paradigm was a dichotomous listening test (see Chapter 19) with random intrusions of noise, a shortening of mouth to cecum transit time was observed (Narducci et al., 1951). These and other observations have clearly demonstrated the influence of emotion on the gastrointestinal tract.

Clinically, the sensitivity of the gastrointestinal tract to emotional stress finds expression in the full gamut of symptomatology normally associated with gastrointestinal disorders, including anorexia, nausea, vomiting, abdominal pain, diarrhea, and constipation. Most studies confirm that abdominal pain and diarrhea, in the absence of physical signs, are common manifestations of stress in the general population. In school-aged children, 10%–12% may suffer recurrent abdominal pain, with no organic cause identifiable in up to 95% of them (Farrell, 1984). This figure may rise to about 25% in children with psychiatric problems (Faull and Nicol, 1986). In a study of adult nonpatients, 70% reported a stress-induced change in bowel habits and more than half reported that stress contributed to abdominal pain (Drossman et al., 1982). Studies of IBS patients similarly demonstrate an impressive correlation between stress and symptoms (Bennett et al., 1998; Dancey et al., 1998; Jarrett et al., 1998; Drossman, 2000).

Psychosocial aspects of irritable bowel syndrome

From population studies we learn that symptomatology typical of IBS occurs quite commonly in the general population. However, only some of those with symptoms actually seek medical help. What determines the *illness behavior* of this group of subjects? It has been suggested that this behavior may be learned through childhood experience (Whitehead et al., 1982). All six of six studies comparing "consulters" with "nonconsulters" for their abdominal symptoms demonstrate that severity of pain is more severe in consultors (Creed, 1997), and Heaton et al. (1991) found a linear relationship between the number of symptoms of IBS and the consulting rate.

It could have at least two possible roots, both of which illustrate that the majority of persistent IBS sufferers have significant emotional problems. In most IBS sufferers, the onset of symptoms is preceded by some additional emotional stress (Almy and Tulin, 1947; Chaudhury and Truelove, 1962; Drossman et al., 1982). Personal, family, financial, or work-related problems were reported in 80% of 130 patients in Chaudhury and Truelove's study. Others have also observed stresses preceding hospitalization (Mendeloff et al., 1970) or illness onset, more often in IBS patients than in other patients or healthy controls.

In attempting to determine why only some patients with IBS symptoms consult their physician, Whitehead et al. (1988) suggested that symptoms of psychological distress are more apparent in those who consult the doctor than in those who do not or in nonsymptomatic controls. These authors concluded, moreover, that the symptoms of psychological distress are unrelated to IBS but do influence which patients consult a doctor. In this sense the patients constitute a self-selected group. Furthermore, there is a widespread clinical perception that patients with IBS are more neurotic, anxious, or depressed than others (Mendeloff et al., 1970; Hislop, 1971; Liss et al., 1973; Palmer et al., 1974). In three separate studies, psychiatric diagnoses were made in 72% (Young et al., 1976), 93% (Liss et al., 1973), and 100% (Latimer et al., 1981) of IBS patients, although in these studies, the very high level of psychiatric diagnosis suggests an ascertainment bias (see Chapter 13). This implies that the very high incidence of psychiatric diagnoses found in these studies resulted from the selection of the most symptomatic and intractable cases of IBS. However, more recent studies similarly confirm a higher incidence of general anxiety, depression, and hypochondriasis in women IBS sufferers according to DSM-IV criteria (Trikas et al., 1999). Most IBS patients have scored in the abnormal range on psychometric tests such as the Minnesota Multiphasic Inventory (MMPI), the Eysenck Personality Inventory (Esler and Goulston, 1973; Palmer et al., 1974; Latimer et al., 1981), and the Hopkins Symptom Checklist (Whitehead et al., 1980). The predominant conditions found were anxiety, depression, and a tendency to present multiple somatic complaints.

Because patients with persistent bowel and abdominal symptoms tend to be referred to a gastroenterologist, other symptoms, which may be less obtrusive, are likely to be overlooked or disregarded. However, some investigators have pointed out that IBS sufferers frequently have symptoms indicative of "heightened emotional arousal" (Almy and Rothstein, 1987). These include anxiety, fatigability, hostile feelings, sadness, and sleep disturbances, as well as palpitations, hand tremor, and fear of serious disease (Svedlund et al., 1985; Whorwell et al., 1986). In addition, anxiety-associated symptoms such as bladder dysfunction (nocturia, frequency and urgency of micturition, and incomplete bladder empty-ing), back pain, an unpleasant taste in the mouth, and dysparunia are also more common (Whorwell et al., 1986). Other authors have also reported headache to be more common in IBS patients (Watson et al., 1978; Crean, 1985). This pat-tern of polysystemic symptomatology, of which the abdominal symptoms are only part, reinforces the impression supported by the literature that the abdomi-nal and bowel symptoms are primarily expressions of unusual emotional tension. It is worth noting that the tendency toward somatization of emotional stress that is seen most frequently in women also finds expression in IBS, where in most of the larger series the majority of patients are women (studies cited in the pre-ceding paragraph; Thompson and Heaton, 1980). In community samples of IBS patients, there is a female-to-male ratio of 2:1 in prevalence of symptoms (Mayer et al., 1999).

Pathophysiology of motility changes in irritable bowel syndrome

Pain, the major symptom in IBS, is induced by intestinal contraction or dis-tention. Altered secretory behavior of the bowel seems to play little part in symp-tom production except in a few patients. In one study, 52% of IBS patients com-plaining of diarrhea as their predominant symptom had a normal stool output of 50–200 g/day (Cann et al., 1983). It seems that many patients may be inappro-priately labeling their urgency and frequency of defecation as "diarrhea." As men-tioned, many of the changes considered typical of IBS have also been observed in normal subjects. The opposite is also true: patients with IBS may show nor-mal motility patterns. As a group, however, IBS patients do exhibit certain char-acteristic functional changes.

Functional changes in irritable bowel syndrome. There have been nu-merous attempts to evaluate the motility and secretory responses of the gas-trointestinal tract in IBS patients. Despite the technical difficulties involved in these studies, a picture of altered intestinal motility (and secretory behavior) has emerged. Although some researchers still remain skeptical, especially with re-gard to the significance of motility changes in the colon (Christensen, 1989), there seems to be general agreement that in most IBS sufferers the bowel be-haves differently than in normals.

Recordings of colonic contraction frequency in normal subjects show two broad ranges, with maximum frequencies of 3–4 contractions/min and 6–9 con-tractions/min (Taylor et al., 1974; Snape et al., 1977; Welgan et al., 1985). The higher frequency range predominates in normal subjects and is present for up to 50% of recording time. In IBS patients the incidence of the slow wave frequency appears to be significantly higher than in controls. Symptoms of IBS are usually episodic, and repeated evaluations of myoelectrical changes with time show a persistence of the slow wave frequency of 2–4 contractions/min during asymptomatic phases (Taylor et al., 1980). These changes are also unrelated to the presence of symptoms or to stool frequency. The predominance of slow wave activity was shown to be as prevalent in a group of psychoneurotic controls as in IBS patients (Latimer et al., 1981), strongly suggesting that this change reflects a particular emotional state.

Random segmental contractions of circular muscle in the colon have the effect of moving luminal contents backward and forward, without progression along the colon. Paradoxically, in constipation this segmental contractile activity of the colon is increased, whereas in diarrhea it is decreased (Connell, 1962). Patients with IBS exhibit similar changes in segmental contractions, depending on whether the predominant symptom is constipation (increased segmental activity) or diarrhea (decreased segmental activity) (Wangel and Deller, 1965).

As with the relay of pain signals at a segmental level of the spinal cord, there is apparently bidirectional communication between the enteric nervous system and the regional ganglia. Centripetal fibers originating in the colon, for example, project to the inferior mesenteric ganglion and there influence synaptic transmission. Studies in the guinea pig have shown that 79% of the neurons tested showed spontaneous activity, presumably coinciding with spontaneous colonic activity. In addition, inhibition of colonic movement with drugs such as papaverine and isoprenaline decreased colonic afferent input to inferior mesenteric ganglia, whereas acetylcholine or pelvic nerve stimulation, which increase colonic activity, increased colonic afferent input to the inferior mesenteric ganglia (Szurszewski and Weems, 1976).

Differences in functional responses of the bowel in IBS patients have been demonstrated in a variety of tests. In normal people, colonic motility increases in response to food, parasympathomimetic drugs, and cholecystokinin (Kock et al., 1968; Harvey and Read, 1973). Patients with IBS have a delayed increase in colonic motility 60–90 minutes after eating a meal (Sullivan et al., 1978; Battle et al., 1980), which may be due to a delay in gastric emptying (Caballero-Plasencia et al., 1999). Small bowel motility may also be altered. Prolonged recording (30 hours) of duodenojejunal motility in 22 IBS patients showed motor abnormalities in 19 following intermittent stress (video games). The changes included total abolition of migrating motor complexes and abnormal irregular contractile activity (Kumar and Windgate, 1985). In 8 of the 22 patients, these irregular contractile episodes coincided with bouts of abdominal pain, their presenting complaint.

Is irritable bowel syndrome a disease? "Until recently, many physicians did not consider IBS to be a disease at all; they viewed it as nothing more than a somatic manifestation of psychological stress . . . The condition is now recognized as a syndrome complex of motor disorders affecting not only the colon but also other areas of the gastrointestinal system" (Chung, 1989). This quotation, taken from a description of IBS in a medical textbook, illustrates the difficulty (and confusion) attending the classification of psychosomatic disorders. The author's meaning, it seems to me, is that since certain specific motility disorders have now been documented in IBS patients (i.e., defined functional responses reflecting specific structure–function changes), the condition need no longer be considered simply as reflecting emotional stress. I believe this statement reiterates a futile though commonly expressed polemic and is not necessarily the view of the writer himself. If we define disease as *Oxford English Dictionary* does—"a condition of the body, or some part or organ of the body, in which its functions are disturbed or deranged"—IBS may certainly be considered a disease insofar as typical cases are characterized by a certain constellation of symptoms and a specific set of abnormal functional responses. The problem here is that the motility and secretory changes which characterize bowel responses in IBS are a matter of degree, not of kind. In other words, all the responses described as typical of IBS also occur but are less pronounced in individuals without IBS. There are no unique functional or morphological changes that characterize the condition. As the preceding quotation implies, however, there is sufficient documentation, both clinical and experimental, of functional change in the motility and secretory behavior of IBS patients for the disorder to qualify as a disease (Talley, 1998).

Management of Patients with Gastrointestinal Symptoms

For some patients, the exclusion of other underlying disease states, especially cancer, is reassuring, allowing patients to adjust to their intermittent gastrointestinal symptoms and tolerate them without undue anxiety or concern. Similarly, the exclusion of a disaccharidase deficiency, such as lactose intolerance, is an important part of the diagnostic workup. For the symptomatic IBS sufferer, bulk purgatives (e.g., psyllium hydrophilic mucilloid), antimotility medications (e.g., mebeverine), or antispasmodic medications (e.g., papaverine) are usually prescribed in various combinations. For the smaller group of persistently symptomatic and suffering patients, however, a more comprehensive evaluation of emotional state is indicated. Psychotherapy is sometimes tried, but there are few reports of well-controlled studies to validate its use in IBS.

Both the efficacy and long-term effectiveness of group cognitive behavioral therapy for patients were evaluated in a group of 25 IBS patients compared to 20 patients who served as waiting list controls (van Dulmen, 1996). Treatment consisted of eight two-hour sessions over a period of 3 months with subsequent follow-up for an average of 2.25 years (range 6 months to 4 years). The abdominal complaints of the treated patients improved significantly more than those of the control group, and on long-term follow-up the treatment group's improvement in symptoms had been maintained. Similarly favorable results have been reported with the use of hypnotherapy in the management of IBS (Whorwell et al., 1987; Houghton et al., 1996; Galovski and Blanchard, 1998). Besides documenting a reduction in pain and suffering, the hypnotherapy was found to improve the patient's quality of life and to reduce absenteeism from work.

A study employing an innovative computerized biofeedback system allowed patients to navigate through a gastrointestinal lumen graphically represented on a computer screen. Increased tension (as reflected in palmar electrodermal changes) was represented graphically as frothy intraluminal secretions with slow forward progress, while increasing relaxation resulted in the clearing of secretions with facilitated passage through the intestinal lumen (Leahy et al., 1998). Of 40 IBS patients refractory to conventional medical treatment, 20 responded well and were able to help diminish the frequency and intensity of their symptoms through biofeedback. The positive outcome of the more rigorous studies quoted in the last two paragraphs provides additional support to a growing literature on the value of cognitive behavioral therapy and biofeedback in the management of psychosomatic conditions. In spite of a favorable outcome for some IBS patients, it should be emphasized too that approximately half of the group in the Leahy et al. (1998) study did not respond to biofeedback. With psychotherapy, too, results have been variable. Talley et al. (1996) found, in a systematic review of the literature, that eight studies reported psychological treatments superior to control treatment, but five failed to detect a significant effect.

THE HEART

A significant minority of patients (20%–25% in most series) who undergo cardiac catheterization in the investigation of unexplained chest pain have normal coronary arteries. Some of these patients may have an equivocal or abnormal electrocardiogram (ECG) on exercise or positive thallium scan, though there is no metabolic or hemodynamic evidence of myocardial ischemia. In patients with chest pain and normal coronary arteries the clinical diagnosis may vary between mitral valve prolapse, microvascular dysfunction (syndrome X), or esophageal motility disorder if the physician is a cardiologist, gastoenterologist, or primary care physician or panic disorder if a psychiatrist.

Based on a series of studies in these patients Cannon (1995) concluded that the chest pain is due to a state of abnormal cardiac pain perception, a condition he called "the sensitive heart." Thus, chest pain was produced in 10 of 11 such patients by catheter movement within the right atrium and by intra-atrial boluses of normal saline, manipulations that were not felt by seven patients with coronary artery disease and nine patients with mitral valve disease (Shapiro et al., 1988). Similar observations were made by Chauhan et al. (1994). Studying 36 patients with chest pain and normal coronary angiograms, Cannon et al. (1990) found that pain could be induced in 86% by right ventricular pacing at a heart rate 5 beats/min faster than their resting heart rate (with the pain worsened by increasing the stimulus intensity). In this same group of patients, pain could be provoked in 56% by injecting contrast medium into the left coronary artery. By contrast, only 2 patients with coronary artery disease out of 42 and none of 10 patients with valvular disease responded with pain to similar maneuvers. Infusion of dipyridamole, which also induces tachycardia, produced pain in 21 of 29 patients with chest pain and normal coronary arteries but in none of 20 healthy controls (Rosen et al., 1994).

It is important to note, too, that patients with this syndrome of "cardiac sensitivity" may show, in fact, a higher than normal tolerance for thermocutaneous pain, suggesting that the visceral sensitivity is not part of a global hypersensitivity to pain (Cannon et al., 1990). A similar dissociation between a normal thermocutaneous tolerance to pain and increased visceral sensitivity has been observed in patients with IBS (Cook et al., 1987; Whitehead et al., 1990). The question why a particular patient will respond with either cardiac or gastrointestinal symptoms has not yet been answered.

Chest Pain in Anxious Patients

The diagnostic dilemma: ischemic versus nonischemic

Chest pain or discomfort is encountered very commonly in general medical practice. The accepted clinical approach is to try to determine, initially according to the medical history, physical examination, and electrocardiograph (ECG), whether the pain is cardiac or noncardiac. In the typical case of cardiac pain, that is, angina pectoris, the history conveys the diagnosis with a considerable degree of certainty; however, there are inevitably patients in whom the precise cause of the pain is uncertain and in whom heart disease cannot confidently be excluded on the basis of clinical evaluation alone. These patients, if subsequently shown to have coronary artery disease, may then be said to be suffering from atypical angina pectoris. Their history may be considered atypical because of the unusual character or location of the pain and because it is not obviously related to common triggers of angina pectoris such as physical exertion, emotional excitement, exposure to cold (air or water), or eating a large meal. Changes in the ECG tracing of the kind shown in Figure 11-1 may add to the uncertainty.

The use of increasingly sophisticated diagnostic tests for ischemic heart disease in cases of uncertainty, including coronary angiography, has served to emphasize the fact that atypical angina pectoris is not a rare event. The diagnostic

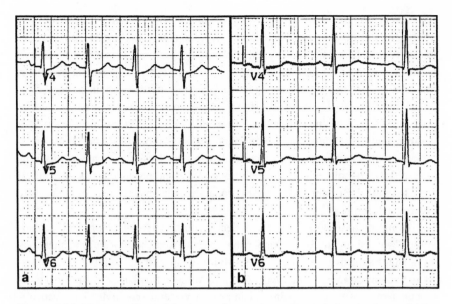

FIGURE 11.1 Electrocardiographic changes in a patient with nonischemic chest pain due to a panic attack. (*a*) During the attack, the pulse rate is 113 beats/min. Note the deep S waves in V4 with ST depression. (*b*) With recovery, the pulse slows to 74 beats/min and there is normalization of the axis and ST changes.

dilemma is compounded by the existence of less common conditions such as Prinzmetal's angina, in which atheromatosis is minimal or absent and the ischemic pain occurs as a result of spasm of the coronary artery. The pointers to Prinzmetal's angina include a history of pain, with ST segment elevation on ECG, that tends to occur at rest, during sleep, after exercise, during emotional excitement, or on arising in the morning (Glazier et al., 1988). Hyperventilation may also predispose to coronary artery spasm.

Coronary angiography is generally considered the most certain method of determining the condition of the coronary arteries in view of the potential implication of significant coronary artery disease, coupled with the unreliability of simpler screening tests. Many physicians prefer to adopt a more aggressive diagnostic approach in patients complaining of chest pain. In the United States estimates of the number of coronary angiograms performed per year vary from half a million (Bass and Wade, 1984; Faxon et al., 1984; Katon et al., 1988; Beitman et al., 1989) to approximately one and a half million (Assey, 1993). As the number of normal angiograms in most series is around 20%–30% (Kemp et al., 1973; Bass and Wade, 1984; Assey, 1993), this means that between 100,000 and 450,000 coronary angiograms showing a normal coronary vasculature are performed each year.

Myocardial Microvascular Disorder

In patients with a history of angina pectoris but normal coronary angiograms some cardiologists think the chest pain results from myocardial arteriolar spasm. This condition has been called syndrome X (Kemp et al., 1973) and should not be confused with the other more recently named syndrome X used to describe patients suffering from insulin resistance, hypertriglyceridemia, low serum high-density lipoprotein levels, hypertension, and an increased risk of coronary artery disease (Reaven, 1988). The characteristic constellation includes symptoms and signs of chest pain with normal coronary arteries but often in addition evidence of myocardial perfusion defects on thallium scintigraphy, which suggests ischemia (Meller et al., 1979; Cannon et al., 1992; Tweddel et al., 1992). Similarly, 50% of patients with chest pain and normal coronary arteries showed abnormalities of myocardial perfusion when studied with positron emission tomography (Geltman et al., 1990). The intramural prearteriolar coronary vessels affected by this disorder are too small to be seen on angiography (Cannon and Epstein, 1988). Electrocardiographic evidence of ischemia may be seen with exercise or cardiac pacing. In normal subjects the myocardial vasculature dilates with increased work demands in order to increase blood flow. It is postulated that these subjects have a limited capacity to respond to work demands with vasodilatation because of an increased tone or resistance of the microvasculature, which results in a state of "vascular insufficiency."

One study suggested that 35% of syndrome X patients may show left ventricular dysfunction on evaluation (Schofield et al., 1986), but subsequent work has challenged these findings and it is now claimed that these patients show neither hemodynamic nor metabolic evidence of ischemia while experiencing pain. Furthermore, the excellent prognosis indicates that no significant myocardial pathology is causing the pain.

Intestinal Motility Disorders

The esophagus can cause chest pain which may be indistinguishable from that due to myocardial ischemia. In general, pain derived from the hollow muscular viscera of the gastrointestinal tract is caused either by spasm (most commonly) or by distension of the smooth muscle wall. Manometric studies of esophageal contractility have shown the distal esophagus in particular to be sensitive to stressful stimuli. Between 18% and 58% of patients with noncardiac chest pain exhibited a variety of esophageal motility disorders, including spasm, peristaltic contractions of very high amplitude (nutcracker esophagus), hypertensive lower esophageal sphincter, and nonspecific motility disorder (Svennson et al., 1978; Patterson, 1982; Richter and Castell, 1984; Katz and Castell, 1985). When patients referred for esophageal manometry were studied by psychiatric evaluation, a psychiatric diagnosis could be made in 84% of those with motility abnormalities (Clouse and Lustman, 1983). In 76% (19 of 25) of these subjects as opposed to 31% (4 of 13) of the patients with the normal manometric patterns, the diagnosis was depression, anxiety disorder (generalized anxiety disorder or panic disorder), or somatization disorder.

Esophageal manometry demonstrated motility disorders in 80% (16 of 20) of mitral valve prolapse (MVP) subjects with chest pain and normal coronary arteries (Koch et al., 1989). An increased frequency of irritable bowel syndrome has also been observed in MVP patients (Sataline, 1985).

These observations have important clinical implications. First, although many chest pain patients with normal coronary arteries have a diagnosable panic disorder, there may be an overlap of clinical features including mitral valve prolapse, syndrome X, and esophageal motility disorders; each of these diagnostic entities may represent a spectrum of visceral responses to a given emotional state. The motility syndromes in these symptomatic patients may reflect a more general disorder of intestinal motility.

Moreover, many patients suffering from coronary angiogram–negative chest pain also have manifestations of increased smooth muscle tone such as systemic hypertension, esophageal contractility problems, and increased bronchospasm in response to methacholine challenge (Cannon et al., 1985; Cannon, 1988). These findings, coupled with an impaired forearm hyperemic response to ischemia in the same type of patients (Sax et al., 1987), suggest the possibility of a generalized increase in smooth muscle tone, which includes a reduction in responsiveness of the myocardial microvasculature at times of increased functional demand. One study has demonstrated a high rate of panic disorder in this group of patients (Roy-Byrne et al., 1989).

Since the radiation of pain in irritable bowel syndrome may extend beyond the abdomen to unusual sites including the chest, in at least some MVP patients complaining of chest pain the source of the pain may be the lower gastrointestinal tract. These and other studies support the possibility that chest pain in patients with normal coronary arteries, with or without MVP, may also originate from the gastrointestinal tract. Furthermore, if the patient also suffers from an esophageal motility disorder of the kind mentioned above, the likelihood of an associated psychiatric diagnosis is extremely high.

Chest pain with normal coronary arteries

The frequent occurrence of chest pain in panic disorder, often with palpitations and mitral valve prolapse on clinical examination and echocardiography, has aroused considerable interest. The picture emerging from numerous studies of this problem may be summarized as follows.

Among patients with chest pain, those with normal coronary arteries are much more likely than those with significant coronary artery stenosis to be suffering from a psychiatric condition of which the most frequently diagnosed are anxiety state and panic disorder (up to 50% in most studies). Most sufferers are women aged between 35 and 50 years. The description of the chest pain is often atypical for angina pectoris, although it may be quite indistinguishable, including referral to the left shoulder or arm with or without a feeling of numbness or tingling.

Patients with recurrent chest pain and normal coronary angiograms have a favorable prognosis. Followed over 10 years, such patients have a 2%–3% chance of a coronary event, as compared to 14% in patients with mild narrowing (<30% stenosis) and 33% in those with moderate narrowing (30%–50% stenosis) (Proudfit et al., 1980; Isner et al., 1981). The Coronary Artery Surgery Study (CASS) Registry shows a seven-year survival rate of 96% in subjects with normal coronary arteriograms (Kemp et al., 1986).

In spite of the reassuring data on prognosis, patients with chest pain and normal coronary arteries often suffer considerable disability. Around 80% of patients have persistent symptoms and more than 50% are limited to the extent of being unable to do physical work (Isner et al., 1981). Up to 40% continue to believe that they suffer from heart disease despite reassurance to the contrary (Lavey and Winkle, 1979; Ockene et al., 1980; Papanicolaou et al., 1986). These patients continue to be major consumers of health care services even after angiograms have proved to be normal (Lavey and Winkle, 1979). It is estimated that each person with noncardiac chest pain spends approximately $3500 a year on symptom management, including an average of one to two prescriptions per month, 2.2 physician or emergency room visits, and one hospitalization per year. This parallels clinical experience with other chronic or recurrent pain syndromes, such as pelvic pain without apparent physical basis and the irritable bowel syndrome, where patients may remain symptomatic for years despite medical and psychiatric care (Waller and Misiewicz, 1969; Henker, 1979).

Patient beliefs in the clinical differentiation of ischemic from nonischemic chest pain

From the standpoint of the medical practitioner, methods are needed to assist in the recognition of chest pain not associated with coronary artery disease. Panic disorder (PD) manifests itself in episodes of acute anxiety without an external precipitating factor, where the patient experiences fear that may be intense and an array of physical symptoms, often including chest pain. Typically, during the attack the patient has a fear of death or of going crazy or losing control.

Fraenkel et al. (1997) suggested that these two cognitive elements of the panic attack—fear of death or of going crazy—may serve as markers for the diagnosis of panic disorder in patients presenting with chest pain and that the presence of one or both of these elements as a predominant presenting symptom, in the absence of objective evidence to the contrary, may be considered to rule out an ischemic event. These authors argued that the main complaint of a patient with coronary artery disease would be a physical complaint such as chest pain or dyspnea and that it is highly improbable that an ischemic event would present primarily as a cognitive disturbance. They studied three groups of patients suffering from confirmed coronary artery disease (CAD+), panic disorder (PD), and chest pain with normal coronary angiograms (CAD−). Information on patients' symptomatology during the acute episode was obtained with a formal panic questionnaire from the Structured Clinical Interview for DSM-IIIR Patients (SCID). The last two items in the questionnaire refer to the patient's thoughts during the chest pain episode: "During the attack, were you afraid you might die?" and the second: "During the attack, were you afraid you are going crazy or might lose control?" Following the symptom inventory, the patient was requested to state which of the symptoms listed in the formal questionnaire were the most disturbing during the acute episode. The answer to this question was then recorded in one of two groups:

> *Physical predominance*, meaning that the patient viewed the episode mainly as an insult to the body and physiological balance and did not experience severe anxiety at the time.

> *Cognitive predominance*, where the patient experienced the episode principally as a frightening cognition of a sense of imminent death, loss of control, or imminent catastrophe.

An inconclusive answer, meaning that the patient could not decide whether cognitive or physical symptoms predominated, was considered for the purpose of analysis to be physical predominance.

The outcome of the survey is illustrated in Figure 11-2. In the CAD+ group, 18% of patients experienced frightening thoughts, but only in 4% (2/66) were they the predominant experience during the chest pain. In contrast, all of the panic disorder patients experienced frightening thoughts and 83% reported that they were the predominant experience. Of the patients in the CAD− group, 48% (23/48) were compatible with panic disorder and 52% (25/48) were not. Half the patients in the CAD− group (24/48) had cognitive symptoms during the chest pain episode and 21% (10/48) described them as predominant. With panic disorder patients, predominance of cognitive symptoms was found to have a diagnostic sensitivity of 83% and a specificity of 97%. Equally important, however, is the *absence of specific cognitions in the CAD+ patients*. "Absence of cognitions" in a subject with chest pain was found to have a diagnostic sensitivity of 82% and a specificity of 100% for CAD. In CAD+ patients, "predominance of physical symptoms" had a diagnostic sensitivity of 97% and a specificity of 83%.

This study indicates that patients' thoughts during episodes of chest pain, as evaluated by three questions, helps to differentiate between the symptoms of true coronary artery disease and those of panic disorder. This claim appears to be particularly valid in the early, uncomplicated stage of the natural history of symptomatic ischemic heart disease. It is precisely this group of patients, with chest

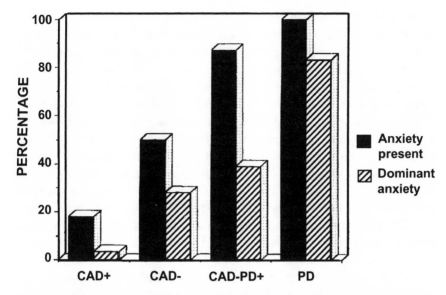

FIGURE 11.2 The relationship of chest pain with anxiety in different clinical groups. CAD+, coronary artery disease positive; CAD−, chest pain with coronary arteries; CAD–PD+, chest pain with normal coronary arteries, panic disorder compatible; PD, panic disorder. (From Fraenkel et al., 1997, with permission of *Depression and Anxiety*.)

pain of recent onset, who often present the greatest dilemma to the examining physician and who may consequently be subjected to cardiac catheterization. For a patient without risk factors such as diabetes mellitus, hypertension, hypercholesterolemia, or cigarette smoking, who presents with chest pain and thoughts of imminent catastrophe, in the absence of objective evidence of ischemia, the next step would be an examination to validate probable panic disorder, before a more detailed cardiac evaluation is done.

The diagnostic challenge: understanding chest pain with intense fear

One of the most persistent misconceptions in clinical practice has to do with anxiety and fear as manifestations of angina pectoris. The notion that marked apprehension is an expected association of angina pectoris has been embedded in the medical literature since the eighteenth-century description of Heberden, who spoke of the "sense of strangling and anxiety with which it is attended" (Heberden, 1771). Similarly, in a landmark review of angina pectoris, Keefer and Resnik (1928) quoted Allbutt, who describes the "anguish" of a typical attack as being "even in slight or incipient cases, an organic dread or sense of ill-omen, as contrasted with rational apprehension, . . . a strange indescribable fear." Physicians understood then the serious implication of the symptom and the overwhelming sense of vulnerability, helplessness, and apprehension felt by a sufferer at a time in which there was no treatment. Keefer and Resnik ominously commented that "the likelihood of sudden death is the one distinguishing feature that differentiates true angina from all forms of false angina." Today, however, intense fear is not an accompaniment of angina pectoris in most patients and certainly not in the earliest attacks (Fraenkel et al., 1997). In fact, the prominent presence of fear during the first attacks of chest pain is the hallmark of a panic attack and, in the absence of objective evidence of myocardial ischemia, it is a strong predictor of normal coronary arteries (Cormier et al., 1988). This means not merely that the patient with panic disorder feel fear but that fear, rather than the actual physical discomfort of the chest pain, is the dominating preoccupation. But in a panic attack, despite the intense fear experience—and here's the catch—the patient is prone to speak only of the chest pain in the belief that the sinister, life-threatening implication of this symptom is commensurate with the intensity of the fear response. It's the chest pain which is going to lead to disability or death, and so it is this that has to be fixed.

In angina pectoris the patient is typically preoccupied with the physical pain, and fear, if present, does not overshadow the patient's preoccupation with the pain. Anxiety may develop in time in patients with ischemic heart disease, particularly in those who undergo a more active course with the need for repeated catheterizations or operation.

Management of patients with chest pain and normal coronary arteries

Since a substantial proportion of patients with chest pain and normal coronary arteries may be diagnosed as suffering from panic disorder, it seems perfectly appropriate *in the absence of objective evidence of ischemia or of recognized risk factors for coronary artery disease*, and in view of the considerable morbidity of these patients, to treat them for panic disorder. Cannon et al. (1994) treated a group of such patients with imipramine, a tricyclic antidepressant used successfully for the treatment of panic disorder, and reported more than a 50% reduction in symptom frequency. Regular follow-up with special attention to the patient's response to the antipanic medication, or cognitive behavioral intervention, will help confirm the diagnosis. The treatment of panic disorder is discussed in detail in the next chapter.

REFERENCES

Accarino AM, Azpiroz F, Malagelada J-R (1994). Cognitive processes have major influence on abdominal symptoms. Gastroenterology 106(suppl): A457. Abstract.

Almy TP, Kern F, Tulin M (1949). Alteration in colonic function in man under stress. II. Experimental production of sigmoid spasm in healthy persons. Gastroenterology 12:425–436.

Almy TP, Rothstein RI (1987). Irritable bowel syndrome: classification and pathogenesis. Ann Rev Med 38:257–265.

Almy TP, Tulin M (1947). Alterations in colonic function in man under stress. I. Experimental production of changes simulating the "irritable colon." Gastroenterology 8:314–318.

Assey ME (1993). The puzzle of normal coronary arteries in the patient with chest pain: what to do? Clin Cardiol 16:170–180.

Barish CF, Castell DO, Richter JE. (1986). Graded esophageal balloon distension: a new provocative test for noncardiac chest pain. Dig Dis Sci 31:1292–1298.

Bass C, Wade C (1984). Chest pain with normal coronary arteries; a comparative study of psychiatric and social morbidity. Psychosom Med 14:51–61.

Battle WM, Cohen S, Snape WJ (1980). Inhibition of postprandial colonic motility after ingestion of an amino acid mixture. Dig Dis Sci 25:647–652.

Beaumont W (1833). Experiments and Observations on the Gastric Juice and the Physiology of Digestion. Plattsburgh, NY: FP Allen, p 107.

Beitman BD, Mukerji V, Lamberti JW, et al. (1989). Panic disorder in patients with chest pain and angiographically normal coronary arteries. Am J Cardiol 63:1399–1403.

Bennett EJ, Tennant CC, Piesse C, et al. (1998). Level of chronic life stress predicts clinical outcome in irritable bowel syndrome. Gut 43:256–261.

Caballero-Plasencia AM, Valenzuela-Barranco M, Herrerias-Gutierrez JM, et al. (1999). Altered gastric emptying in patients with irritable bowel syndrome. Eur J Nucl Med 26:404–409.

Cann PA, Read NW (1985). A disease of the whole gut? In: Read NW, Ed. Irritable Bowel Syndrome. Orlando, Fl: Grune and Stratton, pp 53–63.

Cann PA, Read NW, Brown C, et al. (1983). The irritable bowel syndrome: relationship of disorders in the transit of a single solid meal to symptom patterns. Gut 24:405–411.

Cannon RO (1988). Causes of chest pain in patients with normal coronary angiograms: the eye of the beholder. Am J Cardiol 62:306–308.

Cannon RO (1995). The sensitive heart: a syndrome of abnormal cardiac pain perception. JAMA 273:883–887.

Cannon RO, Benjamin SB (1993). Chest pain as a consequence of abnormal visceral nociception. Dig Dis Sci 38:193–196.

Cannon RO, Camici PG, Epstein SE (1992). Pathophysiological dilemma of syndrome X. Circulation 85:883–892.

Cannon RO, Epstein SE (1988). "Microvascular angina" as a cause of chest pain with angiographically normal coronary arteries. Am J Cardiol 61:1338–1343.

Cannon RO, Leon MB, Watson RM, et al. (1985). Chest pain and "normal" coronary arteries: role of small coronary arteries. Am J Cardiol 55:50B–60B.

Cannon RO, Quyyumi AA, Mincemoyer R, et al. (1994). Imipramine in patients with chest pain despite normal coronary angiograms. N Engl J Med 330:1411–1417.

Cannon RO, Quyyumi AA, Schenke WH, et al. (1990). Abnormal cardiac sensitivity in patients with chest pain and normal coronary arteries. J Am Coll Cardiol 16:1359–1366.

Cannon WB (1902). The movements of the intestines studied by means of the roentgen rays. Am J Physiol 6:251–277.

Cervero F, Laird JMA (1999). Visceral pain. Lancet 353:2145–2148.

Chaudhury NA, Truelove SC (1962). The irritable colon syndrome: a study of the clinical features, presdisposing causes and prognosis in 130 cases. Q J Med 31:307–323.

Chauhan A, Mullins PA, Thuraisingham SI, et al. (1994). Abnormal cardiac pain perception in syndrome X. J Am Coll Cardiol 24:329–335.

Christensen J (1989). Colonic motility. In: Handbook of Physiology. Section 6: The Gastrointestinal System. Bethesda, Md: Americal Physiological Society, pp 939–973.

Chung O (1989). Irritable bowel disease. In: Kelley WN, ed. Textbook of Internal Medicine. Philadelphia: JB Lippincot, pp 519–522.

Clouse RE, Lustman RJ (1983). Psychiatric illness and contraction abnormalities of the esophagus. N Engl J Med 309:1337–1342.

Coffin B, Azpiroz F, Malagelada JR (1994). Somatic stimulation reduces perception of gut distension in humans. Gastroenterology 107:1636–1642.

Connell AM (1962). The motility of the pelvic colon. II. Paradoxical motility in diarrhea and constipation. Gut 3:342–348.

Constantini M, Sturniolo GC, Zaninotto G, et al. (1993). Altered esophageal pain threshold in irritable bowel syndrome. Dig Dis Sci 38:206–212.

Cook IJ, van Eeden A, Collins SM (1987). Patients with irritible bowel syndrome have a greater pain tolerance than normal subjects. Gastroenterology 93:727–733.

Cormier LE, Katon W, Russo J, et al. (1988). Chest pain with negative cardiac diagnostic studies: relationship to psychiatric illness. J Nerv Ment Dis 176:351–358.

Crean GP (1985). Towards a Positive Diagnosis of Irritable Bowel Syndrome. In: Read NW, ed. Irritable Bowel Syndrome. Orlando, Fl: Grune and Stratton, pp 29–42.

Creed FH (1997). Commentary on: Who needs a doctor for IBS? Gut 41:415–416.

Dancey CP, Taghavi M, Fox RJ (1998). The relationship between daily stress and symptoms of irritable bowel: a time-series approach. J Psychosom Res 44:537–545.

Drossman DA (2000). Do psychosocial factors define symptom severity and patient status in irritable bowel syndrome? Am J Med 107(5A):41S–50S.

Drossman DA, Funch-Jensen P, Janssens J, et al. (1990). Identification of subgroups of functional bowel disorders. Gastroenterol Int 3:159–172.

Drossman DA, Li Z, Andruzzi E, et al. (1993). U.S. householder survey of functional GI disorders: prevalence, sociodemography and health impact. Dig Dis Sci 38:1569–1580.

Drossman DA, Powell DW, Sessions JT (1977). The irritable bowel syndrome. Gastroenterology 73:811–822.

Drossman DA, Sandler RS, McKee DC, et al. (1982). Bowel patterns among subjects not seeking health care: use of a questionnaire to identify a population with bowel dysfunction. Gastroenterology 83:529–534.

Esler MD, Goulston KJ (1973). Levels of anxiety and colonic disorders. N Engl J Med 288:16–20.

Farrell MK (1984). Abdominal pain. Pediatrics 74:955–957.

Faull C, Nicol AR (1986). Abdominal pain in six-year olds: an epidemiological study in a new town. J Child Psychol Psychiatry 27:251–260.

Faxon DP, McCabe CH, Kreigel DE, et al. (1984). Therapeutic and economic value of a normal coronary angiogram. Am J Med 75:500–505.

Ferguson A, Sircus W, Eastwood MA (1977). Frequency of "functional" gastrointestinal disorders. Lancet 2:613–614.

Fielding JF (1977). The irritable bowel syndrome. 1. Clinical spectrum. Clin Gastroenterol 6:607–622.

Fraenkel YM, Kindler S, Melmed RN (1997). Differences in cognitions during chest pain of patients with panic disorder and ischemic heart disease. Depress Anxiety 1997:217–222.

Galvoski TE, Blanchard EB (1998). The treatment of irritable bowel syndrome with hypnotherapy. Appl Psychophysiol Biofeed 23:219–232.

Geltman EM, Henes CG, Senneff MJ, et al. (1990). Increased myocardial perfusion at rest and diminished perfusion reserve in patients with angina and angiographically normal coronary arteries. J Am Coll Cardiol 16:586–595.

Glazier JJ, Faxon DP, Melidossian C, et al. (1988). The changing face of coronary artery spasm: a decade of experience. Am Heart J 116:572–576.

Grace WJ, Wolf S, Wolff HG (1951). The Human Colon. New York: Hoeber.

Greenbaum D, Abitz L, VanEgeren L, et al. (1983). Irritable bowel symptom prevalence, rectosigmoid motility and psychometrics in symptomatic subjects not seeing physicians. Gastroenterology 84:1174. Abstract.

Hamm LR, Sorrells SC, Harding JP, et al. (1999). Additional investigations fail to alter the diagnosis of irritable bowel syndrome in subjects fulfilling the Rome criteria. Am J Gastroenterol 94:1279–1282.

Harvey RF, Read AE (1973). Effect of cholecystokinin on colonic motility and symptoms in patients with the irritable bowel syndrome. Lancet 1:1–3.

Harvey RF, Salih SY, Read AE (1983). Organic and functional disorders in 2000 gastroenterology outpatients. Lancet 1:632–634.

Heaton KW, Ghosh S, Braddon FEM (1991). How bad are the symptoms and bowel dysfunction of patients with irritable bowel syndrome? A prospective, controlled study with special reference to stool form. Gut 32:73–79.

Heberden W (1771). Some account of a disorder of the breast. Med Trans R Coll Physicians Lond 2:59, quoted in Keefer CS, Resnik WH. Angina pectoris. A syndrome caused by anoxia of the myocardium. Arch Intern Med 1928; 41:769–807.

Henker FO (1979). Diagnosis and treatment of nonorganic pelvic pain. South Med J 72:1132–1134.

Hewer W, Rost W, Gattaz WF (1995). Cardiovascular effects of fluvoxamine and maprotiline in depressed patients. Eur Arch Psychiat Clin Neurosci 246:1–6.

Hillman LC, Stace NH, Pomare EW (1984). Irritable bowel patients and their long-term response to a high fiber diet. Am J Gastroenterol 79:1–7.

Hislop IG (1971). Psychological significance of the irritable bowel syndrome. Gut 12:452–457.

Holmes KM, Slater RH (1982). Irritable bowel syndrome: a safe diagnosis? Br Med J 285:1533–1534.

Houghton LA, Heyman DJ, Whorwell PJ (1996). Symptomatology, quality of life and economic features of irritable bowel syndrome: the effect of hypnotherapy. Aliment Pharmacol Ther 10:91–95.

Iovino P, Azpiroz F, Domingo E, et al. (1995). The sympathetic nervous system modulates perception and reflex responses to gut distension in humans. Gastroenterology 108:680–686.

Isner JM, Salem DN, Banas JL, et al. (1981). Long term clinical course of patients with normal coronary arteriography: follow-up study of 121 patients with normal or nearly normal coronary arteriograms. Am Heart J 102:645–653.

Jarrett M, Heitkemper M, Cain KC, et al. (1998). The relationship between psychological distress and gastrointestinal symptoms in women with irritable bowel syndrome. Nurs Res 47:154–161.

Katon W, Hall ML, Russo J, et al. (1988). The relationship of psychiatric illness to coronary arteriographic results. Am J Med 84:1–9.

Katz PO, Castell DO (1985). Review: esophageal motility disorders. Am J Med Sci 290:61–69.

Keefer CS, Resnik WH (1928). Angina pectoris: a syndrome caused by anoxia of the myocardium. Arch Intern Med 41:769–807.

Kellow JE, Eckersley CM, Jones MP (1991). Enhanced perception of physiological intestinal motility in the irritable bowel syndrome. Gastroenterology 101:1621–1627.

Kellow JE, Gill RC, Windgate DL (1990). Prolonged ambulant recordings of small bowel motility demonstrate abnormalities in the irritable bowel syndrome. Gastroenterology 98:1208–1218.

Kemp HG Jr, Vokanas PS, Cohn PF, et al. (1973). The anginal syndrome associated with normal coronary arteriograms: report of a six year experience. Am J Med 54:735–742.

Kemp HG, Kronmal RA, Vlietstra RE, et al. (1986). Seven year survival of patients with normal or near normal coronary arteriograms: a CASS registry study. J Am Coll Cardiol 7:479–483.

Kemp HG, Vokonas PS, Cohn PF, et al. (1973). The anginal syndrome associated with normal coronary arteries. Am J Med 54:732–742.

Koch KL, Davidson WR, Day FP, et al. (1989). Esophageal dysfunction and chest pain in patients with mitral valve prolapse: a prospective study utilizing provocative testing during esophageal manometry. Am J Med 86:32–38.

Kock NG, Hulten L, Leandoer L (1968). A study of the motility in different parts of the human colon: resting activity, response to feeding and to prostigmine. Scand J Gastroenterol 3:163–169.

Kumar D, Windgate DL (1985). The irritable bowel syndrome: a paroxysmal motor disorder. Lancet 2:973–977.

Latimer P, Sarna S, Campbell D, et al. (1981). Colonic motor and myoelectric activity: a comparative study of normal subjects, psychoneurotic patients and patients with irritable bowel syndrome. Gastroenterology 80:893–901.

Lavey EB, Winkle RA (1979). Continuing disability of patients with chest pain and normal coronary arteriograms. J Chronic Dis 32:191–196.

Leahy A, Clayman C, Mason I, et al. (1998). Computerised biofeedback games: a new method for teaching stress management and its use in irritable bowel syndrome. J R Coll Physicians Lond 32:552–556.

Leman M, Dederding JP, Flourie B, et al. (1991). Abnormal perception of visceral pain in response to gastric distention in chronic idiopathic dyspepsia. Dig Dis Sci 36:1249–1254.

Liss JL, Alpers D, Woodruff RA (1973). The irritable colon syndrome and psychiatric illness. Dis Nerv System 34:151–157.

Manning AP, Thompson WG, Heaton KW, et al. (1978). Towards positive diagnosis of the irritable bowel. Br Med J 2:653–654.

Mayer EA, Naliboff B, Lee O, et al. (1999). Review article: gender-related differences in functional gastrointestinal disorders. Aliment Pharmacol Ther 13 (suppl 2):65–69.

Meller J, Goldsmith SJ, Rudin A, et al. (1979). Spectrum of exercise thallium-201 myocardial perfusion imaging in patients with chest pain and normal coronary angiograms. Am J Cardiol 43:717–723.

Mendeloff AI, Monk M, Siegel CI, et al. (1970). Illness experience and life stresses in patients with irritable colon and with ulcerative colitis: an epidemiological study of ulcerative colitis and regional enteritis in Baltimore, 1960–1964. N Engl J Med 282:14–17.

Munakata J, Naliboff B, Harraf F, et al. (1997). Repetitive sigmoid stimulation induces rectal hyperalgesia in patients with irritable bowel syndrome. Gastroenterology 112:55–63.

Narducci F, Snape WJ, Battle WM, et al. (1951). Increased colonic motility during exposure to a stressful situation. Dig Dis Sci 30:40–44.

Ockene IS, Shay MJ, Alpert JS, et al. (1980). Unexplained chest pain in patients with normal coronary arteriograms: a follow-up study of functional status. N Engl J Med 303:1249–1252.

Owens DM, Nelson DK, Talley NJ (1995). The irritable bowel syndrome: long-term prognosis and the physician–patient interaction. Ann Int Med 122:107–112.

Palmer RL, Stonehill E, Crisp AH, et al. (1974). Psychological characteristics of patients with the irritable bowel syndrome. Postgrad Med J 50:416–419.

Papanicolaou MN, Califf RM, Hlatky MA, et al. (1986). Prognostic implications of angiographically normal and insignificantly narrowed coronary arteries. Am J Cardiol 58:1181–1187.

Patterson DR (1982). Diffuse oesophageal spasm in patients with undiagnosed chest pain. J Clin Gastroenterol 4:415–417.

Peters LJ, Maas LC, Petty D, et al. (1988). Spontaneous non-cardiac chest pain: evaluation by 24-hour ambulatory esophageal motility and pH monitoring. Gastroenterology 94:878–886.

Prior A, Sorial E, Sun W-M, et al. (1993). Irritable bowel syndrome: differences between patients who show rectal sensitivity and those who do not. Eur J Gastroenterol Hepatol 5:343–349.

Proudfit WL, Bruschke AV, Sones FM Jr (1980). Clinical course of patients with normal coronary arteriography: 10-year follow-up of 521 patients. Circulation 62:712–717.

Reaven G (1988). Role of insulin resistance in human disease. Diabetes 37:1595–1607.

Richter JE, Barish CF, Castell DO (1986). Abnormal sensory perception in patients with esophageal chest pain. Gastroenterology 91:845–852.

Richter JE, Castell DO (1984). Diffuse esophageal spasm: a reappraisal. Ann Intern Med 100:242–245.

Richter JE, Dalton CB, Bradley LA, et al. (1987). Oral nifedipine in the treatment of noncardiac chest pain in patients with the nutcracker esophagus. Gastroenterology 93:21–28.

Ritchie J (1973). Pain from distention of the pelvic colon by inflating a balloon in the irritable colon syndrome. Gut 14:125–132.

Rosen SD, Uren NG, Kaski JC, et al. (1994). Coronary vasodilator reserve, pain perception, and sex in patients with syndrome X. Circulation 90:50–60.

Roy-Byrne PP, Schmidt P, Cannon RO, et al. (1989). Microvascular angina and panic disorder. Int J Psychiat Med 19:312–325.

Roza C, Laird JMA, Cervero F (1998). Spinal mechanisms underlying persistent pain and referred hyperalgesia in rats with experimental ureteric stone. J Neurophysiol 79:1603–1612.

Sataline L (1985). Irritable bowel syndrome and mitral valve prolapse syndrome (letter) JAMA 253:41.

Sax FI, Cannon RO, Hanson C, et al. (1987). Impaired forearm vasodilator reserve in patients with microvascular angina: evidence of a generalized disorder of vascular function? N Engl J Med 317:1366–1370.

Schofield PM, Brooks NH, Bennet DH (1986). Left ventricular dysfunction in patients with angina pectoris and normal coronary angiograms. Br Heart J 56:327–333.

Shapiro LM, Crake T, Poole-Wilson PA (1988). Is altered cardiac sensation responsible for chest pain in patients with normal coronary arteries? Clinical observation during cardiac catheterization. Br Med J 296:170–171.

Silverman DHS, Munakata JA, Ennes H, et al. (1997). Regional cerebral activity in normal and pathological perception of visceral pain. Gastroenterology 112:64–72.

Snape WJ, Carlson GM, Cohen S (1977). Human colonic myoelectric activity in reponse to prostigmine and the gastrointestinal hormones. Am J Dig Dis 22:881–887.

Stewart WF, Liberman JN, Sandler RS, et al. (1999). Epidemiology of Constipation (EPOC) study in the United States: relation of clinical subtypes to sociodemographic features. Am J Gastroenterol 94:3530–3540.

Sullivan MA, Cohen S, Snape WJ (1978). Colonic myoelectrical activity in the irritable bowel syndrome. effect of eating and anticholinergics. N Engl J Med 298:878–883.

Svedlund J, Sjodin I, Dotevall G, et al. (1985). Upper gastrointestinal and mental symptoms in the irritable bowel syndrome. Scand J Gastroenterol 20:595–601.

Svennson O, Stenport G, Tibbling L, et al. (1978). Oesophageal function and coronary angiogram in patients with disabling chest pain. Acta Med Scand 204:173–178.

Swarbrick ET, Hegarty JE, Bat L, et al. (1980). Site of pain from the irritable bowel syndrome. Lancet 2:443–446.

Szurszewski JH, Weems WA (1976). A study of peripheral input to and its control by post-ganglionic neurones of the inferior mesenteric ganglion. J Physiol Lond 256:541–556.

Talley NJ (1998). Irritable bowel syndrome: disease definition and symptom description. Eur J Surg Suppl 583:24–28.

Talley NJ, Owen BK, Boyce P, et al. (1996). Psychological treatments for irritable bowel syndrome: a critique of control treatment trials. Am J Gastroenterol 91:277–283.

Talley NJ, Zinsmeister AR, Melton LJ (1995). Irritable bowel syndrome in a community: symptom subgroups, risk factors, and health care utilization. Am J Epidemiol 142:76–83.

Taylor I, Basu P, Hammond P, et al. (1980). Effect of bile acid perfusion on colonic motor function in patients with the irritable bowel syndrome. Gut 21:843–847.

Taylor I, Duthie HL, Smallwood R, et al. (1974). The effect of stimulation on the activity of the myoelectrical activity of the rectosigmoid in man. Gut 15:599–604.

Thompson WG, Longstreth GF, Drossman DA, et al. (1999). Functional bowel disorders and functional abdominal pain. Gut 45(suppl 2):II43–47.

Thompson WG, Dotevall G, Drossman DA, et al. (1989). Irritable bowel syndrome: guidelines for the diagnosis. Gastroenterol Int 2:92–95.

Thompson WG, Heaton KW (1980). Functional bowel disorders in apparently healthy people. Gastroenterology 79:283–288.

Thompson WR, Heaton KW (1980). Women more frequently complain of IBS symptoms. Gastroenterology 80:283–288.

Thompson WG, Heaton KW, Smyth GT, et al. (2000). Irritable bowel syndrome in general practice: prevalence, characteristics, and referral. Gut 46:78–82.

Trikas P, Vlachonikolis I, Fragkiadakis N, et al. (1999). Core mental state in irritable bowel syndrome. Psychosom Med 61:781–788.

Tweddel AC, Martin W, Hutton I (1992). Thallium scans in syndrome X. Br Heart J 68:48–50.

Van Dulmen AM, Fennis JF, Bleifenburg G (1996). Cognitive-behavioral group therapy for irritable bowel syndrome: effects and long-term follow-up. Psychosom Med 58:508–514.

Waller SL, Misiewicz JJ (1969). Prognosis in the irritable bowel syndrome. Lancet 2:754–756.

Wangel AG, Deller DJ (1965). Intestinal motility in man. III. Mechanisms of constipation and diarrhea with particular reference to the irritable bowel syndrome. Gastroenterology 48:69–84.

Watson WC, Sullivan SN, Corke M, et al. (1978). Globus and headache: common symptoms of the irritable bowel syndrome. Can Med Assn J 118:387–388.

Welgan P, Meshkinpour H, Hoehler F (1985). The effect of stress on colon motor and electrical activity in irritable bowel syndrome. Psychosomat Med 47:139–149.

Whitehead WE, Bosmajian L, Zonderman AB, et al. (1988). Symptoms of psychological distress associated with irritable bowel syndrome. Gastroenterology 95:709–714.

Whitehead WE, Engel BT, Schuster MM (1980). Irritable bowel syndrome: physiological and psychological differences between diarrhea-predominant and constipation-predominant patients. Dig Dis Sci 25:404–413.

Whitehead WE, Holtkotter B, Enck P, et al. (1990). Tolerance for rectosigmoid distension in irritable bowel syndrome. Gastroenterology 98:1187–1192.

Whitehead WE, Winget C, Fedoravicius AS, et al. (1982). Learned illness behavior in patients with irritable bowel syndrome and peptic ulcer. Dig Dis Sci 27:202–208.

Whorwell PJ, Clouter C, Smith CL (1981). Oesophageal motility in the irritable bowel syndrome. Br Med J 282:1101–1102.

Whorwell PJ, McCullum M, Creed FH, et al. (1986). Non-colonic features of irritable bowel syndrome. Gut 27:37–40.

Whorwell PJ, Prior A, Colgan SM (1987). Hypnotherapy in severe irritable bowel syndrome, a further experience. Gut 28:423–425.

Young SJ, Alpers DH, Norland CC, et al. (1976). Psychiatric illness and the irritable bowel syndrome: practical implications for the primary physician. Gastroenterology 70:162–166.

Chapter 12.

PANIC ATTACKS: THE GREAT MIMIC

Panic disorder is a major blind spot in clinical practice. This paradoxical fact stems not from any inherent difficulty in making the diagnosis, because it happens to be one of the easiest of the major psychiatric disorders to identify, but simply because the nonpsychiatric physician too seldom considers it as a diagnostic possibility. Consequently, diagnosis is often delayed, sometimes by a few years, with considerable cost to the patient in needless suffering and disability, and to the medical system through countless, expensive investigations (Ballenger, 1997).

Whereas epidemiological studies have described increased medical service utilization in patients with panic disorder, service use in primary care panic patients relative to other primary care patients is less well characterized. Roy-Byrne et al. (1999) administered a waiting room screening questionnaire in three primary care practices to identify 81 patients with panic disorder (according to DSM-IV criteria) as well as a group of 183 psychiatrically healthy patients, in order to determine their psychiatric comorbidity, panic characteristics, disability, and medical and mental health service use, including medications. A subsample of 41 patients with panic disorder were interviewed 4 to 10 months later to determine the adequacy of treatment received for the panic symptoms. The authors found that 70% of panic patients had a comorbid psychiatric diagnosis. Patients had more disability in the previous month (days missed or reduced activities), as well as greater utilization of emergency room and medical provider visits, and more mental health visits than the nonpatient group. Nevertheless, only 42% received psychotropic medication, 36% psychotherapy, and 64% any treatment. On follow-up, 85% still met diagnostic criteria for panic, and only 22% had received adequate medication and 12% adequate psychotherapy (i.e., cognitive-behavioral therapy).

What tends to most mislead the physician is that the presentation of panic disorder is almost invariably somatic, whether cardiovascular (palpitations, chest pain, flushes), respiratory (dyspnea, sensation of choking), neurological (paresthesias, vertigo), or gastrointestinal (abdominal pain, vomiting, dysphagia, anorexia) (Bridges and Goldberg, 1985). Accurate diagnosis will depend, therefore, on a high index of suspicion and a routine of systematic questioning aimed at identifying features of panic such as *intense anxiety related to the symptoms*, fear *that the symptoms indicate serious and possibly catastrophic illness*, and avoidance behavior and features of agoraphobia (see below). Multiple system complaints are often helpful in suggesting the diagnosis, though sometimes the recurrence of only one or two symptoms such as dizziness, flushes, or palpitations may dominate the clinical picture (Rosenbaum, 1987). Hence systematic questioning is important to rule out panic disorder, particularly where there is a clear discrepancy between the degree of suffering or evident distress and the paucity of objective findings of disease.

THE CLINICAL PICTURE

Panic attacks are characterized by bouts of physical discomfort associated with intense anxiety and apprehension. The onset is sudden, which serves to heighten the anxiety as patients feel they are "losing control" in both a physical and an emotional sense. In most cases the somatic symptoms are localized mainly to the chest, with palpitations and chest pain or discomfort often being the predominant complaint. Symptoms of hyperventilation are frequently present, adding to the feeling of light-headedness and unreality as well as intensifying the physical discomfort. Patients often admit to feeling fearful that something catastrophic is about to happen to them (such as a heart attack or stroke), and they often experience fear of impending death. Hypocapneic ECG changes suggestive of ischemia may add to the physician's uncertainty about the presence of ischemic heart disease. Similarly, the fact that panic attacks may occur during sleep tends to convince the patient that a serious condition underlies the attacks.

Patients who suffer from panic disorder usually consult general physicians and often use the services of the hospital emergency department (Shapiro et al., 1988; Markowitz et al., 1989). Up to 85% of panic disorder patients have their first contact with a health care professional in general medical practice, and almost half of the patients are treated in that setting. Of this group with panic disorder, 43% of patients are first seen by an emergency room physician, and 15% are initially brought to the emergency department in an ambulance (Katerndahl and Realini, 1995). In one study, 70% of patients with panic disorder had consulted an average of 10 physicians (Sheehan et al., 1980). Despite substantial anxiety and fear associated with the symptoms, almost all of these patients tend to emphasize the physical symptoms, as it is these they find most threatening. Furthermore, when pressed about their feelings of anxiety or fear, they will ascribe these to the presence of the symptoms and the presumed implication that they reflect severe underlying disease. While the physician may be well aware of a patient's anxiety, both the seriousness and the particular nature of the problem are usually underestimated. Patients are often referred for tests, including the accepted screening tests for ischemic heart disease such as exercise tests, Holter evaluation, isotope studies of cardiac perfusion, and coronary angiography.

While the information provided by such studies may reassure the physician, a pronouncement of "no disease" does not resolve the uncertainties in the patient's mind. Although patients usually feel some relief on hearing that the tests are normal, they still need an adequate explanation of why the symptoms occurred in the first place. The palpitations, chest pain, vertigo, and light-headedness are so real to the patient that they simply cannot be dismissed by the statement that there is no organic disorder behind them and that "everything is fine." Nor will the frequently administered benzodiazepine tranquilizer help resolve the problem, though it may ease it for a while (Holister, 1980). In addition, such patients are often "locked in" to the cycle of panic attacks and anxiety. Even those subjects who fully understand the irrational nature of the process are helpless to prevent further attacks or an escalation of the condition.

The prevalence of panic attacks as a recurrent lifetime phenomenon has been estimated at 1.6%–2%, though isolated attacks may occur in up to 10% of the population (Weissman, 1988). The rate is slightly higher in women than in men. In a study of 3021 adolescents and young adults aged 14 to 24 years, Reed and Wittchen (1998) found panic symptoms to be quite common in the community (13.1%), with lifetime prevalence of DSM-IV panic disorder at 4.3%. The first attack rarely occurred before puberty. The authors found that "late onset" (i.e., after the age of 18 years) of panic attacks in their population sample was strongly associated with the development of multimorbidity of mental disorders.

In a study of anxiety disorders in an older (55 to 85 year) population in the Netherlands, Beekman et al., (1998) found an overall prevalence of 10%. They based their assessment on a random sample of 3107 adults, stratified for age and sex. Generalized anxiety disorder was the most common condition (7.3%), followed by phobic disorders (3.1%). Both panic disorder (1.0%) and obsessive-compulsive disorder (0.6%) were uncommon. Aging itself did not have any impact on the overall prevalence of anxiety, but panic disorder declined in

TABLE 12–1. DSM-IV Diagnostic Criteria for Panic Disorder

A. At some time during the disturbance, one or more panic attacks (discrete periods of intense fear or discomfort) have occurred that were (1) unexpected (i.e., did not occur immediately before or on exposure to a situation that almost always causes anxiety) and (2) not triggered by situations in which the person was the focus of others' attention.

B. Either four attacks, as defined in criterion A, have occurred within a four-week period, or one or more attacks have been followed by a period of at least a month of persistent fear of having another attack.

C. At least four of the following symptoms developed during at least one of the attacks:*

1. Shortness of breath (dyspnea) or smothering sensations	7. Nausea or abdominal distress
2. Dizziness, unsteady feelings, or faintness	8. Depersonalization or derealization
3. Palpitations or accelerated heart rate (tachycardia)	9. Numbness or tingling sensation (paresthesias)
4. Trembling or shaking	10. Flushes (hot flashes) or chills
5. Sweating	11. Chest pain or discomfort
6. Choking	12. Fear of dying
	13. Fear of going crazy or doing something uncontrolled

D. During at least some of the attacks, at least four of the C symptoms developed suddenly and increased in intensity within 10 minutes of the beginning of the first C symptom noticed in the attack.

E. It cannot be established that an organic factor, e.g., amphetamine or caffeine intoxication or hyperthyroidism, initiated and maintained the disturbance.†

*Attacks involving four or more symptoms are panic attacks; attacks involving fewer than four symptoms are limited-symptom attacks.

†Mitral valve prolapse may be an associated condition, but it does not preclude a diagnosis of panic disorder.

prevalence in the older age group, a finding also supported by other reports (Krasucki et al., 1998). Suggested explanations for this observation include the possibility that panic disorder may be associated with earlier death. However, Flint et al. (1998) observed that following an intravenous injection of a panicogenic agent (cholecystokinin tetrapeptide, CCK-4), normal subjects over 65 years had significantly fewer and less intense anxietylike symptoms than a comparable group of subjects aged 20 to 35 years. This observation strongly points to age-related changes in responsivity to CCK-4, which may be indicative of age-related changes in the CNS that confer a lesser tendency to panic disorder in older people.

Table 12-1 lists the diagnostic criteria for panic disorder according to the DSM-IV criteria, although it should be remembered that patients may present with panic attacks in the medical clinics without fulfilling the criteria for a diagnosis of panic disorder. It would be wise to maintain regular contact with these patients to confirm resolution of their symptoms; if this fails, vigorous treatment of the condition should be undertaken (see below).

ANTICIPATORY ANXIETY AND AGORAPHOBIA

The emotional distress caused by a panic attack is often so marked that the patient retains a residue of anxiety and apprehension at the possibility of further attacks. The resulting tension is reinforced and compounded by each further episode, to the point where the sustained anxiety, the so-called *anticipatory anxiety*, serves to perpetuate the condition. If an attack has occurred in a particular situation, such as driving a car, the subject is likely to experience further attacks while driving. This is much like a classical conditioned response, although the element of anticipation is always present too (Chapter 8).

With repeated attacks, patients may become fearful about going to certain places, usually public venues. Their explanations for this may vary but usually the main reason is the fear of an attack away from home, where they feel much more vulnerable because help may not be available, or in the company of strangers, where patients would perceive their loss of control as seriously humiliating. This *avoidance behavior*, or *phobic avoidance*, may develop into a fear of particular places, or *agoraphobia*. The feared places might be, for example, buses, crowded shops, or theaters. A common feature in most of these situations is fear of being unable to leave the place quickly. Patients may also fear being alone. Partial states are common in the earlier phases of the disorder. Thus, the patient may, with great apprehension, go to the supermarket, but at a time when it is usually relatively free of shoppers. By the time the problem has developed to this extent, the persistent anxiety may have prompted the patient (often in response to the pressure of a family member) to consult a mental health professional for assistance.

PANIC ATTACKS

Specific Vulnerability or Unusual Stress Response?

The question we would like to answer in considering the cause of panic attacks is whether the attacks occur only as the expression of a particular constitutional makeup in certain people or whether everyone could suffer a panic attack with anxiety of sufficient intensity. The studies considered next were undertaken to try to answer that question.

Family studies

The etiological basis of panic disorder is currently a subject of debate. Some workers support a strong biological predisposition or vulnerability, based on family and especially twin studies (Crowe et al., 1980; Pauls et al., 1980). Studies have pointed to a high risk of panic disorder among first-degree relatives (15%–20%) (Crowe et al., 1983; Harris et al., 1983). Perna et al. (1997) interviewed 120 twins recruited from the general population, looking for the presence of anxiety disorders and sporadic panic attacks. A significantly higher concordance for panic disorder was found among monozygotic twins than among dizygotic twins (73% versus 0%) but not for sporadic panic attacks (57% versus 43%). When 90 of the twins were challenged with a one-vital-capacity inhalation of 35% CO_2–65% O_2, a panicogenic stimulus, a significantly higher concordance was found for 35% of CO_2–induced panic attacks among monozygotic (55.6%) than dizygotic (12.5%) twins (Bellodi et al., 1998). These results confirm a genetic role for the development of panic disorder, though not necessarily for sporadic panic attacks.

Genetic studies

The strong pointers in the family and twin studies to an inherited susceptibility suggest that panic disorder may be amenable to more precise genetic analysis. However, studies have failed to demonstrate a definitive Mendelian inheritance (Vieland et al., 1996) and no major gene locus has been unambiguously identified (Knowles et al., 1998). This has led to the suggestion that panic disorder is multifactorial and oligo- or polygenic, with each gene contributing only a small portion of the variance. Thus, studies are under way that are better suited to discover such susceptibility genes with presumably minor but significant effects.

One approach in molecular genetic studies of panic disorder patients is to choose candidate genes on the basis of our knowledge of the molecular mechanisms of drugs that are effective in treating panic disorder or in provoking panic attacks. The effectiveness of the serotonin reuptake inhibitors led to the study of a functional serotonin transporter gene polymorphism (Lesch et al., 1996; Deckert et al., 1997), and the fact that the adenosine receptor antagonist caffeine produces panic attacks led to the study of adenosine receptor genes (Deckert et al., 1998).

Another class of drug used to treat panic disorder consists of inhibitors of monoamine oxidase A, the gene for which is located on chromosome X. Deckert et al. (1999) studied a novel repeat polymorphism in the promoter of the monoamine oxidase A gene in two population samples suffering from panic disorder, 80 German patients and 129 Italian patients. By correlating structural with functional changes of this gene allele in the majority of patients they were able to suggest a specific molecular mechanism possibly contributing to the development of panic disorder. But much more study of potential genetic aberration in panic disorder sufferers will be needed before we reach a clearer understanding of which genetic changes confer a vulnerability for the development of the disorder.

Clinical observations

Panic attacks often begin at times of increased tension or anxiety, whether as a result of unusually hard work, increased responsibility, or adverse life events (Last et al., 1984; Breier et al., 1986; Roy-Byrne et al., 1986). Many months may pass between an attack and the traumatic event that prompted it, such as the death of a parent. Symptoms may therefore develop at a time when the subject is relatively free from overt anxiety or depression, convincing both patient and practitioner of the "spontaneous" nature of the attack. As with other somatic expressions of anxiety, the frequent dissociation between the emotionally stressful event and the onset of physical symptoms may confuse both the practitioner and the patient and delay the true diagnosis. Because of the time lag between the event and the consequences of the emotional response to it, the practitioner is likely to miss the association and overinvestigate the patient's symptoms.

The sudden occurrence of spontaneous panic attacks in certain people, without warning and without apparent cause, may also appear to indicate a biological predisposition. In many cases definite events or thought processes seem related to the panic attack episode (Margraf et al., 1986). Particularly in anxious patients, certain external and internal cues are more likely to be perceived as threatening. Careful history taking may reveal thoughts of death, serious illness, or loss of control at the time of perceiving some bodily sensation (Beck et al., 1974). Experimental studies designed to evaluate the responsiveness of patients suffering from panic disorder have shown that a falsely elevated feedback of their heart rate (i.e., the patients were shown an instrument reading indicating a faster pulse rate than was happening in reality) produced greater anxiety and physiological arousal than in controls or even in a panic attack (Margraf et al., 1987). Similarly, in studies using 24-hour electrocardiograph monitoring, only panic attack patients responded with anxiety to ventricular extrasystoles (Strian, 1987). Significantly, neither normal controls nor asymptomatic mitral valve prolapse patients showed anxiety with extrasystoles. I have observed patients with persistent multiple ventricular extrasystoles, or with runs of supraventricular tachycardia of up to 180 beats/min, in whom the only evident distress was a mildly expressed physical discomfort at the sensation of palpitation.

It is important to note, however, that mistakes may be made in attributing attacks of palpitations to panic attacks when they are in fact due to unrecognized paroxysmal supraventricular tachycardia (PST). Lessmeier et al. (1997) conducted a retrospective survey of 107 consecutive patients suffering from PST and found that 67% of the group fulfilled the criteria for a DSM-IV diagnosis of panic disorder. The PST was unrecognized in 59 (55%) of the group and remained un-recognized for over three years. Physicians (nonpsychiatrists) attributed symp-toms to panic, anxiety, or stress in 32 of the 59 patients, and women were more likely than men to have the symptoms ascribed to a psychiatric condition. These authors stress that the diagnosis of PST is more likely to be made by event mon-itoring rather than the more widely used method of Holter examination, which is indicated when trying to determine whether a patient's symptoms are due to a heart beat irregularity. The Holter monitor provides a continuous recording of electrocardiographic activity over 24 hours. If the patient has no bouts of PST during this time, as often happens, the condition will be missed. In contrast, with event monitoring the patient activates a marker and transmits the cardiograph at the time he or she is having symptoms, or the record is read at a later time.

Hyperventilation: Cause or Consequence?

The universal occurrence of hyperventilation during panic attacks has led some to postulate a causative role for hyperventilation in the development of the at-tack (Lum, 1981; Clark and Helmsley, 1982; Ley, 1985). As expected, panic at-tack patients find that many of their symptoms may be induced by voluntary hy-perventilation. In one study where subjects were requested to take 60 breaths per minute for three minutes, 67% of the panic attack patients were unable to com-plete the test as opposed to 4% of the controls (Bonn et al., 1984). Almost all of the panic attack patients (21 of 22) confirmed that the symptoms were similar to (though less intense than) naturally occurring panic attacks. In another study, the mean resting P_{CO_2} of a group of panic attack patients was significantly lower than that of a matched group of controls, suggesting strongly that these subjects are chronic hyperventilators (Salkovskis et al., 1986). Comparing a group of 17 panic disorder (PD) patients, 18 patients with general anxiety disorder (GAD), and 20 normal controls, Hegel and Ferguson (1997) found that those with PD exhibited significantly lower end–tidal carbon dioxide levels (an indicator of anx-iety-induced hyperventilation) than the GADs and normal controls. This was de-spite of the fact that the PDs were equivalent to GADs on baseline anxiety lev-els. Others, however, have found hypocapnia much more infrequently in panic disorder patients (Hibbert and Pilsbury, 1989; Garssen et al., 1996).

The consensus today seems to be that hyperventilation is not a significant pre-cipitant of panic attacks in most patients with panic disorder. Since anxious peo-ple breathe more rapidly than nonanxious ones (Chapter 14), one would expect some anxious subjects to develop hypocapnia and the symptoms of hyperventi-lation. In addition, given the exaggerated tendency of anxious subjects to inter-pret bodily symptoms and especially discomfort negatively, it seem plausible that hyperventilation may be the trigger for panic attacks in some individuals. As sympathetic activation and respiratory activity are found to be closely integrated under all situations where they have been evaluated together, the argument concerning priority of influence tends to be circular and consequently futile. In all probability, any symptom associated with sympathetic activation or hyperventilation in patients subject to panic attacks may lead to a cascade effect of intensifying symptomatology, with rapidly increasing anxiety and the development of panic.

Induction of Panic Attacks

Panic attacks may be induced in susceptible subjects by a variety of agents, most of which either lead to activation of the sympathetic nervous system or reproduce the cardiovascular and respiratory effects of sympathetic activation. Studies have consistently shown that panic attacks may be induced in about 70% of such patients by lactate infusion (Pitts and McClure, 1967; Fink et al., 1970; Kelly et al., 1971). One of the most widely used agents in the clinical investigation of panic disorder is 0.5M sodium lactate; its mechanism of action, however, is poorly understood. Induction of the panic attack apparently does not depend on the production of a metabolic alkalosis, change in serum pH, reduction in serum calcium levels, or mobilization of catecholamines (Liebowitz et al., 1986). While most thinking has tended to focus on the lactate moiety as the active factor in inducing panic symptoms, Peskind et al. (1998) evaluated whether the large sodium load in the 0.5 mol/L sodium lactate infusion might be involved in panic induction. They found that sodium lactate and hypertonic saline produced the same high incidence of panic and equivalent increases in panic symptoms in the panic disorder subjects, clearly implicating the sodium rather than lactate as the active agent. George et al. (1995), studying a group of 20 patients with panic disorder, found that they were significantly more likely to have a panic attack in response to infusion of lactate dissolved in 0.9% sodium chloride than lactate dissolved in 5% dextrose in water.

Another established technique for the production of panic attacks is the inhalation of 5% CO_2, which is about as effective as lactate for this purpose (Gorman et al., 1984). Carbon dioxide acts as a powerful stimulant of the brain respiratory center and of the locus ceruleus, a major center of influence over of the sympathetic nervous system (Elam et al., 1981). This coupling of enhanced respiratory activity with sympathetic activation is yet another example of the tight linkage between these two processes. It is also possible that lactate infusion may give rise to an increase in cerebral CO_2 levels and thus work in the same way as inhaled CO_2 to bring about sympathetic activation (Carr and Sheehan, 1984; Gorman et al., 1984). However, the fact that lactate infusion causes hyperventilation may be sufficient to explain its other effects here.

The increase in heart rate and blood pressure levels following lactate infusion is similar in panic disorder patients and controls (Ehlers et al., 1986; Yeragani et al., 1989), yet in most cases it is only the patients who respond with panic attacks. A differential sensitivity to the effects of controlled inhalation (a single breath) of 35% CO_2 has also been demonstrated between patients suffering from panic disorder and generalized anxiety disorder in that the latter group tended to respond like the controls with fewer and less intense symptoms (Perna et al., 1999). Thus, any adequate explanation of panic attacks must include a consideration of the physical state, the patient's negative interpretation of body signals, and previous learning experience (Ackerman and Sachar, 1974; Margraf et al., 1986).

In unsuspecting subjects who begin to develop panic attacks after using an agent such as cocaine (Aronson and Craig, 1986), it is unlikely that individual susceptibility alone is operating since panic attacks are reported in 64% of chronic cocaine users (Washton and Gold, 1984). Panic attacks may also be induced by a variety of other substances that promote or enhance sympathetic activity, such as isoproteronol (a nonselective β-receptor agonist) (Easton and Sherman, 1976; Rainey et al., 1984), caffeine (a phosphodiesterase inhibitor) (Charney et al., 1985), yohimbine (a selective alpha-2 antagonist leading to increased central sympathetic activity) (Charney et al., 1984), and cholecystokinin (Bradwejn et al., 1991). Not all laboratory stressors induce panic. Cognitive stress such as mental arithmetic (Kelly et al., 1971), metabolic stress such as hypoglycemia (Uhde et al., 1984; Schweitzer et al., 1986), and pain (Roy-Byrne et al., 1985) do not usually induce panic.

The Neuroanatomical Basis of Panic Attacks

This subject has been critically reviewed by Gorman et al. (1989), who divided panic disorder into three distinct clinical components: the acute panic attack, anticipatory anxiety, and phobic avoidance. Considering the defined clinical nature of each process, it seems logical to assume that they arise from primary activation of three distinct neuroanatomical locations, the brain stem, limbic system, and prefrontal cortex, respectively. Coplan and Lydiard (1998) offered a similar analysis: "When considering the panic neurocircuitry, the 'fear' vs. 'anxiety' vs. 'panic' distinction is an important one."

Panic attacks and the brain stem

Two lines of evidence point to the brain stem as the origin of panic attacks. First, panic attacks are characterized clinically by pronounced autonomic activity. The initial indicators of an attack in the minds of most patients are the distinctive and usually frightening physical sensations mediated by autonomic activity. In contrast to other anxiety states where the affect is described in terms of "worry" or "tension," in this case it is the pronounced physical symptoms that nearly always lead panic disorder patients to a series of consultations with internists or to repeated emergency room visits. Second, the ability to provoke panic attacks in susceptible individuals through the administration of agents that activate or potentiate sympathetic or respiratory activity indicates a primary stimulation of brain stem centers.

The locus ceruleus is considered to be of central importance because its stimulation produces almost all the physiological and autonomic signs of panic. The locus ceruleus is directly innervated by fibers that originate in the periphery and project through the vagus nerve to the nucleus solitarius of the medulla, by fibers from chemosensitive nuclei in the medullary reticulum, including the nucleus reticularis paragigantocellularis, and by descending serotonergic fibers from midbrain raphe nuclei. Serotonergic projections from the dorsal raphe nucleus inhibit the firing of the locus ceruleus neurons, whereas noradrenergic innervation from the locus ceruleus in turn excites dorsal raphe nucleus neurons. Based on the differing projections of the dorsal and median raphe nuclei and their often opposing influences, Grove et al. (1997) postulated that the limbic projections of median raphe nucleus may be important in the modulation of fear and anticipatory anxiety and the autonomic responses associated with panic, whereas the striatal projections of the dorsal raphe nucleus may modulate cognitive and motoric behavioral functions, including the suppression or release of escape or fleeing responses.

Information about heart rate and rhythm and about ventilatory function is conveyed through vagal afferents to the nucleus solitarius (Kalia, 1977). Afferents then pass from the nucleus solitarius to other parts of the brain stem (Beckstead et al., 1980). Gorman et al. (1989) speculated that these brain stem loci may be stimulated into activity, leading to a cascade of events, by a "mismatch" between peripheral autonomic activity and actual metabolic demand. One example is the effect resulting from an isoproteronol infusion, where the cardiovascular system is stimulated in excess of the body's metabolic needs. Normally the rise in pulse rate and cardiac output correlate extremely well with the metabolic demands (especially the increased oxygen utilization) of skeletal muscle activity. While this type of "mismatch" is characteristic of autonomic activation secondary to more intense anxiety states, there is no particular reason to believe that it may cause a panic attack. As mentioned earlier, stresses such as mental arithmetic and pain, which may be expected to induce pulse and blood pressure changes and thus lead to a similar mismatch between cardiovascular activity and metabolic demands, are not known to precipitate panic attacks in susceptible subjects.

Anticipatory anxiety and the limbic lobe

As emphasized by Gorman et al. (1989), patients suffering from panic attacks feel a real dread but are not always able to articulate precisely what they fear. Characteristically, however, they will agree vigorously with the physician's suggestion that they are fearful of further attacks. The presumably identical processes of anticipatory anxiety and symptom anticipation have been dealt with in Chapter 8.

The central role of the limbic system in basic emotions such as fear, rage, and anxiety has been demonstrated in both animals and humans. Lesions in the cingulate portion of the limbic lobe decrease anxiety in humans. The benzodiazepine diazepam may be quite effective in reducing anticipatory anxiety, even though it has little effect on panic attacks and the limbic system of the brain is particularly rich in benzodiazepine receptors. Together with the evidence presented in Chapter 8, this strongly suggests that anticipatory anxiety is a process centered on activity in the limbic lobe.

Phobic avoidance and the prefrontal cortex

Humans tend to avoid adverse situations with much greater persistence than lower animals. In animals, prolonged absence of an adverse stimulus will eventually result in extinction of the avoidance. By contrast, in humans, a single aversion-inducing experience may be enough to trigger phobic avoidance, which may persist for many years or even a lifetime. The prefrontal cortex has extensive anatomical connections with limbic structures (Neutra and Domesick, 1981). The cognitive processes that are associated with panic attacks may be instrumental in inducing them. The typical catastrophic thought content leads to limbic activation, which in turn activates or potentiates hypothalamic–autonomic activity.

Although the schema suggested by Gorman et al. (1989) provided an approximation of the neuroanatomical basis of panic disorder at the time it was proposed, we know now that there are other important parts to this story. This more contemporary understanding has been culled from various sources, including more extensive basic research on fear mechanisms, the probable site of action of medication for panic disorder, and the positron emission tomography (PET) neuroimaging of patients during a panic attack. While there are a number of overlapping theoretical models of panic neurocircuitry, the following summary covers some of the important areas under consideration.

LeDoux (1998) pointed out that fear responses tend to be hard-wired, species typical expressions of fear that are not learned or conditioned. The fear responses that are conditioned (as may occur with panic attacks) thus involve the coupling of new stimuli to preexisting responses. That is, the fear response is triggered by a new repertoire of stimuli through learning. In the context of panic disorder, however, the initial emphasis on brain stem–midbrain axis must now be modified and the central importance of the amygdala integrated with these theories (Coplan and Lydiard, 1998). The amygdala, with rich efferent connections to the brain stem, midbrain, and cortex, is identified today as a key site of fear processing and fear learning. The connections between the amygdala and the hippocampus and its role in contextual conditioning, on one hand, and with the medial prefrontal cortex and its role in extinction, on the other, make it a central part of the fear conditioning apparatus (LeDoux, 1998). The amygdalofugal pathways, with primary connections to the hypothalamus and brain stem, are phylogenetically well conserved in mammalian species. Fear conditioning occurs throughout the phyla, and within the vertebrates it appears that very similar neural mechanisms are involved across the species.

Although amygdaloid structures may not be readily distinguishable on PET scanning, the insular cortex, with its extensive reciprocal connections to the more deeply located lateral nucleus of the amygdala, provides a direct input into the central nucleus of the amygdala (Amaral and Insausti, 1992). The central nucleus of the amygdala has a high concentration of neurons containing corticotropin-releasing factor (CRF), an anxiogenic hormone in animals (Heinrichs et al., 1997). The CRF is localized to other monoamine-containing nuclei in the brain stem as well, such as the dorsal raphe nucleus (DRN), which is rich in serotonin, leading to an interplay ("crosstalk") between CRF and serotonin function. Furthermore, the central nucleus of the amygdala, which receives input from other subnuclei of the amygdala, in turn controls the expression of defense mechanisms, including behavioral, autonomic, and hormonal (hypothalamic–pituitry–adrenal axis) responses. Thus, lesions of the central nucleus of the amygdala interfere with the expression of fear responses of all types (LeDoux, 1998).

On the basis of PET studies in panic disorder patients, Reiman (1997) postulated abnormal function in the anterior insular cortex and anterior temporal regions. What is not resolved by these studies, however, is the source of the primary stimulus, that is, whether to insular cortex from an activated amygdala or the reverse. Nevertheless, studies with functional magnetic resonance imaging have now shown activation of the amygdala during fear imaging (Buchel et al., 1998).

PANIC DISORDER AND MORTALITY: A CAUTIONARY TALE

Unnatural Death

Epidemiological research over the last few years indicates an increased risk of death by suicide among people suffering from panic disorder and attacks. In a survey of 18,011 adults, Weissman et al. (1989) found that 20% of subjects with panic disorder and 12% of those with panic attacks had attempted suicide. Subjects with panic disorder thought more about suicide (suicidal ideation) than did controls. These results could not be explained by the coexistence of major depression, alcoholism, or drug abuse, all of which are more common among panic disorder sufferers (Weissman et al., 1989). This study confirms data obtained from 113 psychiatric inpatients with panic disorder who were followed up over 30–50 years and in whom mortality was significantly higher than in the general population due primarily to suicide and cardiovascular disease (Coryell et al., 1982). It is important to note that a history of suicide attempts is one of the most powerful predictors of subsequent death by suicide. Of people attempting suicide, approximately 1% commit suicide each year during the 10 years after the first attempt. In addition, approximately 35% of people who die by suicide have made a previous attempt (Reich, 1989).

Although a substantial proportion of panic disorder patients (up to 75%) develop depression at some stage, Weissman et al. (1989) excluded depression as a cause of the suicide ideation. Other neuroses may predispose to depression, but none seems to carry the same substantial risk of suicide. Neither obsessive-compulsive disorder nor somatization disorder is associated with a significant risk of suicide (Coryell, 1988; Reiman, 1997). In contrast, about 15% of patients with primary depression die by suicide. In a prospective study of 955 patients with major affective disorder, one of the predictors of early suicide was coexisting panic attacks (Fawcett, 1988). Thus PD appears to carry a special status both as a primary risk factor for suicide and as a condition that may coexist with major depression (Korn et al., 1997; Lecrubier and Ustun, 1998).

Cardiovascular Mortality

The risk of cardiovascular-related death seems to be greater in males suffering from PD than those without PD. In a 35-year follow-up study of inpatients with panic disorder, the risk of cardiovascular mortality was twice that expected from age-specific or sex-specific vital statistics (Coryell et al., 1982). No such excess cardiovascular-related mortality was observed in comparable cohorts with somatization disorder (Coryell, 1981a), obsessive-compulsive disorder (Coryell, 1984), or primary depression (Coryell, 1981b).

The risk factors for coronary artery disease and stroke in panic disorder patients have not yet been systematically evaluated. However, both essential hypertension (Noyes et al., 1978) and heavy smoking are more prevalent in subjects suffering from anxiety neurosis than in the general population (Salmons and Sims, 1981). Since evaluation of a large group (1482) of inpatients with "severe neurosis" showed a similar trend of increased cardiovascular-related mortality in men (Sims, 1984), it seems reasonable to assume that a sex-related risk factor may also prevail in panic disorder patients. Other relevant risk factors in Sims's severe neurosis group include physical inactivity and raised serum cholesterol levels.

The potential implications of the conclusion that panic disorder is associated with increased cardiovascular mortality are considerable. It may introduce a major source of pressure into the minds of people who are already preoccupied with catastrophic thinking, particularly because chest pain is one of the most common expressions of panic attacks and fear of cardiac death often is a major concern during the attacks. As Fleet and Beitman (1998) noted, however, this idea is suggested by studies of certain categories of patients with PD (mostly men late in the course of the disorder), but it does not seem to apply to the majority of panic disorder sufferers (healthy women aged 30 to 55 years). Still, a number of the more persuasive prospective studies have shown an association between phobic anxiety, not specifically PD, and sudden cardiac death (Haines et al., 1987; Kawachi et al., 1994), and in a patient suffering from ischemic heart disease, it would seem plausible that an intense anxiety reaction might trigger a sudden, fatal arrhythmia. Since we have such effective therapy for anxiety disorders, the possible cardiovascular effects make it all the more important that patients at risk be identified.

MANAGEMENT OF PANIC DISORDER

There have been substantial advances in the management of panic disorder and agoraphobia with both drugs that have high efficacy and few side effects (Chapter 17) and cognitive-behavioral techniques. In a meta-analysis of 43 controlled studies that included 76 treatment interventions for panic disorder, Gould et al. (1995) compared the effectiveness of drug, cognitive-behavioral therapy (CBT), and combined drug and cognitive-behavioral treatments. They graded the treatment effects as follows: cognitive-behavioral (effect size = 0.68), combined drug and CBT (effect size = 0.56), and drugs alone (effect size = 0.47). They also noted that there was a much lower dropout rate in patients receiving CBT compared to those receiving drugs. Brown and Barlow (1995) found that while the impact of CBT was sustained over a reasonable period of time, among patients followed for up to two years, about 48% sought no further treatment for panic disorder during this time. This clearly indicates that even with initially effective CBT, patients should be followed for a couple of years at least since PD has a high relapse rate. A one- to two-year follow-up study of 124 consecutive patients treated for panic disorder and social phobia also showed significant improvement during treatment and further significant improvement during follow-up. A quarter of the participants no longer met diagnostic criteria, they had not sought further treatment, and their anxiety had stopped troubling them since the treatment (Hunt and Andrews, 1998). Other authors have emphasized the importance of treating and following agoraphobic avoidance since this may not remit on its own even with successful resolution of the panic attacks (Craske et al., 1991) and have argued that agoraphobic avoidance may be the most significant predictor of long-term outcome (Katschnig et al., 1995).

Cognitive-behavioral therapy may also reduce the panic-inducing effects of a 35% CO_2 challenge in PD patients. Schmidt et al. (1997). assigned 54 patients with panic disorder to one of three groups: CBT with respiratory training, CBT alone, or delayed treatment. Subjects received five repeated vital-capacity inhalations of 35% CO_2 before and following either 12 treatment sessions or a 12-

week waiting session. During the pretreatment assessments, 74% of patients experienced a panic attack during at least one inhalation. Following treatment, only 20% of treated participants compared to 64% of untreated patients panicked in response to the 35% CO_2 challenge. Furthermore, 44% of treated participants, compared with none of the untreated, reported no anxiety during all posttreatment inhalations.

Satisfactory control of panic disorder with medication may today be achieved in many patients suffering from PD. The tricyclic antidepressants (TCAs) are effective in reducing panic attacks and phobic avoidance (Gloger et al., 1981; Ballenger, 1986), as are the selective serotonin reuptake inhibitors (SSRIs) (Evans et al., 1986; Black et al., 1993; Hoehn-Saric et al., 1993) (see Chapter 17). However, the much more favorable tolerance of SSRIs and their generally more rapid onset of action compared to TCAs, as well as their usual once-a-day dosage, have made the SSRIs the preferred treatment (although once-a-day slow-release forms of TCAs are also available). Thus, in a study comparing paroxetine to clomipramine and placebo in 367 patients with DSM-IIIR–defined panic disorder, paroxetine appeared to have a more rapid onset of action than clomipramine in reducing the number of panic attacks to zero, and it was much better tolerated (Lecrubier et al., 1997). The efficacy of both groups of drugs in treating panic disorder is, however, equivalent.

The start of treatment with both groups of drugs may produce what appears to be an exacerbation of the anxiety and panic symptoms. This state usually lasts up to five or seven days, and in most patients resolves with continued treatment. For this reason patients need to be provided with maximum support and easy accessibility to their practitioner in these first few days in order to ensure that they continue with the medication until their situation stabilizes. If these exacerbated symptoms prove to be a real obstacle to the continued drug management of the patient, the problem may be handled either by stopping the medication for a few days until the symptoms subside and then beginning again with lower doses, raising the dose only when the medication is tolerated, or by the additional administration of a benzodiazepine such as alprazolam, which may be discontinued gradually as the SSRI clinical effectiveness improves over about two to four weeks (Ballenger et al., 1988). General practitioners should be aware, however, of a considerable tendency of alprazolam to be associated with dependency if administered over an extended period.

The foregoing discussion has centered on the management of PD, a diagnosis that implies the recurrence of panic attacks or panic attacks associated with persistent anxiety about further attacks (see Table 12-1). It is much more common in medical practice, however, to hear patients describe episodic panic attacks, usually at times of stress, and often simple reassurance dealing with the specific fears about the assumed significance of the attack is sufficient to allay anxiety. One of the principal objectives in managing the problem is to educate the patient to understand the association of panic attacks with anxiety or stress states—to learn to see it as part of that state—as well as providing reassurance that nothing harmful will actually happen no matter how bad the patient feels during the attack, as in many cases the patient may be in good health. Relaxation therapy during which the details of a typical attack are invoked often helps the patient lose the fear of attacks (Chapter 19), and a program of physical activity may help reduce the frequency and intensity of anxiety attacks (Chapter 13). Limited behavioral interventions and guidance regarding life-style such as a regular exercise program are often preferred by patients over the taking of drugs for an extended period.

REFERENCES

Ackerman SH, Sachar EJ (1974). The lactate theory of anxiety: a review and reevaluation. Psychosom Med 36:69–81.

Amaral DG, Insausti R (1992). Retrograde transport of D-[3H]-aspartate injected into the monkey amygdaloid complex. Exp Brain Res 88:375–388.

American Psychiatric Association (1994). Diagnostic and Statistical Manual of Mental Disorders, 4th ed. Washington, DC: Author.

Aronson TA, Craig TJ (1986). Cocaine precipitation of panic disorder. Am J Psychiatry 143:643–645.

Ballenger JC (1986). Pharmacotherapy of the panic disorders. J Clin Psychiatry 47(suppl 6):27–32.

Ballenger JC (1997). Panic disorder in the medical setting. J Clin Psychiatry 58(suppl 2):13–17.

Ballenger JC, Burrows G, Dupont RL, et al. (1988). Alprazolam in panic disorder and agoraphobia: results from a multicenter trial: 1. Efficacy in short-term treatment. Arch Gen Psychiatry 45:413–422.

Beck AT, Laude R, Bohnert M (1974). Ideational components of anxiety neurosis. Arch Gen Psychiatry 31:319–325.

Beckstead RM, Morse JR, Norgren R (1980). The nucleus of the solitary tract in the monkey: projections to the thalamus and brain stem nuclei. J Comp Neurol 190:259–282.

Beekman AT, Bremmer MA, Deeg DJ, et al. (1998). Anxiety disorders in later life: a report from the Longitudenal Aging Study Amsterdam. Int J Geriatr Psychiatry 13:717–726.

Bellodi L, Perna G, Caldirola D, et al. (1998). CO_2-induced panic attacks: a twin study. Am J Psychiatry 155:1184–1188.

Black DW, Wesner R, Bowers W, et al. (1993). A comparison of fluvoxamine, cognitive therapy, and placebo in the treatment of panic disorder. Arch Gen Psychiatry 50:44–50.

Bonn JA, Readhead CP, Timmons BH (1984). Enhanced adaptive behavioral response in agoraphobic patients pretreated with breathing retraining. Lancet 2:665–669.

Bradwejn J, Koszycki D, Bourin M (1991). Dose ranging study of the effects of cholecystokinin in healthy volunteers. J Psychiatry Neurosci 16:91–95.

Breier A, Charney DS, Heninger GR (1986). Agoraphobia with panic attacks: development, diagnostic stability, and course of illness. Arch Gen Psychiatry. 43:1029–1036.

Bridges KW, Goldberg BP (1985). Somatic presentation of DSM-III psychiatric disorders in primary care. J Psychosom Res 29:563–569.

Brown TA, Barlow DH (1995). Long-term outcome in cognitive-behavioral treatment of panic disorder: clinical predictors and alternative strategies for assessment. J Consult Clin Psychol 63:754–765.

Buchel C, Morris J, Dolan RJ, et al. (1998). Brain systems mediating aversive conditioning: an event-related fMRI study. Neuron 20:947–957.

Carr DB, Sheehan DV (1984). Panic anxiety: a new biological model. J Clin Psychiatry 45:323–330.

Charney DS, Heninger GR, Breier A (1984). Noradrenergic function in panic anxiety: effects of yohimbine in healthy subjects and patients with agoraphobia and panic disorder. Arch Gen Psychiatry 41:751–763.

Charney DS, Heninger GR, Jatlow PI (1985). Increased anxiogenic effects of caffeine in panic disorders. Arch Gen Psychiatry 42:233–243.

Clark DM, Hemsley DR (1982). The effects of hyperventilation; individual variability and its relation to personality. J Behav Ther Exp Psychiatry 13:41–47.

Coplan JD, Lydiard RB (1998). Brain circuits in panic disorder. Biol Psychiatry 44:1264–1276.

Coryell W (1981a). Diagnosis-specific mortality: primary unipolar depression and Briquet's syndrome (somatization disorder). Arch Gen Psychiatry 38:939–942.

Coryell W (1981b). Obsessive-compulsive disorder and primary unipolar depression: comparisons of background, family history, course, and mortality. J Nerv Ment Dis 169:220–224.

Coryell W (1984). Mortality after thirty to forty years: panic disorder compared to other psychiatric illnesses. In: Grinspoon L, ed. Psychiatric Update, The American Psychiatric Association Annual Review, Vol III.

Coryell W (1988). Panic disorder and mortality. Psychiatr Clin North Am 11:433–440.

Coryell W, Noyes R, Clancy J (1982). Excess mortality in panic disorder: a comparison with primary unipolar depression. Arch Gen Psychiatry 39:701–703.

Craske MG, Brown TA, Barlow DH (1991). Behavioral treatment of panic: a two-year follow-up. J Behav Ther 22:289–304.

Crowe RR, Noyes R Jr, Pauls DL, et al. (1983). A family study of panic disorder. Arch Gen Psychiatry 40:1065–1069.

Crowe RR, Pauls DL, Slymen DJ, et al. (1980). A genetic study of anxiety neurosis. Arch Gen Psychiatry 37:77–79.

Deckert J, Catalano M, Heils A, et al. (1997). Functional promoter polymorphism of the human serotonin transporter: lack of association with panic disorder. Psychiatr Genet 7:45–47.

Deckert J, Catalano M, Syagailo YV, et al. (1999). Excess of high activity monoamine oxidase A gene promoter alleles in female patients with panic disorder. Hum Mol Genet 8:621–624.

Deckert J, Nothen MM, Franke P, et al. (1998). Systematic mutation screening and association study of the A1 and A2a adenosine receptor genes in panic disorder suggest a contribution of the A2a gene to the development of disease. Mol Psychiatry 3:81–85.

Easton JD, Sherman DG (1976). Somatic anxiety attacks and propranolol. Arch Neurol 33:689–691.

Ehlers A, Margraf J, Roth WT, et al. (1986). Lactate infusions and panic attacks: do patients and controls respond differently? Psychiatr Res 17:295–308.

Elam M, Yoa T, Thoren, P, et al. (1981). Hypercapnia and hypoxia: chemoreceptor-mediated control of locus ceruleus, neurons and splanchnic sympathetic nerves. Brain Res 222:373–381.

Evans L, Kenardy J, Schneider P, et al. (1986). Effect of a selective serotonin uptake inhibitor in agoraphobia with panic attacks. Acta Psychiatr Scand 73:49–53.

Fawcett J (1988). Predictors of early suicide: identification and appropriate intervention. J Clin Psychiatry 49(suppl):7–8.

Fink M, Taylor MA, Volovka J (1970). Anxiety precipitated by lactate [letter]. N Engl J Med 281:1129.

Fleet RP, Beitman BD (1998). Cardiovascular death from panic disorder and panic-like anxiety: a critical review of the literature. J Psychosom Res 44:71–80.

Flint AJ, Koszycki D, Vaccirino FJ, et al. (1998). Effect of aging on cholecystokinin-induced panic. Am J Psychiatry 155:283–285.

Garssen B, Buikhuisen M, van Dyck R (1996). Hyperventilation and panic attacks. Am J Psychiatry 153:513–518.

George DT, Lindquist T, Nutt DJ, et al. (1995). Effects of chloride or glucose on the incidence of lactate-induced panic attacks. Am J Psychiatry 52:692–697.

Gloger S, Grunhaus L, Birmacher B, et al. (1981). Treatment of spontaneous panic attacks with clomipramine. Am J Psychiatry 138:1215–1217.

Gorman JM, Ashkenazi J, Liebowitz MR, et al. (1984). Response to hyperventilation in a group of patients with panic disorder. Am J Psychiatry 141:857–861.

Gorman JM, Liebowitz MR, Fyer AJ, et al. (1989). A neuroanatomical hypothesis for panic disorder. Am J Psychiatry 146:148–161.

Gould RA, Otto MW, Pollack MH (1995). A meta-analysis of treatment outcome for panic disorder. Clin Psychol Rev 15:819–844.

Grove G, Coplan JD, Hollander E (1997). The neuroanatomy of 5-HT dysregulation and panic disorder. J Neuropsychiatry Clin Neurosci 9:198–207.

Haines AP, Imeson JD, Meade TW (1987). Phobic anxiety and ischemic heart disease. Br Med J 295:297–299.

Harris EL, Noyes R Jr, Crowe RR, et al. (1983). Family study of agoraphobia: report of a pilot study. Arch Gen Psychiatry 40:1061–1064.

Hegel MT, Ferguson RJ (1997). Psychophysiological assessment of respiratory function in panic disorder: evidence for a hyperventilation subtype. Psychosom Med 59:224–230.

Heinrichs SC, Lapsansky J, Lovenberg TW, et al. (1997). Corticotrophin-releasing factor CRF1, but not CRF2, receptors mediate anxiogenic-like behavior. Regul Pept 71:15–21.

Hibbert GA, Pilsbury D (1989). Hyperventilation: is it a cause of panic attacks? Br J Psychiatry 155:805–809.

Hoehn-Saric R, McLeod DR, Hipsley PA (1993). Effect of fluvoxamine in panic disorder. J Clin Psychopharmacol 13:321–326.

Holister L (1980). A look at the issues: use of minor tranquilizers. Psychosomatics 21:4–6.

Hunt C, Andrews G (1998). Long-term outcome of panic disorder and social phobia. J Anxiety Dis 12:395–406.

Kalia M (1977). Neuroanatomical organization of the respiratory centers. Fed Proc 36:2405–2411.

Katerndahl DA, Realini JP (1995). Where do panic sufferers seek care? J Fam Pract 40:237–243.

Katschnig H, Amering A, Stolk JM, et al. (1995). Long-term outcome in panic disorder. Br J Psychiatry 167:487–494.

Kawachi I, Colditz GA, Ascherio A, et al. (1994). Prospective study of phobic anxiety and risk of coronary heart disease in men. Circulation 89:1992–1997.

Kelly D, Mitchell-Heggs N, Sherman D (1971). Anxiety and the effects of sodium lactate assessed clinically and physiologically. Br J Psychiatry 119:129–141.

Knowles JA, Fyer AJ, Vieland VJ, et al. (1998). Results of a genome-wide genetic screen for panic disorder. Am J Med Genet 81:139–147.

Korn ML, Plutchik R, Van Praag HM (1997). Panic-associated suicide and aggressive ideation and behavior. J Psychiatr Res 31:481–487.

Krasucki C, Howard R, Mann A (1998). The relationship between anxiety disorders and age. Int J Geriatr Psychiatry 13:79–99.

Last CG, Barlow DH, O'Brien GT (1984). Precipitants of agoraphobia: role of stressful life events. Psychol Rep 54:567–570.

Lecrubier Y, Bakker A, Dunbar G, et al. (1997). A comparison of paroxetine, clomipramine and placebo in the treatment of panic disorder. Acta Psychiatr Scand 95:145–152.

Lecrubier Y, Ustun TB (1998). Panic and depression: a worldwide primary care perpective. Int Clin Psychopharmacol 13 (suppl 4):S7–11.

Ledoux J (1998). Fear and brain: where have we been, and where are we going? Biol Psychiatry 44:1229–1238.

Lesch KP, Bengel D, Heils A, et al. (1996). Association of anxiety-related traits with a polymorphism in the serotonin transporter gene regulatory region. Science 274:1483–1487.

Lessmeier TJ, Gamperling D, Johnson-Liddon V, et al. (1997). Unrecognized paroxysmal supraventricular tachycardia: potential for misdiagnosis as panic disorder. Arch Intern Med 157:537–543.

Ley R (1985). Blood, breath and fears: a hyperventilation theory of panic attacks and agoraphobia. Clin Psychol Rev 5:79–81.

Liebowitz MR, Gorman JM, Fyer A, et al. (1986). Possible mechanisms for lactate's induction of panic. Am J Psychiatry 143:495–502.

Lum LC (1981). Hyperventilation and anxiety state. J R Soc Med 74:1–4.

Margraf J, Ehlers A, Roth WT (1986). Biological models of panic disorder and agoraphobia: a review. Behav Res Ther 24:553–567.

Margraf J, Ehlers A, Roth WT (1987). Panic attack associated with perceived heart rate acceleration: a case report. Behav Ther 18:84–89.

Markowitz JS, Weissman MM, Ouellettte R, et al. (1989). Quality of life in panic disorder. Arch Gen Psychiatry 46:984–992.

Neutra WJH, Domesick VB (1981). Ramifications of the limbic system. In: Matthysse S, ed. Psychiatry and the Biology of the Human Brain. New York: Elsevier.

Noyes R, Clancy J, Hoenck CR, et al. (1978). Anxiety neurosis and physical illness. Compr Psychiatry 19:407–413.

Pauls DL, Bucher KD, Crowe RR, et al. (1980). A genetic study of panic disorder pedigrees. Am J Hum Genet 32:639–644.

Perna G, Bussi R, Allevi L, et al. (1999). Sensitivity to 35% carbon dioxide in patients with generalized anxiety disorder. J Clin Psychiatry 60:379–384.

Perna G, Caldirola D, Arancio C, et al. (1997). Panic attacks: a twin study. Psychiatr Res 66:69–71.

Peskind ER, Jensen CF, Pascualy M, et al. (1998). Sodium lactate and hypertonic sodium chloride induce equivalent panic incidence, panic symptoms, and hypernatremia in panic disorder. Biol Psychiatry 44:1007–1016.

Pitts FN Jr, McClure JN Jr (1967). Lactate metabolism in anxiety neurosis. N Engl J Med 277:1329–1336.

Rainey JM Jr, Pohl RB, Williams M, et al. (1984). A comparison of lactate and isoproterenol anxiety states. Psychopathology 17(suppl 1):74–82.

Reed V, Wittchen HU (1998). DSM-IV panic attacks and panic disorder in a community sample of adolescents and young adults: how specific are panic attacks? J Psychiatr Res 32:335–345.

Reich P (1989). Panic attacks and the risk of suicide [editorial]. N Engl Med 321:1260–1261.

Reiman EM (1997). The application of positron emission tomography to the study of normal and pathological emotions. J Clin Psychiatry 58(suppl 16):4–12.

Rosenbaum JF (1987). Limited-symptom panic attacks. Psychosomatics 28:407–412.

Roy-Byrne PP, Geraci M, Uhde TW (1986). Life events and course of illness in patients with panic disorder. Am J Psychiatry 143:1033–1035.

Roy-Byrne PP, Stein MB, Russo J, et al. (1999). Panic disorder in the primary care setting: comorbidity, disability, service utilization, and treatment. J Clin Psychiatry 60:492–499.

Roy-Byrne PP, Uhde TW, Post RM, et al. (1985). Normal pain sensitivity in patients with panic disorder. Psychiatr Res 14:75–82.

Salkovskis PM, Jones DRO, Clark DM (1986). Respiratory control in the treatment of panic attacks: replication and extension with concurrent measurement of behavior and pCO_2. Br J Psychiatry 148:526–532.

Salmons P, Sims A (1981). Smoking profiles of patients admitted for neurosis. Br J Psychiatry 139:43–.

Schmidt NB, Trakowski JH, Staab JP (1997). Extinction of panicogenic effects of a 35% CO2 challenge in patients with panic disorder. J Abnorm Psychol 106:630–638.

Schweitzer E, Winokur A, Rickels K (1986). Insulin-induced hypoglycemia and panic attacks. Am J Psychiatry 143:654–655.

Shapiro S, Skinner EA, Kessler LG, et al. (1988). Utilization of health and mental health services: three epidemiological Catchment Area sites. Arch Gen Psychiatry 49(suppl): 7–8.

Sheehan DV, Ballenger J, Jacobsen G (1980). Treatment of endogenous anxiety with phobic, hysterical, and hypochondriacal symptoms. Arch Gen Psychiatry 37:51–59.

Sims A (1984). Neurosis and mortality: investigating and association. J Psychosom Res 28:353.

Strian F (1987). Psychiatrische Aspektes des Mitralklappenprolapse-Syndroms. In: Nutzinger DO, Pfersman D, Welan T, Zapatoczky H-G, eds. Die Herzphobie. Stuttgart: Enke, pp 66–74.

Uhde TW, Vittone BJ, Post RM (1984). Glucose tolerance testing in panic disorder. Am J Psychiatry 141:1461–1463.

Vieland VJ, Goodman DW, Chapman T, et al. (1996). New segregation analysis of panic disorder. Am J Med Genet 67:147–153.

Washton AM, Gold MS (1984). Chronic cocaine abuse: evidence for adverse effects on health and functioning. Psychiatr Ann 14:733–739.

Weissman MM (1988). The epidemiology of panic disorder and agoraphobia. In: Hales RE, Frances AJ, eds. Review of Psychiatry, vol 7. Washington, DC: American Psychiatric Press, pp 54–66.

Weissman MM, Klerman GL, Markowitz JS, et al. (1989). Suicidal ideation and suicide attempts in panic disorder and attacks. N Engl J Med 321:1209–1214.

Yeragani V, Balon R, Pohl R (1989). Lactate infusions in panic disorder patients and normal controls: autonomic measures and subjective anxiety. Acta Psychiatr Scand 79:32–40.

Chapter

13

CARDIOVASCULAR CHANGES IN ANXIETY: A LESSON IN INTEGRATIVE PSYCHOPHYSIOLOGY

We have previously analyzed in some detail the way that emotional factors may interplay with, and negatively influence, some clinical disorders. The mechanisms presented in Chapter 8 describe the interplay of the nervous system with specific disease processes and are therefore largely directed at particular organs or tissue functions. The processes presented in this chapter, by contrast, are physical changes of a general kind that may occur as a result of anxiety in particular but also depression, and that may in turn aggravate or perpetuate the emotional condition. The extreme degrees of physical unfitness often associated, for example, with more persistent states of anxiety may have profound consequences on cardiovascular, respiratory, and nervous (particularly autonomic) function. Understanding the processes involved allows the practitioner to evaluate more comprehensively patients whose clinical conditions have a significant affective component, and the knowledge gained often offers additional, valuable therapeutic options for the management of these cases.

We also consider here the related clinical entity of symptomatic primary mitral valve prolapse (MVP). In this condition, symptoms such as palpitations, breathlessness, or chest pain, or some combination of them, are associated with the auscultatory or echocardiographic finding of MVP. The usual assumption is that the mitral valve prolapse, the organic finding, causes the symptoms, the functional component. In those cases where mitral valve prolapse is associated with hemodynamically significant mitral incompetence, this may be true. These cases usually involve abnormal valve morphology (Nishimura et al., 1985; Marks et al., 1989) and are associated with either connective tissue disorders (see below) or localized degeneration of the valve, mostly in older men (Duren et al., 1988). However, there is a larger group of patients who suffer similar symptoms and who are shown to have MVP without significant insufficiency or abnormal valve morphology. In this group, the MVP and the symptoms may each be independently associated with a particular emotional state. The processes contributing to this state are elaborated in this chapter.

ANXIETY AND PHYSICAL ACTIVITY

The Cardiovascular Effects

Clinical experience has confirmed the frequently documented observation that patients suffering from chronic anxiety states and particularly panic disorder are disinclined to exercise: This is generally attributed to lack of energy and also to the fact that exercise-induced palpitations tend to increase anxiety. As a result, symptomatically anxious patients are almost invariably physically unfit (Jones and Mellersh, 1946; Crowe et al., 1979). In the presence of sustained anxiety, even mild exercise or transient emotional stimuli may induce striking tachycardia, more forceful ventricular contraction, and increased cardiac output (Wolf and Wolff, 1946; Hickam et al., 1948), and tolerance for more demanding effort may be considerably reduced. Lassitude (lack of energy), which may be extreme, is a common complaint. Ambulatory electrocardiographic monitoring of 67 patients with neurocirculatory asthenia (an older designation, seldom used today, for a clinical state corresponding to the chronic fatigue syndrome), compared with 33 healthy controls, showed a tendency to sinus tachycardia (>120 beats/min) unrelated to effort in 60 of the patients: 35 had frequent episodes of pronounced sinus arrhythmia, 16 showed transient ST depression, and 6 showed transient ST elevation (Tzivoni et al., 1980). In addition, ventricular premature beats were much more common in the patients than in controls.

Physical inactivity over prolonged periods may produce significant changes in blood volume and cardiac dynamics. With lack of physical activity like prolonged bed rest for at least two or three weeks, blood volume contracts by up to 15%–18%. This seems to occur consistently regardless of the cause of confinement to bed (Rutstein et al., 1945; Taylor et al., 1945; Meneely et al., 1947; Convertino, 1997). These blood volume changes may play a role in the classical complaints of patients convalescing from chronic illness, which are remarkably similar to the symptoms of panic disorder and symptomatic MVP patients: palpitations, tachycardia, postural dizziness, and dyspnea (Meneely et al., 1947). Conversely, expansion of blood volume is relatively easily achieved through moderate exercise programs, which also improve orthostatic tolerance (Mtinangi and Hainsworth, 1998), increase left ventricular stroke and end-diastolic volumes (Mier et al., 1997; Hagberg et al., 1998), and enhance the inotropic response to β-adrenergic stimulation (Mier et al., 1997).

The observed reduction in left ventricular end-diastolic volume in the upright position in MVP patients, both at rest and during exercise, supports the idea that decreased ventricular filling in the upright position may contribute to the pathophysiology of this state, particularly in the more symptomatic patients, who may complain of palpitations and dizziness and sometimes syncope when standing. Furthermore, reduced circulating blood volume is a potent stimulus to sympathetic activation, particularly in the standing position, as is the acidosis produced by anaerobic muscle activity. At the start of physical activity there is a rapid decrease of vagal tone, followed by an increase in sympathetic discharge as the physical activity continues (Victor et al., 1987). The natural tendency for the heart rate to increase when physical activity begins is mediated by these reflexes, which in the unfit symptomatic patient may easily lead to palpitations that cause emotional distress, thus discouraging continuation of the exercise.

When a person stands up, the cardiac output drops by about 20% with the pooling of blood in the veins of the legs, producing a sudden hypovolemic state (Sannerstedt et al., 1970). The fall in blood pressure stimulates carotid and aortic arch baroreceptor activation of sympathetic activity, resulting normally in a rapid restoration of blood pressure through an increase in vascular resistance (Julius, 1988). It is possible that sustained or recurrent sympathetic activation with frequent vasoconstriction, as occurs in anxiety and panic disorder patients, may be sufficient to produce a state of hypovolemia (Gaffney et al., 1983). In panic disorder patients the fall in blood pressure on standing (orthostatic drop) is greater than in controls and persists into remission of the PD (Middleton, 1990). The cardiovascular and autonomic changes described in populations of patients with panic disorder or MVP are remarkably similar to the condition termed idiopathic hypovolemia (Jacob et al., 1997; Kuchel and Leveille, 1998). Here patients suffer from episodic hypertension, hypotension, or orthostatic intolerance (dizzyness or fainting on standing for a few minutes), tachycardia, anxiety, and flushing. As the name implies, these symptoms are attributed to a state of hypovolemia. Although anxiety is listed by both Jacob et al. and by Kuchel and Leveille as one of the prominent symptoms, they emphasize instead other elements of the condition such as patterns of hormone secretion, especially catecholamines and renin-angiotensin.

In the chronic fatigue syndrome (CFS) (see Chapter 15), a condition characterized by extremes of physical unfitness, symptoms of orthostatic intolerance such as disabling fatigue, dizziness, diminished concentration, and tremulousness are often evident. Cardiovascular deconditioning has been proposed as the basis for this state, but viral neuropathy and "a partial autonomic defect" have also been suggested as possible mechanisms (Schondorf et al., 1999; Stewart et al., 1999). The efficacy of programs of graded exercise in improving cardiovascular function in CFS patients strongly supports the deconditioning hypothesis (Mc-Cully et al., 1996; Fulcher and White, 1997). Stewart et al. (1999) studied the blood pressure and heart rate responses to head-up tilting of 26 adolescents aged 11 to 19 years with CFS compared to 13 normal healthy control children of similar age and 26 adolescence who had had a simple faint. Of the 26 CFS subjects, 25 experienced severe orthostatic symptoms, associated with syncope in 7, orthostatic tachycardia and hypotension in 15, and tachycardia alone in 3 subjects. A total of 4 of the 13 controls and 18 of 26 simple faint patients experienced typical faints with an abrupt blood pressure and heart rate decrease associated with loss of consciousness.

If the presence of MVP reflects a reduction of left ventricle volume, then we may ask whether a reduced intravascular volume is also a characteristic of MVP patients who are asymptomatic. This may be suggested by a study of asymptomatic pilots with stringently confirmed MVP and normal psychiatric status (Whinnery, 1986). Abnormal acceleration tolerance, manifesting as loss of consciousness, was documented in 15% of 78 U.S. Air Force pilots with MVP, as opposed to 7% of 1126 without MVP. This study shows that in healthy, asymptomatic subjects the presence of MVP may be associated with subtle differences in circulatory responses, presumably due to changes in blood volume and autonomic control. For asymptomatic MVP subjects, however, these differences are of no clinical significance in the usual repertoire of day-to-day activities, since the autonomic reflexes and circulatory adjustments that occur are adequate for the demands.

The Metabolic Effects

The tendency to unfitness in these and other anxious subjects is associated with a reduced maximum oxygen uptake (Vo_2max) (Convertino, 1997), an increased oxygen demand by skeletal muscles, and a greater tendency to produce lactate on exertion (Saltin et al., 1968; Holloszy and Booth, 1976). Excessive lactate production on standard exercise has been reported in patients with "anxiety neurosis" (Jones and Mellersh, 1946; Linko, 1950; Holmgren and Strom, 1959). Similar metabolic changes have also been documented in the chronic fatigue syndrome, another condition in which patients show a pronounced intolerance to physical exertion (Lloyd et al., 1988; Riley et al., 1990).

Intravenous infusion of lactate is a well-known inducer of panic attacks, which suggests that its enhanced endogenous production may be yet another mechanism underlying panic attacks in a susceptible person. But in a study of blood lactate increases induced in panic disorder sufferers by either infusion or strenuous exercise, panic occurred in 16 of 24 patients after infusion but only in 1 of the group following strenuous exercise (Martinsen et al., 1998). The blood lactate levels observed after exercise (ave 10.7 mmol/L) were much higher than those obtained after infusion (ave 5.5 mmol/L). A plausible explanation for this differential effect is provided by the observation that it is probably the sodium rather than the lactate in the sodium lactate infusion which is the active factor in inducing panic symptoms (Peskind et al., 1998) (see Chapter 12).

Autonomic Lability

More elaborate evaluation of MVP patients, with a variety of tests of autonomic responses, reveals a much wider variability of response in most parameters tested compared to controls. For example, MVP patients showed a much greater oscillation of the heart rate in the upright position as well as an exaggerated and prolonged bradycardia during the recovery phase of the Valsalva maneuver and after their return to recumbency in the postural test (Coghlan, 1988). Greater catecholamine response in MVP patients on standing, coupled with a decreased stroke volume on measurement of cardiac output, strongly suggests that these patients have a reduced blood volume (Gaffney et al., 1983).

As with other categories of anxious patients (Lader and Wing, 1964), physiological studies of autonomic activation show that panic disorder patients with agoraphobia exhibit clear signs of increased autonomic activation. Their most consistent differences from normal controls are tonically elevated levels of skin conductance and heart rate (Roth et al., 1986). Surprisingly, when these patients were exposed to sudden loud noise of controlled intensity and duration, there was no difference in the responsiveness of patients and controls as measured by heart rate change. Other studies of anxious patients have actually demonstrated less responsiveness of the heart rate to the stress of mental arithmetic than in control subjects (Kelly et al., 1970). Only certain measures of autonomic activity thus appear to be increased on a chronic basis in panic disorder patients. Furthermore, it is clear from these studies that the lability of autonomic activity exhibited by most of these patients is not generalized to all stimuli. Certain subgroups of PD patients exhibit striking autonomic dysfunction, mostly in the direction of sympathetic hyperresponsivity, although some studies also indicate excessive vagal tone and responsiveness. Patients with panic disorder may show increased resting and standing plasma catecholamines compared to control subjects (Pasternac et al., 1982; Gaffney et al., 1983), a factor that may contribute to a vigorous physical response and intensified panic symptoms during attacks.

Changes at the Membrane Level: Receptor Hyperresponsivity

The possibility that the exaggerated autonomic responses reported in MVP patients may result from β-adrenergic hypersensitivity was investigated by Davies et al. (1987). In this study, isoproteronol was infused in order to either increase the heart rate by 25 beats/min or reduce the blood pressure by 20 mm Hg. The dose required for these effects was significantly less in the MVP patients than in controls. These authors proposed a state of "supercoupling" of the β-adrenergic receptor with the selective agonist, isoproteronol. This conclusion was supported by *in vitro* observations on the interaction of isoproteronol with neutrophil membranes, where despite similar receptor numbers and comparable binding affinities in both groups, about twice as much cyclic AMP (cAMP) was produced in membranes derived from the MVP patients as in those from controls.

This enhancement of β-adrenergic responses to agonist stimulation is reminiscent of corticosteroid-induced effects seen in the same system: marked potentiation of the production of cAMP by adenylate cyclase following receptor-mediated agonist stimulation. The increase in cAMP production following corticosteroid administration may be as much as a hundredfold more than the untreated condition (Davies and Lefkowitz, 1980; Davies and Lefkowitz, 1981). Panic disorder patients may manifest a basal hypercortisolism similar to that seen in depression and some other psychiatric disorders (Avery et al., 1985; Roy-Byrne et al., 1986). The increased circulating cortisol may enhance β-adrenergic responsiveness to endogenous catecholamines, thereby contributing to a hyperresponsive state. However, the probable operation of additional mechanisms at the cell membrane level is suggested by the observation that some depressed patients, despite their tendency to basal hypercortisolism, show impaired β-adrenergic sensitivity to agonist stimulation (Pandey et al.,1979; Mann et al., 1985). This occurs in spite of an adenylate cyclase system that could be activated by bypassing this receptor mechanism, suggesting the operation of a modulating process between adenylate cyclase and the ligand–receptor complex in the plasma membrane.

MITRAL VALVE PROLAPSE

I have suggested that the symptomatic patient with MVP is in effect suffering principally from an anxiety syndrome with an associated MVP, and because many of the changes described in the previous section for patients with anxiety syndromes occur as well in symptomatic MVP patients, we now look more closely at MVP.

Mitral valve prolapse may occur as part of a generalized connective tissue disorder such as Marfan's or Ehlers-Danlos syndrome, or in other inherited disorders such as polycystic kidney disease, Klinefelter syndrome, and genetic disorders of the myocardium. It may also result from a localized myxomatous degeneration of the mitral valve. These cases are usually classified as secondary forms of the disorder and occur much more rarely in the general population than the comparatively common and predominant primary form. Marfan's syndrome, one of the best documented of the secondary forms, accounts for only about 1 in 500 cases of MVP (Roman et al., 1989).

Echocardiography, which visualizes the anatomical structure and function of the heart valves, remains the most objective and now widely accepted way of diagnosing the abnormality. There has been a tendency to overdiagnose the defect by echocardiography due to a faulty appreciation of the appropriate diagnostic criteria (Levine and Weyman, 1984). This led to the view that MVP occurs in as much as 20% of the population (Markiewicz et al., 1976). In recent years the overall prevalence of MVP in the general population was estimated, however, to be closer to 5% (Savage et al., 1983; Bryhn and Persson, 1984). With greater refinement of the diagnostic criteria, the estimate dropped even further. In the Framingham Heart Study of a community-based sample of 1845 women and 1646 men, 2.4% had "classic" prolapse—a superior displacement of the mitral leaflets of more than 2 mm during systole and a maximum leaflet thickness of at least 5 mm during diastasis—and 1.3% had nonclassic prolapse—a displacement of more than 2 mm and a maximum thickness of less than 5 mm (Freed et al., 1999). Using comparable diagnostic criteria, Gilon et al. (1999) found a similar prevalence in a population of patients aged 45 or less (213 patients and 263 controls) who had suffered from stroke. With this categorization, our primary group would be mostly classified as nonclassic MVP.

Although the precise cause of primary MVP is not known, the evidence favors a role for inherited factors, with an autosomal dominant expression. Sex, age, and body build appear to be important factors in the primary expression of MVP. The incidence of MVP used to be considered greatest in women between the ages of 20 and 50 years. There may be an up to 50% expression of MVP in adult female first-degree relatives; adult men, older women (over 50 years), and children of both sexes show a lower level of expression (Devereux et al., 1982a). Thin, slightly built people have a greater tendency to MVP (Devereux et al., 1982b; Cohen et al., 1987; Flack et al., 1999; Freed et al., 1999).

Mitral valve prolapse is associated characteristically with midsystolic clicks and late-systolic murmurs on auscultation of the heart (Barlow et al., 1963). Typically, the midsystolic clicks shift their timing in relation to the first and second heart sounds with maneuvers that alter the relationship between the size (volume) of the left ventricle in relation to the mitral valve annulus (Perloff and Child, 1987). With maneuvers that reduce ventricle size, such as sitting and standing, the systolic click is heard earlier in systole and the systolic murmur is prolonged, that is, the defect is exaggerated. Squatting, which increases chamber size and diminishes the severity of the defect, results in a late systolic click and a shorter systolic murmur.

Several authors have emphasized the variability of these clinical signs. A study in which 137 subjects with echocardiographically demonstrated MVP were examined twice in a standardized protocol at a mean interval of four years confirmed that auscultatory findings change with time, at least slightly, in most individuals (Devereux et al., 1987). Some authors have emphasized that prolapse of the anterior cusp represents the more benign form of the disorder, and one study found that approximately 20% of anterior cusp MVP patients remitted spontaneously (Kamei et al., 1999). The disappearance of MVP has been documented in panic attack patients in remission for more than six months (Gorman, 1986), as well as in treated patients suffering from anorexia nervosa (Meyers et al., 1986). This variability is characteristic of MVP and probably accounts for the reported discordance of findings between different diagnostic modalities (Barron et al., 1988). These observations strengthen the view that the mobility of the mitral valve cusps and their position in relation to the atrioventricular annulus during ventricular systole are part of a physiological continuum. Left ventricular volume is influenced by posture, circulating blood volume, and sympathetic stimulation of myocardial contractility, all of which seem to play a role in the genesis of MVP.

The Clinical Picture

One of the enduring controversies in clinical cardiology, from the time MVP was first described as a clinical entity (Barlow et al., 1963) and for almost 30 years thereafter, concerns the range of symptoms attributable to the presence of MVP (Retchin et al., 1986). Following the first reports of MVP as a defined clinical entity, a number of studies emphasized that nonanginal chest pain, dyspnea, and anxiety-related symptoms were commonly associated with MVP. Controlled studies performed in tertiary care hospitals have tended to confirm such an association (Devereux et al., 1986; Retchin et al., 1986). But because it is only symptomatic patients, and in particular those who are most distressed by their symptoms, who are admitted to hospitals and subjected to the most intense clinical scrutiny, an *ascertainment bias* is clearly operative in many of the studies reported (Motulsky, 1978). An asymptomatic individual in whom MVP is discovered during a routine physical or echocardiographic examination is unlikely to arouse clinical curiosity. As a result, unless evaluation is performed in an unselected population (matched for age and sex), an inevitable bias results from introducing the most symptomatic patients into the study. In the community-based study by Freed et al. (1999) cited earlier, no difference between those with and without MVP was observed in the frequency of chest pain, dyspnea, or syncope. A series of studies addressing this problem (reviewed by Devereux et al. [1989]) indicate that nonanginal chest pain, dyspnea, anxiety symptoms, and prolongation of the electrocardiographic QT interval occur with equal frequency in patients with MVP and in cardiovascularly normal individuals evaluated in the same clinical setting.

Morbidity and Mortality of Mitral Valve Prolapse

The presence of MVP, like that of any other mitral valve malfunction, may also predispose the individual to a number of other disorders. The two most common complications of MVP are transient ischemic attacks and bacterial endocarditis.

Transient ischemic attacks (TIAs) are strokes due to the embolization of cerebral or retinal vessels by very small platelet and thrombus particles that become detached from the prolapsed valve. Clinically, this process of microembolization produces transient neurological or visual disturbances such as weakness in a limb or amaurosis fugax. Amaurosis fugax designates the painless, transient loss of vision in one eye. In relation to MVP, it is assumed to be due to retinal ischemia resulting from a small fibrin-platelet thrombus occluding the retinal artery or one of its branches.

Bacterial endocarditis is a complication that may develop on a prolapsed mitral valve. Prophylactic antibiotics to prevent endocarditis following dental treatment or colonic studies such as barium enema or colonoscopy may be as important here as in patients with rheumatic valvular disease (Clemens et al., 1982). The reported incidence with bacterial endocarditis on prolapsed mitral valves varies between 1% and 10% (Allen et al., 1974; Bisset et al., 1980), although these figures probably relate to patients with anatomical changes of the valve cusps.

It must be stressed that the most recent studies indicate that the primary or nonclassic MVP we are considering here is extremely unlikely to lead to any significant complication (Freed et al., 1999; Nishimura and McGoon, 1999). In one study of a group of 60 patients under 45 years old who had suffered TIAs, using early echocardiographic criteria which increased the number of false positives, 40% were found to have MVP in the absence of any other condition that may have predisposed them to the development of the emboli. The control subjects had a 10% incidence of MVP (Barnett et al., 1980). However, in a case-control study of 213 consecutive patients 45 years of age or younger with documented ischemic stroke or transient ischemic attacks, MVP was present in 1.9% compared to 2.7% of 263 control subjects (Gilon et al., 1999). The latter study used stricter echocardiographic criteria for MVP than had earlier studies. Thus, primary MVP seems to pose no special risk of stroke or TIA. Similarly, the overall mortality of MVP patients is not significantly different from that of age- and sex-matched controls. Sudden death, presumably from ventricular arrhythmia, has been reported in MVP patients, but it is rare. Most of the reported cases seem to involve a small subset of women with abnormal resting electrocardiograms, prolonged QT intervals, a family history of sudden death, or compex ventricular ectopic beats (Devereux et al., 1976; Chesler et al., 1983).

Mitral Valve Prolapse and Anxiety

When patients with panic disorder (with or without agoraphobia) are evaluated for the presence of MVP, most studies show that its incidence is higher than in the general population. In a review of 12 studies incorporating observations on a total of 490 panic disorder patients, an average of 28% (range 0–50%) were found to have MVP (Crowe, 1988), as opposed to an average incidence of less than 5% in the general population. In addition, as pointed out first by Wooley (1976) and subsequently by others (e.g., Crowe, 1988), the major symptoms of panic disorder and MVP are almost identical: palpitations, chest pain, dyspnea, fatigue, dizzyness, syncope, and anxiety symptoms. The remarkable overlap of clinical symptomatology between these two conditions suggests that the most symptomatic MVP patients are those who are in fact suffering from an anxiety state or panic disorder and that MVP does not *in itself* create a predisposition to panic attacks (Margraf et al., 1988). Supporting this hypothesis is the fact that not only the symptoms, as mentioned above, but also the major epidemiological features of MVP and panic disorder are almost identical. Both affect about 3%–5% of the population, females about twice as frequently as males, and both have strong familial associations.

Whether the combined presence of panic attacks and MVP represents comorbidity is also uncertain. One alternative possibility is that chronically anxious persons, especially those suffering from panic attacks, may develop cardiovascular changes, including MVP. Surprisingly, this possibility that chronic anxiety or panic disorder may predispose to the development of MVP (and not the reverse) has not yet been seriously considered in the literature. This could result from the physical consequences of the emotional state, namely, an extreme lack of physical fitness with its attendant effects on the cardiovascular and autonomic nervous systems, as described previously. This is characterized by greater autonomic lability, with an exaggerated expression of sympathetic activity for any given level of stimulation. Lack of physical fitness and autonomic lability are interrelated and tend to promote each other. Either or both may promote the development of MVP. Another possibility is that there is a shared constitutional predisposition to both anxiety disorder and mitral valve prolapse.

REVERSING THE PROCESS

As promised at the start of this chapter, a clear view of the integrated psychophysiology of anxiety states could lead us to formulate a program of management that represents the logical response geared to reversing many of the key clinical features of MVP. Thus, if the physical inactivity associated with anxiety states in particular leads to contraction of blood volume, a reduced left ventricle volume, MVP, autonomic lability, and increased fatigability, then a structured fitness program could conceivably reverse these changes. Does this actually happen? The answer is yes, and it is worth first considering the effects of physical activity and fitness on the cardiovascular system (see Table 13-1).

It is well-established that athletes, in particular middle- and long-distance runners, tend to have an increased plasma volume and a borderline low hemoglobin count compared to the general population (Dill et al., 1974; Brotherhood et al., 1975; Lindemann, 1978; Convertino et al., 1980). The heart responds adaptively to the demands of regular physical activity. In trained athletes the mean left ventricle diastolic volume and mass increase (Morganroth et al., 1975); the blood volume increase tends to counteract the development of functional MVP. Furthermore, metabolic adaptations to increased physical activity lead to enhanced oxygen utilization by the skeletal muscles and lower production of lactate for any given level of activity (Klausen et al., 1974; Magel et al., 1978). In addition, the secretion of catecholamines is less pronounced in physically fit than in unfit individuals (Hartley et al., 1972) and autonomic responses are much more stable. These observations clearly have therapeutic implications for patients suffering from anxiety.

TABLE 13-1. Physiological Consequences of Fitness Status and the Relationship to Panic Disorder and Mitral Valve Prolapse

PHYSICALLY FIT SUBJECTS	PANIC DISORDER/MVP PATIENTS
Stable cardiovascular responses	Labile cardiovascular responses
Mild sympathetic responses	Exaggerated sympathetic responses
Slow pulse	Rapid pulse
Increased blood volume	Reduced blood volume
Increased left ventricular diastolic volume	Reduced left ventricular diastolic volume producing MVP
Good effort tolerance, decreased fatigability	Poor effort tolerance, increased fatigability
Reduced O_2 utilization for a given effort	Increased O_2 utilization for a given effort
Reduced lactate production	Increased lactate production

THE IMPACT OF EXERCISE ON PSYCHOLOGICAL WELL-BEING

Where tested, exercise programs have proved to be valuable in improving the psychological and physical well-being of patients with chronic conditions. In a study of panic disorder patients comparing the therapeutic benefits of a 10-week running program to clomipramine or placebo, the reduced endurance capacity of the patients was improved by the exercise, as were their anxiety symptoms (Meyer et al., 1998). Running was more efficient than placebo in improving the panic symptoms, though clomipramine was better than either running or placebo. In a 16-week randomized control trial of 156 patients with major depression, Blumenthal et al. (1999) similarly showed that although the antidepressant sertraline produced a quicker response, after 16 weeks exercise was equally effective in reducing depression.

Emery et al. (1998) compared the impact of education (i.e., lectures on pulmonary physiology, blood gases, and pathophysiology of chronic obstructive lung disease [COPD]) and stress management to that of exercise along with education and stress management and to that of waiting without intervention on 79 adults with COPD randomly assigned to one of these groups. Those patients exposed to the program that included all three elements experienced changes not seen in the patients who received only education and stress management or those who received nothing. The improvement was measurable in physical endurance, reduced anxiety, and improved cognitive performance. Grant et al. (1987) showed that in COPD patients with mild hypoxemia, tests of cognitive function are impaired as compared to age- and sex-matched controls. With the exercise program in the Emery et al. (1998) study, it is reasonable to assume that the improved cognitive function was related to improved brain oxygenation associated with increased cardiorespiratory fitness. In contrast to this positive outcome, a study by Madden et al. (1989) on the effects of a 16-week structured aerobic exercise program in 85 healthy adults aged between 60 and 83 years showed that although there were significant increases in cardiorespiratory fitness, no improvement was observed in cognitive functions. Thus, when a reduction in cognitive function occurs because of age-related changes in the brain, as occurred in the Madden et al. study, the process is uninfluenced by increased fitness.

A relatively low-intensity exercise program has had a significant impact on emotional and physical well-being even in exceptionally high-stress situations, such as during radiotherapy for breast cancer. In a study by Mock et al. (1997), 46 women were assessed before and after radiation treatment for breast cancer and were randomly assigned to either an individualized, self-paced, home-based walking program or a control group that received the usual care. The exercise group scored significantly better on physical functioning and symptom intensity, particularly fatigue, anxiety, and difficulty sleeping.

Other psychological benefits attributed to physical activity include enhanced mental performance and concentration (Emery and Gatz, 1990), unless there is a loss of brain substance, which occurs with aging, improved self-image, and feelings of confidence and control (Ossip-Klein et al., 1989; Emery and Gatz, 1990), better sleep (Brassington and Hicks, 1995), and a reduction in feelings of anger, time urgency, and time pressure (Blumenthal et al., 1988). Graded aerobic exercise programs have also proved beneficial in chronic somatic conditions usually associated with severe restriction in physical activity, such as chronic back pain (Frost et al., 1995), chronic fatigue syndrome (McCully et al., 1996; Fulcher and White, 1997), COPD (Grant et al., 1987) and fibromyalgia (McCain et al., 1988).

Although not all studies have found exercise to increase psychological well-being, every study included in the review by Byrne and Byrne (1993) that documented fitness gains after exercise showed concurrent improvement in psychological outcomes (i.e., depression, anxiety, and other mood states). Reviewers of this literature, however, have pointed to at least three limitations of the published studies (Brown, 1992; LaFontaine et al. 1993; Byrne and Byrne, 1993; Wykoff, 1993):

1. Many studies have not used a control group, making it difficult to differentiate between spontaneous changes in mood over time.
2. Some studies have not monitored the impact of the exercise on fitness, assuming that participation in an exercise program implied increase in fitness. However, in these studies it is still possible to examine the psychological effects of participation in an exercise program independent of changes in fitness.
3. Most studies have evaluated the effect of exercise on psychological outcomes over limited periods of time. Very few studies have examined the long-term effects of exercise after completion of the intervention phase. Doyne et al. (1987) reported sustained improvement in depression in clinically depressed women 12 months after participating in either an 8-week aerobic exercise program or an 8-week weight training program. Similarly, DiLorenzo et al. (1999) found, in a study of 82 healthy adults who participated in a 12-week aerobic fitness program with confirmed increases in fitness, that an initial significant improvement in mood state was also evident at the end of one year. Assessment of mood in this study included both anxiety (State-Trait Anxiety Inventory) and depression mood scales (Beck Depression Inventory).

SUMMARY

In chronic anxiety syndromes, the loss in physical fitness due to self-enforced inactivity may be responsible for an additional overlay of debilitating symptoms such as extreme fatigability and postural dizziness. These symptoms as well as the greater tendency to lability of pulse and blood pressure with changes in posture and on minimal exertion will tend to cause palpitations as well, and, with the other physical symptoms, work to enhance the anxiety symptoms. The main objective in this chapter has been to review the physical changes associated with anxiety and to describe as well clinical conditions that have overlapping features with this state. The best known of these is primary MVP with symptoms long regarded as a primarily cardiac condition.

Rigid echocardiographic diagnostic criteria and comprehensive population studies have assisted in helping to define the true clinical significance of primary MVP. It appears that symptoms in the presence of MVP, where the mitral valve is normal morphologically and the degree of prolapse is hemodynamically insignificant (as in the majority of patients considered here), should be assessed independently for an anxiety state including panic disorder. It is suggested that in many patients, both the MVP and the symptoms may be an expression of the same psychophysiological processes associated with the anxiety state. In essence, the MVP may be part of the cardiovascular adaptation to more extreme limitations of physical activity, though this is not intended to imply that all primary MVP cases have this pathogenesis.

The therapeutic implications of these observations are clear, and graduated programs of physical activity may be a useful adjunct to the management of patients with prominent anxiety or fatigue syndromes, as described in the previous section. Guiding patients to such a program has the important effect of not only improving their mood but also enhancing their feelings of self-control and efficacy in the management of their problems as well as helping to reduce their dependency on medication. This particular clinical situation represents one of the clearest examples of how a mind–body approach offers the best chances for the cure or, at least, substantial alleviation of what may often be an incapacitating state.

REFERENCES

Allen H, Harris A, Leatham A (1974). Significance and prognosis of an isolated late systolic murmur: a 9- to 22-year follow-up. Br Heart J 36:525–532.

Avery DH, Osgood TB, Ishiki DM, et al. (1985). The DST in psychiatric outpatients with generalized anxiety disorder, panic disorder, or primary affective disorder. Am J Psychiatry 142:844–848.

Barlow JB, Pocock WA, Marchand P, et al. (1963). The significance of late systolic murmurs. Am Heart J 66:443–452.

Barnett HJ, Boughner DR, Taylor DW, et al. (1980). Further evidence relating mitral-valve prolapse to cerebral ischemic events. N Engl J Med 302:139–144.

Barron JT, Manrose DL, Liebson PR (1988). Comparison of auscultation with two-dimensional and Doppler echocardiography in patients with suspected mitral valve prolapse. Clin Cardiol 11:401–406.

Bisset GS, Schwartz DC, Meyer RA, et al. (1980). Clinical spectrum and long-term follow-up of isolated mitral valve prolapse in 119 children. Circulation 62:423–429.

Blumenthal JA, Babyack MA, Moore KA, et al. (1999). Effects of exercise training on older patients with major depression. Arch Intern Med 159:2349–2356.

Blumenthal JA, Emery CF, Walsh MA, et al. (1988). Exercise training in healthy type A middle-aged men: effects on behavioral and cardiovascular responses. Psychosom Med 50:418–433.

Brassington GS, Hicks RA (1995). Aerobic exercise and self-reported sleep quality in elderly individuals. J Aging Phys Activity 3:120–134.

Brotherhood J, Brosovic B, Pugh LG (1975). Hematological status of middle- and long-distance runners. Clin Sci Mol Med 48:139–145.

Brown DR (1992). Physical activity, ageing, and psychological well-being: an overview of the research. Can J Sports Sci 17:185–193.

Bryhn M, Persson S (1984). The prevalence of mitral valve prolapse in healthy men and women in Sweden: an echocardiographic study. Acta Med Scand 215:157–160.

Byrne A, Byrne DG (1993). The effects of exercise on depression, anxiety and other mood states: a review. J Psychosom Res 37:565–574.

Chesler E, King RA, Edwards JE (1983). The myxomatous mitral valve and sudden death. Circulation 67:632–639.

Clemens JD, Horwitz RI, Jaffe CC, et al. (1982). A controlled evaluation of the risk of bacterial endocarditis in persons with mitral-valve prolapse. N Engl J Med 307:776–781.

Coghlan HC (1988). Autonomic dysfunction in the mitral prolapse syndrome: the brain–heart connection and interaction. In: Boudoulas H, Wooley CF eds. Mitral Valve Prolapse and Mitral Valve Prolapse Syndrome. New York: Futura Publishing Co, pp 389–426.

Cohen JL, Austin SM, Segal KR, et al. (1987). Echocardiographic mitral valve prolapse in ballet dancers: a function of leanness. Am Heart J 113:341–344.

Convertino VA (1997). Cardiovascular consequences of bed rest: effect on maximal oxygen uptake. Med Sci Sports Exerc 29:191–196.

Convertino VA, Brock PJ, Keil LC, et al. (1980). Exercise training-induced hypervolemia: role of plasma albumin, renin, and vasopressin. J Appl Physiol 48:665–669.

Crowe RR (1988). Mitral valve prolapse and anxiety. In: Boudoulas H, Wooley CF, eds. Mitral Valve Prolapse and the Mitral Valve Prolapse Syndrome. New York: Futura Publishing Co, pp 511–523.

Crowe RR, Pauls DL, Vankatesh A, et al. (1979). Exercise and anxiety neurosis: comparison of patients with and without mitral valve prolapse. Arch Gen Psychiatry 36:652–653.

Davies AO, Lefkowitz RJ (1980). Corticosteroid-induced differential regulation of beta-adrenergic receptors in circulating human polymorphonuclear leukocytes and mononuclear leukocytes. J Clin Endocrinol Metab 51:599–605.

Davies AO, Lefkowitz RJ (1981). Agonist-promoted high affinity state of the beta-adrenergic receptor in human neutrophils: modulation by corticosteroids. J Clin Endocrinol Metab 53:703–708.

Davies AO, Mares A, Pool JL, et al. (1987). Mitral valve prolapse with symptoms of beta-adrenergic hypersensitivity: beta 2-adrenergic receptor supercoupling with desensitization on isoproterenol exposure. Am J Med 82:193–201.

Devereux RB, Brown WT, Kramer-Fox R, et al. (1982a). Inheritance of mitral valve prolapse: effect of age and sex on gene expression. Ann Intern Med 97:826–832.

Devereux RB, Brown WT, Lutas EM, et al. (1982b). Association of mitral-valve prolapse with low body-weight and low blood pressure. Lancet 2:792–795.

Devereux RB, Kramer-Fox R, Brown WT, et al. (1986). Relation between clinical features of the mitral valve prolapse syndrome and echocardiographically documented mitral valve prolapse. J Am Coll Cardiol 8:763–772.

Devereux RB, Kramer-Fox R, Kligfield P (1989). Mitral valve prolapse: causes, clinical manifestations, and management. Ann Intern Med 111:305–317.

Devereux RB, Kramer-Fox R, Shear MK, et al. (1987). Diagnostic and classification of severity of mitral valve prolapse: methodological, biologic and prognostic considerations. Am Heart J 113:1265–1280.

Devereux RB, Perloff JK, Reichek N, et al. (1976). Mitral valve prolapse. Circulation 54:3–14.

Dill DB, Braithwaite K, Adams WC, et al. (1974). Blood volume of middle distance runners: effect of 2,300-m altitude and comparison with non-athletes. Med Sci Sports 6:1–7.

DiLorenzo TM, Bargman EP, Stucky-Ropp R, et al. (1999). Long-term effects of aerobic exercise on psychological outcomes. Prev Med 28:75–85.

Doyne EJ, Ossip-Klein DJ, Bowman ED, et al. (1987). Running versus weight lifting in the treatment of depression. J Consult Clin Psychol 55:748–754.

Duren DR, Becker AE, Dunning AJ (1988). Long-term follow-up of idiopathic mitral valve prolapse in 300 patients: a prospective study. J Am Coll Cardiol 11:42–47.

Emery CF, Gatz M (1990). Psychological and cognitive effects of an exercise program for community-residing older adults. Gerontologist 30:184–188.

Emery CF, Schein RL, Hauck ER, et al. (1998). Psychological and cognitive outcomes of a randomized trial of exercise among patients with chronic obstructive pulmonary disease. Health Psychol 17:232–240.

Flack JM, Kvasnicka JH, Gardin JM, et al. (1999). Anthropomorphic and physiological correlates of mitral valve prolapse in a bioethnic cohort of young adults: the CARDIA study. Am Heart J 138:486–492.

Freed LA, Levy D, Levine RA, et al. (1999). Prevalence and clinical outcome of mitral-valve prolapse. N Engl J Med 341:1–7.

Frost H, Klaber Moffett JA, Moser JS (1995). Randomized control trial for evaluation of fitness programme for patients with chronic lower back pain. Br Med J 310:151–154.

Fulcher KY, White PD (1997). Randomized control trial of graded exercise in patients with the chronic fatigue syndrome. Br Med J 314:1647–1652.

Gaffney FA, Bastian BC, Lane LB, et al. (1983). Abnormal cardiovascular regulation in the mitral valve prolapse syndrome. Am J Cardiol 52:316–320.

Gilon D, Buonanno FS, Joffe MM, et al. (1999). Lack of evidence of an association between mitral-valve prolapse and stroke in young patients. N Engl J Med 341:8–13.

Gorman JM (1986). Panic disorder: focus on cardiovascular status. Paper presented at the 139th Annual Meeting of the American Psychiatric Association , Washington, DC.

Grant I, Prigatano GP, Heaton RK, et al. (1987). Progressive neuropsychologic impairment and hypoxemia. Arch Gen Psychiatry 44:999–1006.

Hagberg JM, Goldberg AP, Lakatta L, et al. (1998). Expanded blood volume contribution to the increased cardiovascular performance of endurance-trained older men. J Appl Physiol 85:484–489.

Hartley LH, Mason JW, Hogan RP, et al. (1972). Multiple hormone responses to prolonged exercise in relation to physical training. J Appl Physiol 33:607–610.

Hickam JB, Cargill WH, Golden A (1948). Cardiovascular reactions to emotional stimuli and effect on cardiac output, A-V oxygen differences, arterial pressure and peripheral resistance. J Clin Invest 27:290–.

Holloszy JO, Booth FW (1976). Biochemical adaptations to endurance exercise in muscle. Ann Rev Physiol 38:263–291.

Holmgren A, Strom G (1959). Blood lactate concentration in relation to absolute and relative work load in normal men, and in mitral stenosis, atrial septal defect and vasoregulatory asthenia. Acta Med Scand 163:185–193.

Jacob G, Robertson D, Mosqueda Garcia R, et al. (1997). Hypovolemia in syncope and orthostatic intolerance role of renin-angiotensin system. Am J Med 103:128–133.

Jones M, Mellersh V (1946). A comparison of the exercise response in anxiety states and normal controls. Psychosom Med 8:180–187.

Julius S (1988). Editorial review: the blood pressure seeking properties of the central nervous system. J Hypertension 6:177–185.

Kamei F, Nakahara N, Yuda S, et al. (1999). Long-term site-related differences in the progression and regression of the idiopathic mitral valve prolapse syndrome. Cardiology 91:161–168.

Kelly D, Brown CC, Shaffer JW (1970). A comparison of physiological and psychological measurements on anxious patients and normal controls. Psychophysiology 6:429–441.

Klausen K, Rasmussen B, Clausen JP, et al. (1974). Blood lactate from exercising extremities before and after arm and leg training. Am J Physiol 227:67–72.

Kuchel O, Leveille J (1998). Idiopathic hypovolemia: a self-perpetuating autonomic dysfunction? Clin Auton Res 8:341–346.

Lader MH, Wing L (1964). Habituation of the psycho-galvanic reflex in patients with anxiety states and in normal subjects. J Neurol Neurosurg Psychiatry 27:210–218.

Lafontaine TP, DiLorenzo TM, Frensch PA, et al. (1993). Aerobic exercise and mood: a brief review, 1985–1990. Sports Med 13:160–170.

Levine RA, Weyman RA (1984). Mitral valve prolapse: a disease in search of, or created by its definition. Echocardiography 1:3–15.

Lindemann R (1978). Low hematocrits during basic training: athlete's anemia? N Engl J Med 299:1191–1192.

Linko E (1950). Lactic acid response to muscular exercise in neurocirculatory asthenia. Ann Med Intern Fenniae 39:161–176.

Lloyd AR, Hales JP, Gandevia SC (1988). Muscle strength, endurance and recovery in the post-infection fatigue syndrome. J Neurol Neurosurg Psychiatry 51:1316–1322.

Madden DJ, Blumenthal JA, Allen PA, et al. (1989). Improving aerobic capacity in healthy older adults does not necessarily lead to improved cognitive performance. Psychol Aging 4:307–320.

Magel JR, McArdle WD, Toner M, et al. (1978). Metabolic and cardiovascular adjustments to arm training. J Appl Physiol 45:75–79.

Mann JJ, Brown RP, Halper JP, et al. (1985). Reduced sensitivity of lymphocyte beta-adrenergic receptors in patients with endogenous depression and psychomotor agitation. N Engl J Med 313:715–720.

Margraf J, Ehlers A, Roth WT (1988). Mitral valve prolapse and panic disorder: a review of their relationship. Psychosom Med 50:93–113.

Markiewicz W, Stoner J, London E, et al. (1976). Mitral valve prolapse in one hundred presumeably healthy young females. Circulation 53:464–473.

Marks AR, Choong CY, Sanfilippo AJ, et al. (1989). Identification of high-risk and low-risk subgroups of patients with mitral-valve prolapse. N Engl J Med 320:1031–1036.

Martinsen EW, Raglin JS, Hoffart A, et al. (1998). Tolerance to intensive exercise and high levels of lactate in panic disorder. J Anxiety Disord 12:333–342.

McCain GA, Bell DA, Mai FM, et al. (1988). A controlled study of the effects of a supervised cardiovascular fitness training program on the manifestations of primary fibromyalgia. Arthritis Rheum 31:1135–1141.

McCully K, Sisto S, Natelson B (1996). Use of exercise for treatment of chronic fatigue syndrome. Sports Med 21:35–48.

Meneely GR, Segloff A, Wells EB (1947). Circulatory dynamics in the basal state observed during convalescence: changes in body weight, blood volume and venous pressure. J Clin Invest 26:320–328.

Meyer T, Broocks A, Bandelow B, et al. (1998). Endurance training in panic patients: spiroergometric and clinical effects. Int J Sports Med 19:496–502.

Meyers DG, Starke H, Pearson PH, et al. (1986). Mitral valve prolapse in anorexia nervosa. Ann Intern Med 105:384–386.

Middleton HC (1990). Cardiovascular dystonia in recovered panic patients. J Affect Disord 19:229–236.

Mier CM, Turner MJ, Ehsani AA, et al. (1997). Cardiovascular adaptations to 10 days of cycle exercise. J Appl Physiol 83:1900–1906.

Mock V, Dow KH, Meares CJ, et al. (1997). Effects of exercise on fatigue, physical functioning and emotional distress during radiation therapy for breast cancer. Oncol Nurs Forum 24:991–1000.

Morganroth J, Maron BJ, Henry WL, et al. (1975). Comparative left ventricular dimensions in trained athletes. Ann Intern Med 82:521–524.

Motulsky AG (1978). Biased ascertainment and the natural history of diseases. N Engl J Med 298:1196–1197.

Mtinangi BL, Hainsworth R (1998). Increased orthostatic tolerance following moderate exercise training in patients with unexplained syncope. Heart 80:596–600.

Nishimura RA, McGoon MD (1999). Perspectives on mitral-valve prolapse [editorial]. N Engl J Med 341:48–50.

Nishimura RA, McGoon MD, Shub C, et al. (1985). Echocardiographically documented mitral-valve prolapse: long-term follow-up of 237 patients. N Engl J Med 313:1305–1309.

Ossip-Klein DJ, Doyne EJ, Bowman ED, et al. (1989). Effects of running or weight lifting on self-concept in clinically depressed women. J Consult Clin Psychol 57:158–161.

Pandey GN, Dysken MW, Garver DL, et al. (1979). Beta-adrenergic receptor function in affective illness. Am J Psychiatry 136:675–678.

Pasternac A, Tabau JF, Puddu PE, et al. (1982). Increased plasma catecholamine levels in patients with symptomatic mitral valve prolapse. Am J Med 73:783–790.

Perloff JK, Child JS (1987). Clinical and epiodemiologic issues in mitral valve prolapse: overview and perspective. Am Heart J 113:1324–1332.

Peskind ER, Jensen CF, Pascualy M, et al. (1998). Sodium lactate and hypertonic sodium chloride induce equivalent panic incidence, panic symptoms, and hypernatremia in panic disorder. Biol Psychiatry 44:1007–1016.

Retchin SM, Fletcher RH, Earp J, et al. (1986). Mitral valve prolapse: disease or illness? Arch Intern Med 146:1081–1084.

Riley MS, O'Brien CJ, McCluskey DR, et al. (1990). Aerobic work capacity in patients with chronic fatigue syndrome. Br Med J 301:953–956.

Roman MJ, Deveruex RB, Kramer-Fox R, et al. (1989). Comparison of cardiovascular and skeletal features of primary mitral valve prolapse and Marfan syndrome. Am J Cardiol 63:317–321.

Roth WT, Telch MJ, Barr Taylor C, et al. (1986). Autonomic characteristics of agoraphobia with panic attacks. Biol Psychiatry 21:1133–1154.

Roy-Byrne PP, Uhde TW, Post RM, et al. (1986). The corticotropin-releasing hormone stimulation test in patients with panic disorder. Am J Psychiatry 143:896–899.

Rutstein DD, Thompson KJ, Tolmach DM, et al. (1945). Plasma volume and "extra vascular thiocyanate space" in pneumococcal pneumonia. J Clin Invest 24:11–20.

Saltin B, Blomqvist B, Mitchell JH, et al. (1968). Response to submaximal and maximal exercise after bedrest and training. Circulation 38 (suppl 7):1–78.

Sannerstedt R, Julius S, Conway J (1970). Hemodynamic response to tilt and beta-adrenergic blockade in young patients with borderline hypertension. Circulation 42:1057–1064.

Savage DD, Garrison RJ, Devereux RB, et al. (1983). Mitral valve prolapse in the general population. 1. Epidemiological features: the Framingham Study. Am Heart J 106:571–576.

Schondorf R, Benoit J, Wein T, et al. (1999). Orthostatic intolerance in the chronic fatigue syndrome. J Auton Nerv Syst 75:192–201.

Stewart JM, Gewitz MH, Weldon A, et al. (1999). Orthostatic intolerance in adolescent chronic fatigue syndrome. Pediatrics 103:116–121.

Taylor HL, Erickson L, Henschel A, et al. (1945). The effect of bed rest on the blood volume of normal young men. Am J Physiol 144:227–232.

Tzivoni D, Stern Z, Keren A, et al. (1980). Electrocardiographic characteristics of neurocirculatory asthenia during everyday activities. Br Heart J 44:426–432.

Victor RG, Seals DR, Mark AL (1987). Differential control of heart rate and sympathetic nerve activity during dynamic exercise. J Clin Invest 79:508–516.

Whinnery JE (1986). Acceleration tolerance of asymptomatic aircrew with mitral valve prolapse. Aviat Space Environ Med 57:986–992.

Wolf GA Jr, Wolff HG (1946). Studies on the nature of certain symptoms associated with cardiac disorders. Psychosom Med 8:293–.

Wooley CF (1976). Where are the diseases of yesteryear? Da Costa's syndrome, soldiers heart, the effort syndrome, neurocirculatory asthenia—and the mitral valve prolapse syndrome. Circulation 53:749–751.

Wykoff W (1993). The psychological effects of exercise on non-clinical and clinical populations of adult women: a critical review of the literature. Occup Ther Ment Health 12:69–106.

RESPIRATORY EFFECTS OF ANXIETY: HYPERVENTILATION

THE CLINICAL PICTURE

Hyperventilation is an important key to anxiety. Anxiety is almost always associated with an increased respiratory rate, tachypnea. Characteristically, subjects are not aware that respiratory activity has changed; their attention is focused entirely on the somatic response to the anxiety.

Hyperventilation produces significant clinical effects only when associated with hypocapnia, a fall in alveolar and arterial PCO_2. The hypocapneic symptoms are often distressing in their intensity. They include feelings of dizziness or lightheadedness, sometimes described as "a feeling of unreality," weakness, palpitations, chest pain of varying intensity, air hunger, and sighing respiration (i.e., the feeling that a deeper breath has to be taken because the lungs are not being completely filled by each normal breath). Tension-producing challenges that do not produce hypocapnia, such as a stressful mental tasks, may result in similar symptom patterns (Hornsveld et al., 1990; Roll and Zetterquist, 1990). In severe cases of hypocapnia, paresthesia and carpopedal spasm may develop in association with respiratory alkalosis and tetany.

The sudden, unexpected development of any of these symptoms may induce a feeling of intense anxiety and apprehension. In some persons, the emotional reaction may constitute a full-blown panic attack. However, hyperventilation may not be a prominent component of panic attacks, and if present it can be very transient (Hibbert and Pilsbury, 1989; Garrsen et al., 1996). Furthermore, a growing body of research seems to suggest that hyperventilation should not be considered a discrete clinical entity (Bass, 1997), though as a manifestation of anxiety it may indeed produce symptoms that will serve to intensify the anxiety state. As with many other conditions in the field of psychophysiology, an appropriately high "index of suspicion," coupled with knowledge of the potential mechanisms involved, assists in accurate clinical evaluation and management.

Whereas the clinical picture of acute hyperventilation is easily diagnosed according to the classical symptoms described above, subacute and chronic hyperventilation states are often unrecognized. The obvious hyperventilation seen in acutely distressed or anxious persons is not necessarily evident in chronic hyperventilators. This is mainly because a state of hypocapnia, once established, may be maintained with just an occasional deep, sighing breath (Saltzman et al., 1963). Frequent sighing or the complaint of shortness of breath, characterized by the feeling that the lungs are insufficiently filled upon normal inspiration, almost invariably points to tension or anxiety and may also be an important clue to a state of chronic hyperventilation. Symptomatic hyperventilation should be similarly suspected in anxious or depressed patients with somatic symptoms that are not easily explained on an organic basis. Other suggestive mannerisms include a dry, nonproductive cough, repeated clearing of the throat, and frequent moistening of lips (Magarian, 1982). However, although many somatic symptoms have been attributed to hyperventilation, they may in fact be expressions of anxiety, of which hyperventilation itself is usually one manifestation. In one study of 500 consecutive patients attending a gastroenterology clinic, 29 (5.8%) were found to be symptomatic hyperventilators (McKell and Sullivan, 1947). The authors attributed the hyperventilation in these patients to the anxiety generated by attacks of abdominal pain, but an equally valid interpretation is that both the abdominal pain and the hyperventilation may have resulted from anxiety. Similarly, in patients who are known or suspected to have asthma, breathlessness even after exercise may be due to anxiety-associated hyperventilation rather than asthma (Lowhagen et al., 1999; Ringsberg and Akerlind, 1999).

CASE REPORT: EPISODIC DIZZYNESS AND FAINTNESS

A 31-year-old woman complained of suffering two episodes of dizziness and faintness during the month before examination. On each occasion she thought she was going to faint but did not do so. Two days before the examination she had a similar episode, but on this occasion she also experienced a "floating feeling." She had been examined in the emergency room by a neurologist, who tried to reassure her that there was "nothing to worry about." An electrocardiograph performed on the same visit was reported to be normal, but despite reassurances the patient insisted that she did not feel well. On systematic questioning, she said that she was to be married in two weeks time and had developed apprehension about falling during the ceremony in light of the symptoms she was suffering. She also commented that she felt faint during the course of our conversation. Further conversation revealed signs of anxiety in recent weeks: she had been feeling tired, was working poorly, and suffered occasional palpitations associated with a slight feeling of panic. This troubled her particularly as she was normally energetic and tended to work hard. The patient described herself as very sensitive and a worrier but had no insight into any tension at the time her symptoms developed.

The physical examination revealed no abnormalities. Her blood count, thyroid function, and routine biochemical measures (including renal and liver function) were all within normal limits. The patient was diagnosed as suffering from an anxiety state with hyperventilation. I explained the nature of the problem to her and encouraged her to take four or five very deep breaths in the consulting room. She soon developed familiar symptoms of faintness, slight palpitations, and anxiety and in this way the association between her main symptoms and hyperventilation was demonstrated to her. Further discussion centered around life-style issues, with an emphasis on reducing her workload by taking a complete vacation from work in order to prepare herself for her upcoming wedding. She later told me that she had recovered, that she had been fine during the wedding, and had a return to her normal routine but with greater self-awareness.

This case illustrates a number of important clinical points characteristic of hyperventilating patients:

1. The patient, though very intelligent and self-aware to a certain extent ("sensitive and a worrier"), nevertheless did not link her clinical symptoms to her state of increased anxiety. Because of this, the discomfort associated with the hyperventilation had an alarming impact.
2. The neurologist who examined her suspected an anxiety state but tried to reassure her, after his examination, by telling her that "she had nothing to worry about." This reassurance did nothing for her because it failed to explain where her symptoms were coming from. Even if the neurologist had suspected that she was hyperventilating, he did not mention this possibility to her.
3. Reproducing the symptoms under my supervision by encouraging her to hyperventilate impressed her and helped to eliminate her anxiety by increasing her awareness of the source of her symptoms.

NORMAL CONTROL OF RESPIRATION

Differences in the control of both respiratory activity and breathing pattern are observed at rest and when exercising, talking, eating, and sleeping. As emphasized by von Euler (1981), the simple act of breathing, like walking, belies an exceedingly intricate mechanism involving the interaction of neural control systems at many levels of the nervous system. These control mechanisms are responsive to the physiological state and confer appropriate intensity and duration on a rhythmical breathing pattern. Optimal performance of the respiratory system is critically dependent on a variety of different reflexes and sensory feedback loops. These in turn respond to the continually changing requirements for gas exchange as well as many different demands for nonmetabolic functions such as sniffing, chewing, and swallowing.

Chemical Mechanisms

Respiratory control is mediated by three main mechanisms, chemical, mechanical, and cerebral. Chemoreceptors in the periphery (especially the carotid body and aortic arch) and in the brain stem respond to variations in blood gas (CO_2 and O_2) and hydrogen ion (pH) levels.

The carbon dioxide concentration in the arterial blood is a major stimulus to the brain stem centers (in the pons and medulla oblongata) that control the *respiratory rate* (the number of breaths per minute) and the *tidal volume* (volume of air per breath). The *minute volume* (volume of air breathed per minute) is determined by multiplying the tidal volume by the respiratory rate. Most of the evidence favors the existence of a special chemoceptive system on the ventral surface of the medulla, which is particularly sensitive to the influence of carbon dioxide and hydrogen ions (Loschcke et al., 1979; Schlaefke et al., 1979).

Both hypocapnia and hyperoxia reduce ventilatory activity. Hypocapnia is almost invariably a result of hyperventilation, in which the respiratory rate is incongruously fast for the level of metabolic activity. This results in the removal of carbon dioxide from the lungs and therefore from the blood at a much faster rate than it is produced in the tissues. As a result, there is a drop in the blood carbon dioxide level, or P_{CO_2}. Hyperoxia results only from administration of oxygen at high concentration through a mask. The point at which all rhythmic respiratory output from the CNS ceases is called the *apnea threshold*. Conversely, raised blood P_{CO_2} or reduced blood oxygen levels (P_{O_2}) stimulate respiratory activity.

Mechanical Mechanisms

Nerve signals are transmitted from the lung tissue, where stretch receptors signal an inflationary state of the lung (Younes et al., 1974). There is very little evidence, however, that the proprioceptive afferent input from the lungs via the vagus nerve controls breathing in man with normal lungs and at rest (Guz, 1997), making this mechanism of little relevance to this discussion.

Cerebral Mechanisms

Signals from higher centers, both psychogenic (Lin et al., 1974) and neurogenic (Plum et al., 1962), may influence the depth and rate of respiration. Positron emission tomography (PET), using radioactive water ($H_2^{15}O$) to monitor areas of brain activity through increases in regional blood flow associated with neuronal activation, as well as functional magnetic resonance imaging (fMRI) have been helpful in identifying areas of brain activity associated with volitional control of respiration (Colebatch et al., 1991; Fink et al., 1996; Evans et al., 1999). The areas found were, bilaterally in the primary motor cortex, in the right premotor cortex and in the supplementary motor area, and in the cerebellum. Interestingly, these results are analogous to what has been found with similar studies in voluntary limb movement. Horn and Waldrop (1998) point out that the centers above the level of the pons that are active in respiration are not crucial in respiratory control, but more in the modulation of respiration during various conditions such as locomotion, hypoxia, hypercapnia, and emotional excitement. Corefield et al. (1998), by using transcranial magnetic stimulation of the motor cortex to induce contraction of the diaphragm in human volunteers, provided evidence to suggest that the cortical control of the diaphragm does in fact bypass the brain stem respiratory centers.

The following discussion is limited to mechanisms of specific relevance for psychophysiological states of clinical importance.

VOLUNTARY CONTROL OF BREATHING

In contrast to other vital functions, respiratory activity may be voluntarily influenced to a considerable degree. However, one could never voluntarily completely stop breathing for an extended period. This is because the buildup of carbon dioxide in the blood would eventually trigger the midbrain respiratory centers, which would override the voluntary resistance and force a person to take a breath. The areas of neuronal activation identified with elevated end-tidal P_{CO_2} raised from 40 to 50 mm Hg include centers in the upper brain stem, up through the midbrain, hypothalamus, and thalamus in humans (Corefield et al., 1995). In addition, activation of the limbic system is present, and this may be relevant to the unpleasantness of the sensation of air hunger induced by the hypercarpnia (Guz, 1997). In the unlikely event of actually losing consciousness because of anoxia to the brain, as may occur in children during a breath-holding spell (Gauk et al., 1963), the buildup of carbon dioxide levels with the anoxia would trigger the respiratory activity and normal respiration would be reestablished.

Apnea may also be induced by vigorous hyperventilation, especially passive hyperventilation in anesthetized or conscious individuals. In the vast majority of cases hyperventilation-induced apnea is of limited duration and of little clinical significance; occasionally, however, extended, vigorous hyperventilation may lead to prolonged apnea and the development of dangerous cerebral anoxia (Haldane and Poulton, 1908; Henderson, 1910; Bates et al., 1966; MacDonald et al., 1976).

In the conscious individual, however, vigorous hyperventilation is rarely followed by apnea, though if its duration is short (two or three deep breaths), hypopnea usually results. Even when a striking degree of hypocapnia results from prolonged hyperventilation, some mechanism within the respiratory control system, independent of the chemical drive mechanism, is responsible for the absence of apnea. Furthermore, the majority of studies on voluntary hyperventilation show that most subjects undergo a phase of hyperpnea following hyperventilation (Tawadrous and Eldridge, 1974); that is, an increased minute volume is sustained for a variable period after the phase of active hyperventilation ends.

By increasing either the rate or the depth of respiration, voluntary hyperventilation blows off carbon dioxide, producing hypocapnia and alkalosis. A number of significant physiological consequences of this state underlie the usually disquieting and sometimes distressing symptomatology. These are summarized in the following section.

HYPERVENTILATION

Blood Gas and Metabolic Changes

The normal range of P_{CO_2} in arterial blood is between 30 and 45 mm Hg. A modest increase in ventilation, like one to two deep sighing breaths, may reduce the blood P_{CO_2} to around 25 mm Hg. Symptoms usually occur when the P_{CO_2} is in the 16–25 mm Hg range. The intensity of the symptoms of hypocapnia is largely a function of the speed with which the hypocapnia is produced; that is, it reflects the intensity of hyperventilation. This may best be quantified by measuring the arterial blood gas content with the Astrup machine, or the end-tidal P_{CO_2} (which is very close to arterial P_{CO_2} in a patient with normal lungs) with the capnograph or mass spectrometer, or by continuous sampling from a fine catheter taped 2–4 mm inside the nostril (Bass and Gardner, 1985). The fall in P_{CO_2} is associated with the development of a metabolic state of respiratory alkalosis, the effects of which are described below. The hypocapnea is associated with an arterial blood pH above 7.4. Characteristically, there is also a reduction in the serum inorganic phosphorus level. This has been ascribed to muscular exertion (from hyperventilation), which is known to produce such changes (Havard and Reay, 1926; Paleologos et al., 2000). Gorman et al. (1986) observed that patients with panic disorder who were chronic hyperventilators had hypophosphatemia. Contrary to popular belief, total serum calcium and serum magnesium do not usually change. Another explanation must therefore be found for the tetany that develops in some persons with hyperventilation (Saltzman et al., 1963).

Cerebral Blood Flow and Metabolism

As the most striking clinical symptoms of hyperventilation are psychological, it is worth considering the cerebral circulatory and electroencephalographic (EEG) changes observed. Cerebral arterial blood flow is extremely sensitive to P_{CO_2} levels, and a number of studies have demonstrated a striking reduction in cerebral blood flow and an increase in cerebral vascular resistance associated with hypocapnia. Cerebral blood flow may decrease by as much as 40% with hypocapnia (Kety and Schmidt, 1948; Wasserman and Patterson, 1961; Raichle and Plum, 1972). In a study of regional cerebral blood flow changes during hyperventilation in eight healthy volunteers by using $H_2^{15}O$ and positron emission tomography, Ishii et al. (1998) observed a decrease in total cerebral blood flow in the hypocapneic state, especially in blood flow to the temporal, occipital, and parietal lobes. This finding may help explain the feelings of dizziness and unreality that usually accompany hyperventilation. This decrease in cerebral blood is not a global effect, however, and Ishii et al. also observed in the same group significant activation in the primary motor and premotor cortices, cortical areas normally activated by respiratory activity (Colebatch et al. 1991; Fink et al. 1996; Evans et al., 1999).

In human subjects, the characteristic high-voltage, slow-wave EEG associated with hyperventilation has been correlated with a constriction of cerebral blood vessels and a marked reduction in jugular P_{O_2}. This effect is much more striking in persons under the age of 35 than in those over the age of 35 (Gotoh et al., 1965). When the conditions of hyperventilation are not standardized, EEG changes do not occur in every person (four out of seven in one study), they take a variable time to appear, and they may remain for varying periods (Saltzman et al., 1963). Zwiener et al. (1998), however, standardized the conditions of hyperventilation in 18 healthy volunteers by maintaining the end-tidal P_{CO_2} at 15 mm Hg and found a consistent slowing of the EEG in all with maximum topographical changes.

Do these alterations in cerebral blood flow and electrical activity resulting from hypocapnia affect cerebral function? Half a century ago studies designed to evaluate psychomotor performance (including arithmetic, motor coordination, and reaction time tests) during hypocapnia showed reduced performance below a P_{CO_2} of 25 mm Hg. Psychomotor performance declined to 85% of the pre- and posthyperventilation controls at an average arterial P_{CO_2} of 20–25 mm Hg and to approximately 70% at an average P_{CO_2} of about 14 mm Hg (Rahn et al., 1946; Balke and Lillehei, 1956).

Cardiovascular Changes

Electrocardiographic (ECG) changes induced by hyperventilation have been documented by numerous groups over many years (Thompson, 1943; Scherf and Schlakman, 1947; Wasserburger et al., 1956). The changes mainly affect the ST segment and T wave and may sometimes be indistinguishable from ischemic changes (Jacobs et al., 1974; Lary and Goldschlager, 1974). However, angiographic studies were normal in a group of patients with ST and T wave changes suggestive of ischemia on both exercise testing and hyperventilation. While coronary angiography may exclude significant coronary artery disease, it does not necessarily rule out the possibility of reversible coronary artery spasm in some subjects. In one study, for example, coronary blood flow during hyperventilation was significantly reduced in association with a striking reduction in coronary sinus O_2 and CO_2 tensions (Rowe et al., 1962). The best explanation for this finding is that, as with the cerebral circulation, hypocapnia may induce spasm of the coronary arteries or arterioles. It should be remembered, however, that the ECG changes observed during hyperventilation occur in only about 15% of normal subjects tested (Lary and Goldschlager, 1974). That hypocapnia is the factor inducing the ECG changes in these persons was confirmed by a study of 12 subjects who were known to develop ECG T-wave changes with hyperventilation. The T-wave change was equal to or greater than 1.5 mm and was either depressed (six subjects) or elevated (six subjects). Regardless of direction, the change reverted to normal when the subjects hyperventilated into a mixture of 4.5% CO_2 and air, a maneuver that prevents the development of hypocapnia (Golden et al., 1975).

RESPIRATORY ALKALOSIS AND ARTERIAL SPASM

The development of respiratory alkalosis, which is an integral part of the hypocapnic state, seems to be of major importance in mediating the tendency to arterial spasm observed in both the cerebral and coronary arterial circulations. Experiments *in vitro* have shown that alkalosis (increasing pH, as in respiratory alkalosis) is associated with increased vascular tone, which is thought to result from an enhanced influx of Ca^{2+} into the vascular smooth muscle cells (Hirofumi et al., 1981). Contraction of vascular smooth muscle depends on the presence of Ca^{2+}. In a physiological context, hydrogen ions compete with calcium for the same active sites both at the cell membrane transport system and within the cell (van Breemen et al., 1972; Mrwa et al., 1974). Vasoconstriction occurs when calcium ion concentration increases or hydrogen ion concentration decreases, as in alkalotic states. This mechanism has been shown to operate clinically in a group of patients suffering from Prinzmetal's angina (angina pectoris resulting from spasm, often in an atheroma-free coronary artery). These patients were first given an infusion of tris-buffer (pH 10) and then encouraged to hyperventilate vigorously for five minutes. In eight of the nine patients, chest pain with ischemic changes in the ECG occurred during this procedure or within five minutes after it ended. In four of the patients, coronary artery spasm was demonstrated angiographically. Significantly, in five of the patients given 90 mg diltiazem (a calcium channel blocker) two hours before the procedure, the arterial spasm was prevented (Yasue et al., 1978).

Another issue of clinical relevance is whether hypocapnia predisposes patients with established coronary artery disease to coronary spasm. There is increasing evidence that spasm of atheromatous coronary arteries is a mechanism of considerable importance in the genesis of both angina pectoris and myocardial infarction (Maseri et al., 1977, 1978; Yasue et al., 1979; Oliva and Breckenridge, 1977). Many patients with angina pectoris are understandably anxious because of their condition and therefore are potential hyperventilators. With refinement of the degree of hyperventilation required, for example, approximately 30 respiratory cycles/minute for five minutes, Morales et al. (1993) found under echocardiographic monitoring that hyperventilation in 104 hospitalized patients had a sensitivity of 84% and a specificity of 100% in identifying vasospastic myocardial ischemia. Using hyperventilation alone (for six minutes in the early morning), Nakao et al. (1997) found a sensitivity of 62% and a specificity of 100% in identifying coronary artery spasm in a group of 206 patients in whom coronary spasm had been confirmed on angiography. In a similar study of a much smaller group of 13 patients with coronary artery disease who were asked to hyperventilate for seven minutes, in all subjects coronary blood flow decreased and coronary arterio-venous O_2 difference widened, indicating reduced myocardial perfusion (Weill and Hattenhauer, 1975). Taken together, these studies point to a role for hyperventilation-induced blood gas and pH changes in the genesis of angina pectoris through spasm of the diseased artery. An additional mechanism that could aggravate the effect of the arterial spasm is the increased affinity of hemoglobin for oxygen in hyocapneic alkalosis (Wyman, 1964). Thus, not only is the blood flow decreased, but the oxygen conveyed to the tissues is less available. In situations where the blood flow is compromised to begin with, this may contribute to the development of significant tissue anoxia.

HYPERVENTILATION AND SYMPATHETIC ACTIVATION

The normal integration of ventilatory and autonomic sympathetic activity underlies much of the somatic expression of both hyperventilation and panic attacks. Similarly, the emotional expression of anxiety states is integrated with sympathetic activation and respiratory activity. Furthermore, as described above, hyperventilation that leads to significant hypocapnia may also lead to anxiety as

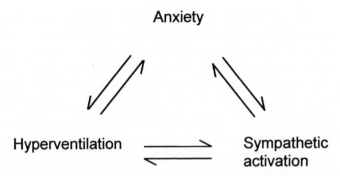

FIGURE 14.1 Diagrammatic representation of the interrelationship between anxiety, sympathetic activation, and hyperventilation.

well as to sympathetic activation. Thus, each element may be viewed as forming an apex of an equilateral triangle in which the flow of interaction is bidirectional (see Figure 14-1).

Cardiorespiratory control mechanisms are tightly integrated in the central nervous system to ensure that arterial concentrations of oxygen, carbon dioxide, and hydrogen ions are maintained within narrow physiological levels, while cardiovascular activity is continuously modified to furnish an adequate supply of oxygen to peripheral tissues and organ systems (Spyer, 1996). The central control mechanisms for respiratory and cardiovascular activity are thus tightly coupled, being sensitive to the same reflex inputs and participating in the expression of behavioral activities in a fully coordinated way (Spyer, 1995). In addition, a tight coupling or respiratory activity, especially inspiration, with sympathetic discharge has been demonstrated in humans to be independent of blood gases (Baron et al., 1996; Wallin et al., 1998). Emotional events such as fear, surprise, anxiety, and anger will trigger both respiratory and cardiovascular symptoms such as "difficulty in breathing," a choking feeling, chest pain, and palpitations. These symptoms are mediated mainly through activation of autonomic centers, and only when the reaction is sufficiently intense are other systems, such as release of adrenal medullary chatecholamines, engaged.

Effects of Sympathomimetic Agents on Emotion and Respiration

"Physiological arousal" is a term used in the psychology literature to describe a physical state that results from autonomic activation. Most episodes of acute anxiety or sudden emotional stress are characterized by symptoms that presumably represent sympathetic activation, such as palpitations, tremor, and perspiration. Over the years, psychophysiologists have been interested in determining the part played by physiological arousal in evoking emotional states appropriate to the stimuli.

The classical experiment of Schachter and Singer (1962) indicated that physiological arousal, without an alternative explanation, would be interpreted in emotional terms with the character of the emotional experience being suggested to the experimental subject by actors playing defined character parts. Thus, if the test subject was with a euphoric person, when aroused the experience would be labeled as "euphoric," and with an angry person the same physiological arousal would be labeled "anger." Subsequent work, however, has tended to contradict the original conclusions of Schachter and Singer by showing that unexplained arousal, produced either by hypnotic suggestion or by an intravenous injection of epinephrine, is mostly associated with negative emotional reactions (Marshall and Zimbardo, 1979; Maslach, 1979). Earlier work had also suggested that the physical state produced by epinephrine injection in experimental subjects was associated in some with feelings of anxiety, fear, tenseness, or worry (Cantril and Hunt, 1932). The physical experience was compatible with the emotional state described, though some of the subjects were aware of the incongruousness of the emotional state at the time that it was experienced.

Research on the emotional associations of physiological arousal has tended to focus on cardiovascular stimulation, with less attention given in the same studies to the respiratory aspects. It was found, however, that hyperventilation was induced in subjects by intravenous administration of the sympatheticomimetic agent isoproterenol (Lockhart et al., 1967; Stone et al., 1970). Both epinephrine and norepinephrine have a similar stimulatory effect on respiratory rate (Whelan and Young, 1953). It therefore seems that activation of ventilatory as well as sympathetic activity is tightly integrated and that in a clinical real-life context, as suggested above, the activation of one is associated with activation of the other.

The emotions evoked by either hyperventilation or sympathetic activation depend on an individual's basic emotional state and previous experience. In a tense or anxious personality the experience of physical arousal may generate extreme concern or apprehension, particularly when unexpected. In more extreme cases it may lead to the development of panic attacks. Several groups have shown that intravenous infusions of isoproterenol precipitate panic attacks much more frequently in subjects known to suffer from them than in controls (Frohlich et al., 1969; Boudoulas et al., 1984; Rainey et al., 1984).

BREATHLESSNESS AND ANXIETY

The Relationship between Hyperventilation and Panic Attacks

Panic attacks are discussed in greater detail in Chapter 12, as they often give rise to clinical problems that have to be evaluated medically. It is clear, however, that many of the somatic symptoms of panic attacks are similar to those experienced with hyperventilation. Thus, it may be assumed that some panic attacks are precipitated by the effects of hyperventilation. It is unlikely, however, that all panic attacks have this origin, as some have suggested (Lum, 1981; Clark and Hemsley, 1982; Ley, 1985). For one thing, some patients insist that they were feeling perfectly relaxed or "unstressed" in the moments preceding an attack. It would also be difficult to invoke hyperventilation as an etiological factor in the case of panic attacks that occur during sleep, as they quite commonly do. Nevertheless, it seems probable that the hyperventilation associated with the considerable apprehension characteristically experienced in a panic attack may serve to intensify the symptoms of the attack.

A number of other clinical conditions may be characterized by breathlessness and anxiety. The first and most common is asthma, and the second is a condition that often simulates asthma, vocal cord dysfunction.

Asthma, Chronic Obstructive Pulmonary Disease, and Mood

The experience of true "air hunger," or dyspnea, is the cardinal symptom of asthma. The feeling of not getting sufficient air with each breath challenges the very act that most symbolizes in our minds the process of being alive—breathing—and thus is a potent stimulus of anxiety. It is not surprising that asthma, like other chronic respiratory conditions characterized by airway obstruction, is associated with an increased incidence of affective disorders such as anxiety states, panic disorder, and depression (Carr, 1998; Lehrer, 1998). Carr (1999) claims that the presence of asthma is a risk factor for the development of panic disorder. A survey of 155 asthmatic children who completed an anxiety questionnaire after an attack of asthma revealed that almost two-thirds of the group had experienced panic (Butz and Alexander, 1992), and similar results have been reported for adult asthmatics (Gift, 1991). While almost all asthmatics experience dyspnea, many more experience panic with some attacks, than actually develop panic disorder. Nevertheless, the incidence of panic disorder in asthmatics is around 10%, which is at least twice that of the general population. Similarly, in a meta-analysis of 60 studies of depression among children with chronic medical problems, Bennett (1996) reported elevated levels of depression among both asthmatic children and their parents.

The case report in Chapter 4 of a patient who suffered repeated bouts of status asthmaticus dramatically demonstrates that significant emotional factors may predispose to recurrent, severe, life-threatening attacks of asthma. In a study of 44 patients who died from asthma and of 19 other patients who had suffered 23 episodes of near-fatal asthma (NFA), Innes et al. (1998) found major psychosocial factors to account for the tendency to severe asthma attacks in the vast majority of these cases. An NFA attack usually is defined by the presence of one or more of the following: respiratory arrest, alteration in consciousness, need for mechanical ventilation, $Paco_2 > 50$ mm. In the Innes study denial was the most frequent psychological factor; domestic, financial, or employment stress and smoking or passive smoking were the most common adverse social factors. Only two patients with NFA and seven who died had no recorded adverse psychological or social conditions. Another study contradicted this conclusion, however. In a group of 17 asthma patients who had suffered near-fatal attacks, Rocco et al., (1998) found no psychiatric or personality characteristics that distinguished them from 17 control subjects. The patients had been interviewed about their personal and family psychiatric history and had been tested with the Hamilton and Zung scales for anxiety and depression and the Minnesota Multiphasic Personality Inventory. What this study was clearly unable to rule out, however, is that the NFA attacks occurred with the intensity they did because the patient was anxious at the time of the attack, though it also indicates that other factors were involved. The intensity of any specific attack of asthma may be a function of a number of processes, such as a sudden release of mediators of inflammation in response to some antigenic stimulus. But repeated attacks raise, in addition, the possibility of anxiety driving the process. Even when asthma has a proven basis of hypersensitivities, a complicating state of anxiety or depression may still be the process that leads to a deteriorating clinical condition with recurrent attacks of asthma or status asthmaticus. Only by attending to the emotional cues can one get a clear idea of the extent to which they are operative in any particular situation.

Patients with advanced lung disease face innumerable challenges to their functional independence, self-esteem, and quality of life (Wingate and Hansen-Flaschen, 1997). Work capacity and social interaction may be severely diminished. Sleep, eating, and sexual intimacy are disrupted. Coughing becomes a major physical ordeal and social embarrassment. Ordinary activities require extra planning and time. No wonder that problems of anxiety and depression are much more common. One study found that as many as 45% of patients with moderate to severe chronic obstructive pulmonary disorder (COPD) suffer from depression (Light et al., 1985), a higher rate that that observed in chronically ill populations in general and substantially higher than the 6%–17% prevalence of depression observed in adult primary care settings. In patients with chronic obstructive lung disease, there is also a tendency toward frequent anxiety and panic disorder (Yellowlees et al., 1987; Porzelius et al., 1992; Pollack et al., 1996).

Various treatment modalities may be considered for the management of these patients. It is often appropriate to prescribe medication such as SSRIs or benzodiazepines for the treatment of an anxiety state, depression, or panic disorder (see Chapter 17). Cognitive-behavioral therapy, which includes education about illness, addressing specific fears, and relaxation training or mindful meditation, may also be appropriate (see Chapters 18 and 19); in addition, a graduated physical fitness program could be considered (see Chapter 13). The latter two options have the added benefit, as in all chronic medical conditions, of enhancing the patient's feelings of self-control in that they are directed toward encouraging self-reliance and independence. Attention to this facet of the patient's emotional struggle may substantially contribute to his or her rehabilitation.

Vocal Cord Dysfunction

Vocal cord dysfunction is an underdiagnosed condition. It is almost invariably diagnosed initially as stridor or assumed to be an exacerbation of preexisting asthma (Barnes et al., 1986). It often presents as a medical emergency, and the patients may be managed with endotracheal intubation or tracheostomy (Patterson et al., 1974; Rogers and Stell, 1978; Cormier et al., 1981; Shafei et al., 1997; Murray and Lawler, 1998). I have seen patients with this condition receive subcutaneous adrenaline injections in the emergency room or an extended course of high-dose steroids with serious side effects for treatment of repeated episodes of acute breathlessness. In both cases it was assumed that the patients were suffering from uncontrolled or steroid-resistant asthma, an observation that parallels the experience of others (Christopher et al., 1983; Rodenstein et al., 1983; Thomas et al., 1999). Thomas et al. (1999) suggest that the differential diagnosis of steroid-resistant asthma should include gastroesophageal reflux, hyperventilation, vocal cord dysfunction, and sleep apnea (see Chapter 15).

It is only an awareness of functional vocal chord dysfunction and an appropriate level of suspicion during physical examination that will facilitate accurate diagnosis. The wheezing in these patients has a definite inspiratory component suggesting stridor, which does not occur in a typical asthma attack. Other clues suggesting this diagnosis include the ability to finish complete sentences, a very difficult task in a true asthma attack, as well as momentary improvement after coughing and panting (McFadden, 1987; Selner et al., 1987) and disappearance of the symptoms during sleep (Kattan and Ben-Zvi, 1985; Martin et al., 1987) or with intubation (Murray and Lawler, 1998). In addition, there are none of the characteristic laboratory or radiological findings of asthma such as a decrease in expiratory flow rates, altered blood gases (especially changes in the alveolar-arterial oxygen tension gradient and the partial arterial carbon dioxide pressure), or hyperinflated lungs. Laryngoscopy in these patients typically shows persistent adduction of the vocal cords during both inspiration and expiration. If the patient is asked to count during examination, however, the vocal cords will move normally.

Most authors report the successful management of cases of vocal cord dysfunction through supportive short-term psychotherapy and, where necessary, speech training. While many patients with this disorder are suffering mainly from an anxiety state (Gavin et al., 1998), more intractable problems sometimes have the character of a true conversion disorder and these patients may be extremely refractory to management. None of these patients should be thought to be willfully creating the problem; rather, the functional disorder represents an inadequate response to stress and therefore some kind of supportive intervention is strongly indicated.

SUMMARY

Hyperventilation that occurs in the absence of a metabolic or respiratory cause has two main clinical implications.

First, respiratory rate is tightly coupled to autonomic activity, in particular sympathetic activity, so tachypnea is usually a concomitant of anxiety states. Conversely, any intervention that slows the rate of breathing in a stressed person will reduce sympathetic activity and in turn the level of anxiety or tension. The functional interplay between respiratory rate and sympathetic activity is exploited in the behavioral therapeutic techniques used in the management of anxiety states such as meditation and deep relaxation, described in Chapter 19.

Second, an increase in respiratory activity may lead to hypocapnia, with consequent effects on cardiovascular and nervous function. Clinically, this process may be subtle and because the patient is not obviously hyperventilating, the symptoms are often misinterpreted by the physician. The patient is likely to stress the somatic symptoms, thus obscuring the real issue of anxiety, and possibly panic disorder. The symptoms, often distressing in their intensity, include feelings of dizziness or light-headedness sometimes described as "a feeling of unreality," weakness, palpitations, chest pain of varying intensity, air hunger, and sighing respiration. It is often the latter that leads to a suspicion of the true diagnosis.

Disorders characterized by breathlessness, such as asthma and chronic obstructive lung disease, may be complicated by affective reactions to the stressful experience of the disease. The emotional state may significantly aggravate the pulmonary condition, leading to the erroneous conclusion that the underlying disease process is progressing. Thus, patients with obstructive lung disease of any kind, whose clinical deterioration is not adequately explained by a pathological condition such as bronchitis or pneumonia, may benefit from an intervention directed at anxiety or depression.

In addition to the association of anxiety states with breathlessness, the possibility of functional vocal cord dysfunction should also be considered. This condition usually presents clinically as an apparent deterioration in the patient's asthma, or as stridor of recent onset. The correct diagnosis is usually fairly simple to make at the bedside, once it has been thought of, saving the patient the consequences of potentially traumatic interventions such as intubation or tracheostomy or the side effects of drugs such as steroids. In most cases it should be viewed as a distress call, and it is usually responsive to supportive psychotherapy.

REFERENCES

Balke B, Lillehei JP (1956). Effect of hyperventilation on performance. J Appl Physiol 9:371–374.

Barnes SD, Grog CS, Lachman BS, et al. (1986). Psychogenic upper airway obstruction presenting as refractory wheezing. J Pediat 109:1067–1070.

Baron R, Habler HJ, Heckmann K, et al. (1996). Respiratory modulation of blood flow in normal and sympathectomized skin in humans. J Auton Nerv Syst 60:147–153.

Bass C (1997). Hyperventilation syndrome: a chimera? J Psychosom Res 42:421–426.

Bass C, Gardner WN (1985). Respiratory and psychiatric abnormalities in chronic symptomatic hyperventilation. Br Med J 290:1387–1390.

Bates JH, Adamson JS, Pierce JA (1966). Death after voluntary hyperventilation. N Engl J Med 274:1371–1372.

Bennett DS (1996). Depression among children with chronic medical problems: a meta-analysis. J Pediat Psychol 19:149–169.

Boudoulas H, King BD, Wooley CF (1984). Mitral valve prolapse: a marker for anxiety or overlapping phenomenon? Psychopathology 17 (suppl 1):98–106.

Butz AM, Alexander C (1992). Anxiety in children with asthma. J Asthma 30:199–209.

Cantril H, Hunt WA (1932). Emotional effects produced by the injection of adrenalin. Am J Psychol 44:300–307.

Carr RE (1998). Panic disorder and asthma: causes, effects and research implications. J Psychosom Res 44:43–52.

Carr RE (1999). Panic disorder and asthma. J Asthma 36:143–152.

Christopher KL, Wood RP, Eckert C, et al. (1983). Vocal-cord dysfunction presenting as asthma. N Engl J Med 308:1566–1570.

Clark DM, Hemsley DR (1982). The effects of hyperventilation; individual variability and its relation to personality. J Behav Therap Exp Psychiatry 13:41–47.

Colebatch JG, Adams L, Murphy K, et al. (1991). Regional cerebral blood flow during volitional breathing in man. J Physiol 443:91–103.

Corfield DR, Fink JR, Ramsay SC, et al. (1995). Evidence for limbic system activation during CO_2-stimulated breathing in man. J Physiol 488:77–84.

Corfield DR, Murphy K, Guz A (1998). Does the motor cortical control of the diaphragm "bypass" the brain stem respiratory centres in man? Respir Physiol 114:109–117.

Cormier YF, Camus P, Desmeules MJ (1981). Non-organic acute upper airway obstruction: description and a diagnostic approach. Am Rev Respir Dis 121:147–150.

Evans KC, Shea SA, Saykin AJ (1999). Functional MRI localisation of central nervous system regions associated with volitional inspiration in humans. J Physiol 520:383–392.

Fink GR, Corfield DR, Murphy K, et al. (1996). Human cerebral activity with increasing inspiratory force: a study using positron emission tomography. J Appl Physiol 81:1295–1305.

Frohlich ED, Tarazi RC, Dustan HP (1969). Hyperdynamic beta-adrenergic circulatory state: increased beta-receptor responsiveness. Arch Intern Med 123:1–7.

Garssen B, Buikhuisen M, Van Dyck R (1996). Hyperventilation and panic attacks. Am J Psychiatry 153:513–518.

Gauk EW, Kidd L, Pritchard JS (1963). Mechanism of seizures associated with breath-holding spell. N Engl J Med 268:1436–.

Gavin LA, Wamboldt M, Brugman S, et al. (1998). Psychological and family characteristics of adolescents with vocal cord dysfunction. J Asthma 35:409–417.

Gift AG (1991). Psychological and physiological aspects of acute dyspnoea in asthmatics. Nurs Res 40:196–199.

Golden GS, Golden LH, Beerel FR (1975). Hyperventilation-induced T-wave changes in the limb lead electrocardiogram. Chest 67:123–125.

Gorman JM, Cohen BS, Liebowitz MR, et al. (1986). Blood gas changes and hypophosphatemia in lactate-induced panic. Arch Gen Psychiatry 43:1067–1071.

Gotoh F, Meyer JS, Takagi Y (1965). Cerebral effects of hyperventilation in man. Arch Neurol 12:410–423.

Guz A (1997). Brain, breathing and breathlessness. Respir Physiol 109:197–204.

Haldane JS, Poulton EP (1908). The effects of want of oxygen on respiration. J Physiol 37:390–407.

Havard RE, Reay GA (1926). Influence of exercise on inorganic phosphates of blood and urine. J Physiol 61:35–48.

Henderson Y (1910). Acapnia and shock. IV. Fatal apnoea after excessive ventilation. Am J Physiol 25:310–333.

Hibbert GA, Pilsburg D (1989). Hyperventilation: is it a cause of panic attacks? Br J Psychiatry 155:805–809.

Hirofumi Y, Omote S, Takizawa A, et al. (1981). Alkalosis-induced coronary vasoconstriction: effects of calcium, diltiazem, nitriglycerin, and propanolol. Am Heart J 102:206–210.

Horn EM, Waldrop TG (1998). Suprapontine control of respiration. Respir Physiol 114:201–211.

Hornsveld H, Garssen B, Fiedeldij DOP M, et al. (1990). Symptom reporting during voluntary hyperventilation and mental load: implications for diagnosing syndrome. J Psychosom Res 34:687–697.

Innes NJ, Reid A, Halstead J, et al. (1998). Psychosocial risk factors in near-fatal asthma and in asthma deaths. J R Coll Physicians Lond 32:430–434.

Ishii K, Sasaki M, Yamaji S, et al. (1998). Cerebral blood flow changes in the primary motor and premotor cortices during hyperventilation. Ann Nucl Med 12:29–33.

Jacobs WF, Battle WE, Ronan JA Jr (1974). False-positive ST-T-wave changes secondary to hyperventilation and exercise: a cineangiographic correlation. Ann Intern Med 81:479–482.

Kattan M, Ben-Zvi Z (1985). Stridor caused by vocal cord malfunction associated with emotional factors. Clin Pediatr 24:158–159.

Kety SS, Schmidt CF (1948). Effects of altered arterial tensions of carbon dioxide and oxygen on cerebral blood flow and cerebral oxygen consumption in normal man. J Clin Invest 27:484–492.

Lary D, Goldschlager N (1974). Electrocardiographic changes during hyperventilation resembling myocardial ischemia in patients with normal coronary anteriograms. Am Heart J 87:383–390.

Lehrer PM (1998). Emotionally triggered asthma: a review of research literature and some hypotheses for self-regulation therapies. Appl Psychophysiol Biofeedback 23:13–41.

Ley R (1985). Blood, breath and fears: a hyperventilation theory of panic attacks and agoraphobia. Clin Psychol Rev 5:79–81.

Light R, Merrill E, Despars J (1985). Prevalence of depression and anxiety in patients with COPD. Chest 87:35–38.

Lin YC, Lally DA, Moore TO, et al. (1974). Physiological and conventional breath-hold breaking points. J Appl Physiol 37:291–296.

Lockhart A, Lissac J, Salmon D, et al. (1967). Effects of isoproterenol on the pulmonary circulation in obstructive airways disease. Clin Sci 32:177–187.

Loschcke HH, Schlaefke ME, See WR, et al. (1979). Does CO_2 act on the respiratory centers? Pflugers Arch 381:249–254.

Lowhagen O, Arivdsson M, Bjarneman P, et al. (1999). Exercise-induced respiratory symptoms are not always asthma. Respir Med 93:734–738.

Lum LC (1981). Hyperventilation and anxiety state. J R Soc Med 74:1–4.

MacDonald KF, Bowers JT, Flynn RE (1976). Posthyperventilation apnea associated with severe hypoxemia. Chest 70:554–557.

Magarian GJ (1982). Hyperventilation syndromes: infrequently recognized common expressions of anxiety and stress. Medicine 61:219–236.

Marshall GD, Zimbardo PG (1979). Affective consequences of inadequately explained physiological arousal. J Person Soc Psychol 37:970–988.

Martin RJ, Blager FB, Gay ML, et al. (1987). Paradoxical vocal cord motion in presumed asthmatics. Sem Resp Med 8:332–337.

Maseri A, L'Abbate A, Baroldi G, et al. (1978). Coronary vasospasm as a possible cause of myocardial infarction: a conclusion derived from the study of "preinfarction" angina. N Engl J Med 299:1271–1277.

Maseri A, Pesola A, Marzilli M, et al. (1977). Coronary vasospasm in angina pectoris. Lancet i:713–717.

Maslach C (1979). Negative emotional biasing of unexplained arousal. J Person Soc Psychol 37:953–969.

McFadden ER Jr (1987). Glottic function and dysfunction [editorial]. J Allergy Clin Immunol 79:707–710.

McKell TE, Sullivan AJ (1947). The hyperventilation syndrome in gastroenterology. Gastroenterology 9:6–16.

Morales MA, Reisenhofer B, Rovai D, et al. (1993). Hyperevntilation-echocardiography test for the diagnosis of myocardial ischemia at rest. Eur Heart J 14:1088–1093.

Mrwa U, Achtig I, Ruegg JC (1974). Influences of calcium concentration and pH on the tension development and ATPase activity of the arterial actomyosin contractile system. Blood Vessels 11:277–286.

Murray DM, Lawler PG (1998). All that wheezes is not asthma: paradoxical vocal cord movement presenting as severe acute asthma requiring ventilatory support. Anaesthesia 53:1006–1011.

Nakao K, Ohgushi M, Yoshimura M, et al. (1997). Hyperventilation as a specific test for diagnosis of coronary artery spasm. Am J Cardiol 80:545–549.

Oliva PB, Breckenridge JC (1977). Arteriographic evidence of coronary arterial spasm in acute myocardial infarction. Circulation 56:366–374.

Paleologos M, Stone E, Braude S (2000). Persistent, progressive hypophosphatemia after voluntary hyperventilation. Clin Sci (Colch) 98:619–625.

Patterson R, Schatz M, Horton M (1974). Munchausen's stridor: non-organic laryngeal obstruction. Clin Allergy 4:307–310.

Plum F, Brown HW, Snoep E (1962). Neurological significance of posthyperventilation apnoea. JAMA 12:1050–1055.

Pollack MH, Kradin R, Otto MW, et al. (1996). Prevalence of panic in patients referred for pulmonary function testing at a major medical center. Am J Psychiatry 153:110–113.

Porzelius J, Vest M, Nochomovitz M (1992). Respiratory function, cognitions, and panic in chronic obstructive pulmonary patients. Behav Res Ther 30:75–77.

Rahn H, Otis AB, Hodge M, et al. (1946). The effects of hypocapnia on performance, J Aviation Med 17:164–172.

Raichle ME, Plum F (1972). Hyperventilation and cerebral blood flow. Stroke 3:566–575.

Rainey M Jr, Ettedgui E, Pohl B, et al. (1984). The beta-receptor: isoproterenol anxiety states. Psychopathology 17 (supp 3):40–51.

Ringsberg KC, Akerlind I (1999). Presence of hyperventilation in patients with asthma-like symptoms but negative asthma test responses: provocation with voluntary hyperventilation and mental stress. J Allergy Clin Immunol 103:601–608.

Rocco PL, Barboni E, Balestrieri M (1998). Psychiatric symptoms and psychological profile of patients with near fatal asthma: absence of positive findings. Psychother Psychosom 67:105–108.

Rodenstein DO, Francis C, Stanescu DC (1983). Emotional laryngeal wheezing: a new syndrome. Am Rev Respir Dis 127:354–356.

Rogers JH, Stell PM (1978). Paradoxical movement of the vocal cords as a cause of stridor. J Laryngol Otol 92:157–158.

Roll M, Zetterquist S (1990). Acute chest pain without obvious organic cause before the age of 40 years: response to forced hyperventilation. J Intern Med 228:223–228.

Rowe GG, Castillo CA, Crumpton CW (1962). Effects of hyperventilation on systemic and coronary hemodynamics. Am Heart J 63:67–77.

Saltzman HA, Heyman A, Sieker HO (1963). Correlation of clinical and physiological manifestations of sustained hyperventilation. N Engl J Med 268:1431–1436.

Schachter S, Singer JE (1962). Cognitive, social and physiological determinants of emotional state. Psychol Rev 69:379–399.

Scherf D, Schlachman M (1947). The electrocardiographic changes caused by hyperventilation. Am J Med Sci 213:342–349.

Schlaefke ME, See WR, Herker-See A, et al. (1979). Respiratory response to hypoxia and hypercapnia after elimination of central chemosensitivity. Pflugers Arch 381:241–248.

Selner JC, Staudenmayer H, Koepke JW, et al. (1987). Vocal cord dysfunction: the importance of psychological factors and provocation challenge testing. J Allergy Clin Immunol 79:726–733.

Shafei H, El Kholy A, Azmy S, et al. (1997). Vocal cord dysfunction after cardiac surgery: an overlooked complication. Eur J Cardiothorac Surg 11:564–565.

Spyer KM (1995). Central nervous mechanisms responsible for cardio-pulmonary homeostasis. In: Kappagoda CT, Kaufman MP, eds. Control of the Cardiovascular and Respiratory Systems in Health and Disease. New York: Plenum, pp 73–79.

Spyer KM (1996). Central nervous integration of cardiorespiratory control. In: Greger R, Windhorst U, eds. Comprehensive Human Physiology, Vol 2. Berlin: Springer-Verlag Berlin, pp 2129–2144.

Stevenson I, Ripley HS (1952). Variations in respiration and in respiratory symptoms during changes in emotion. Psychosom Med 14:476–490.

Stone DJ, Zaldivar C, Keltz H (1970). The effects of very low doses of nebulized isoproterenol, nebulized saline, and intravenous isoproterenol on blood gases in patients with chronic bronchitis. Am Rev Resp Dis 101:511–517.

Tawadrous FD, Eldridge FL (1974). Posthyperventilation breathing patterns after active hyperventilation in man. J Appl Physiol 37:353–356.

Thomas PS, Geddes DM, Barnes PJ (1999). Pseudo-steroid resistant asthma. Thorax 54:352–356.

Thompson W (1943). The electrocardiogram in the hyperventilation syndrome. Am Heart J 25:372–390.

Van Breemen C, Farinas BR, Gerba P, et al. (1972). Excitation–contraction coupling in rabbit aorta studied by the lanthanum method for measuring cellular calcium influx. Circ Res 30:44–54.

Von Euler C (1981). The contribution of sensory inputs to the pattern generation of breathing. Can J Physiol Pharmacol 59:700–706.

Wallin BG, Batelsson K, Kienbaum P, et al. (1998). Two neural mechanisms for respiration-induced cutaneous vasodilatation in humans? J Physiol 513:559–569.

Wasserburger RH, Siebecker KL, Lewis WC (1956). The effect of hyperventilation on the normal adult electrocardiogram. Circulation 13:850–855.

Wasserman AJ, Patterson JL Jr. (1961). The cerebral vascular reponse to reduction in arterial carbon dioxide tension. J Clin Invest 40(ii):1297–1303.

Weill WA, Hattenhauer M (1975). Impairment of myocardial oxygen supply due to hyperventilation. Circulation 52:854–858.

Whelan RF, Young IM (1953). The effect of adrenaline and noradrenaline infusions on respiration in man. Br J Pharmacol 8:98–102.

Wingate BJ, Hansen-Flaschen J (1997). Anxiety and depression in advanced lung disease. Clin Chest Med 18:495–505.

Wyman J Jr (1964). Linked functions and reciprocal effects in hemoglobin: a second look. Adv Protein Chem 19:223–286.

Yasue H, Nagao M, Omote S, et al. (1978). Coronary arterial spasm and Prinzmetal's variant form of angina induced by hyperventilation and tris-buffer infusion. Circulation 58:56–62.

Yasue H, Omote S, Takizawa A, et al. (1979). Exertional angina pectoris caused by coronary artery spasm: effects of various drugs. Am J Cardiol 43:647–652.

Yellowlees PM, Aplers JH, Bowden JJ, et al. (1987). Psychiatric morbidity in patients with chronic airflow obstruction. Med J Aust 147:349–352.

Younes M, Vaillancourt P, Milic-Emili J (1974). Interaction between chemical factors and duration of apnea following lung inflation. J Appl Physiol 36:190–201.

Zwiener U, Lobel S, Rother M, et al. (1998). Quantitative topographical analysis of EEG during nonstandardized and standardized hyperventilation. J Clin Neurophysiol 15:521–528.

Chapter
15

CHRONIC FATIGUE

Fatigue is one of the complaints encountered most frequently in medical practice. Primary care studies in the United States indicate that approximately 20% of patients report feelings of fatigue to their doctors (Buchwald et al., 1987; Kroenke et al., 1988) and 14% present with fatigue as their main or secondary complaint (Cathebras et al., 1992). In the United Kingdom David (1991) found that 10% of 770 patients seen in general practice had chronic fatigue. In a review of 14 large American and British community studies of the prevalence of fatigue, Lewis and Wessely (1992) found that about 19% (a range of 7% to 33%) of males and 25% (11% to 46%) of females experienced fatigue. There was little variation with age, and complaints of fatigue were almost twice as frequent in females in most of the studies they reviewed.

Fatigue of recent onset (suggesting the presence of a newly developed, undiagnosed disease) differs considerably in its possible clinical implications from a complaint of chronic fatigue lasting longer than six months. It is worth noting, however, that in a study at a primary care clinic where patients with fatigue were followed over a one-year period, only 10% were found to have a disease that explained their symptom (Kroenke and Mangelsdorff, 1989).

Definitions of fatigue depend on the vantage point of the definer. The exercise physiologist may view fatigue as the failure to maintain a required or expected force in static contractions or power output during dynamic exercise (Edwards, 1978); others see this as exhaustion (Lewis and Haller, 1991). Some prefer the definition of "a decreased force-generating capacity," which does not prejudge the circumstances in which this state develops (Bigland-Ritchie, 1981; Vollestad and Sejersted, 1988). Clinically, fatigue tends to be seen as a global condition that may best be subjectively defined as "an overwhelming sustained sense of exhaustion and decreased capacity for physical and mental work" (Piper, 1989). This definition helps emphasize the complexity of the state by encompassing its behavioral, biological, and phenomenological aspects. The state is usually verbalized as lack of energy and an inability to maintain usual routines. The problem of chronic fatigue in clinical practice has come to occupy such a defined position that when persistent—lasting for more than six months—and in the absence of any recognizable physical illness or psychiatric diagnosis, it is called the chronic fatigue syndrome (CFS).

DIAGNOSTIC CRITERIA OF CHRONIC FATIGUE SYNDROME

Groups working at the Centers for Disease Control (CDC) in the United States (Holmes et al., 1988) and groups in Britain (Sharpe et al., 1991) proposed specific criteria for the diagnosis of CFS. Although there are differences between the two groups, the following criteria are common to both:

- Any medical illness capable of producing similar symptoms must be excluded.
- The symptom of fatigue should represent a new problem in the sense that there is no lifelong history of fatigue. It should have existed for at least six months (this helps to exclude postviral infection states of fatigue of relatively short duration) and should be present at least 50% of the time or limit performance below 50% of the patient's previous activity level.
- Myalgia and disturbances of mood and sleep, which also characterize the condition of fibromyalgia, are common. Numerous clinical surveys document the coexistence of CFS with fibromyalgia (Buchwald et al., 1987; Goldenberg et al., 1990; Aaron et al., 2000; White et al., 2000). Holmes et al. (1988) describe a number of other accompaniments: mild fever, sore throat, painful lymph nodes (cervical and axillary), headaches, migratory arthralgia, irritability, forgetfulness, difficulty in concentrating, and depression (when judged to be a reaction to the state of fatigue and general disability).
- Chronic psychiatric disorders, such as schizophrenia, substance abuse, and bipolar illness, must be excluded. In the British guidelines, however, depressive illness and anxiety disorder are not necessarily exclusion criteria.

- Physical signs are generally absent or, if present, unremarkable. Some patients may present tenderness of the upper cervical lymph nodes, a mild nonexudative pharyngitis, and/or low-grade fever ($<38.6°C$ orally). There are no characteristic laboratory features and the hematological, biochemical, and immunological changes reported in the literature are variable, generally minor, and mostly of uncertain significance (Komaroff, 1993).

These criteria tend to be restrictive and therefore CFS in the United States, when diagnosed according to the CDC criteria, accounts for fewer than 3% of all cases of fatigue (Manu et al., 1988). This point was confirmed in a study by Bates et al. (1994) which found that in a group of 805 patients with debilitating fatigue without apparent etiology, 61% met the CDC criteria and 55% the British criteria of CFS. These authors made a plea for more inclusive case definitions of CFS.

An important factor complicating attempts to produce a comprehensive definition of CFS centers on the question, previously discussed in relation to IBS (see Chapter 11), of whether CFS is a disease per se (say an idiosyncratic immune reaction to a persistent viral infection) or a psychosomatic disorder. The protagonists of the distinct disease theory, to explain the various clinical and laboratory manifestations of the disorder, see CFS as a disease affecting principally immune and central nervous systems (Komaroff, 2000). Others (Manu, 2000), as do I, see CFS as a psychosomatic condition and contend that all the clinical and laboratory changes of CFS may be adequately explained by psychosomatic mechanisms. These include the extensively investigated immune changes in CFS and the cardiovascular consequences of extreme loss of physical conditioning (Chapter 13). The considerable clinical overlap in CFS patients with other common psychosomatic disorders such as fibromyalgia (see below), temperomandibular disorder (Aaron et al., 2000), and IBS (Gomborone et al., 1996), as well as the general efficacy of cognitive behavior therapy in its management (Price and Couper, 2000), further strengthen this impression.

THE CLINICAL SIGNIFICANCE OF FATIGUE

The development of fatigue depends on cerebral processes, anatomical structures, physiological events, and energy transduction processes. The mechanism of fatigue may be well-defined in certain disease states, such as myasthenia gravis, where there is destruction or blocking of acetylcholine receptors by autoantibodies at the postsynaptic muscle membrane. Here, however, we are most interested in the more general problem: the interplay between undefined central mechanisms that determine the feeling of fatigue and the physiological consequences of physical inactivity, often over extended periods, which aggravate the symptom.

A tendency of CFS patients to exaggerate their disability has been demonstrated in studies showing a discrepancy between performance as measured objectively under control conditions and the patients' perception of performance. Riley et al. (1990), while confirming that 13 CFS patients had a lower exercise capacity than 13 normal controls and 7 patients with irritable bowel syndrome, found that they also had a different perception of their degree of physical exertion: compared to the other groups, the CFS patients perceived their workload, a standardized exercise protocol, to be significantly greater. This is in line with the experience of other researchers (Woods et al., 1987). Using standard neuropsychological tests to assess attention, concentration, and abstraction skills in 21 patients with CFS, Altay et al. (1990) found that they scored significantly better than age-matched controls. Here too there was a clear discrepancy between subjective complaints (of cognitive impairment) and objective test results in the CFS patients. A similar tendency of exaggerated disability was observed in 10 patients suffering from CFS by Sacco et al. (1999), who demonstrated an exercise-related diminution in central motor drive associated with an increased perception of effort as compared to a healthy control group.

This same tendency to exaggerate fatigue occurs in fibromyalgia, a condition of pain and tenderness of the muscles that often coexists with CFS (see below). Elert et al. (1989) studied the perception of fatigue in patients suffering from fibromyalgia. Isokinetic muscular strength, the ability to perform repeated dynamic work, and the perception of muscle fatigue were tested in 10 patients with fibromyalgia and in 10 healthy controls. All performed 100 maximal isokinetic shoulder flexions. There were no differences between patients and controls with respect to amount of work and mean power frequency of the electromyogram at the initial contractions or during the terminal contractions. However, the fibromyalgia patients rated the perception of muscle fatigue as 10 on a 0 to 10 scale after only 20 to 30 contractions. The controls never reached a maximal perception of fatigue. The pronounced tendency to fatigue in fibromyalgia is considered to be mediated mostly by a central mechanism (Henriksson and Bengtsson, 1991) and is expressed through a diminished work capacity. Cathey et al. (1988) compared the work capacity of fibromyalgia patients with those suffering from rheumatoid arthritis and with healthy controls. All were given five standardized work tasks. The fibromyalgia patients performed 59% and the rheumatoid arthritis patients 62% of as much work as the controls.

EVALUATION OF THE PATIENT SUFFERING FROM FATIGUE

In the clinical assessment of a patient whose main symptom is fatigue, one first tries to place the symptom in the context of a recognized disease. Fatigue may appear as a symptom in every major category of disease affecting all systems of the body.

Frequently, however, the underlying disorder is not immediately apparent and may be diagnosed only after a routine examination points to the need for more specific investigations. Certain disorders should nevertheless always be borne in mind, either because they are common or because their prompt diagnosis and treatment may obviate serious complications (they may in fact be easily managed). The following should be routinely sought: an elevated plasma thyrotropin-stimulating hormone (TSH) level, indicating hypothyroidism; anemia, pointing to iron deficiency, chronic renal failure, pernicious anemia, or a blood dyscrasia; an elevated erythrocyte sedimentation rate that indicates an inflammatory process (infective or noninfective); a positive human immunodeficiency virus (HIV) test; and disturbed liver function tests, which may indicate acute or chronic hepatitis. Ischemic heart disease, in the absence of chest pain or signs of cardiac failure, may also present simply as fatigue. This partial list indicates that diseases causing significant fatigue may not be immediately apparent clinically and laboratory tests will be needed to uncover or confirm the diagnosis.

In a comprehensive evaluation, special attention should also be given to three major aspects, drug, sleep, and work history.

Drug History

Certain drugs induce lethargy and fatigue as prominent side effects. These include psychotropic drugs, in particular nocturnal sedatives (sleeping tablets) and antidepressants, antihistamines, β-receptor blockers, cimetidine, and potassium-wasting medicaments (especially diuretics). In the absence of an adequate explanation for the fatigue, any drugs taken by the patient should be viewed with suspicion. The physician might decide to discontinue a medication for a trial period if the clinical state permits, and if not, to substitute another drug with a similar action. It may also be appropriate to inquire into the use of illicit drugs.

Sleep History and Sleep Apnea

A detailed sleep history should be obtained from the patient and if possible from a spouse, parent, or close companion. The patient should be asked about difficulty in falling asleep and very early awakening, which may indicate depression, or frequent awakenings during the night, which could point to bouts of sleep apnea.

Sleep apnea, or sleep-disordered breathing (meaning bouts of either apnea or hypopnea, incomplete cessation of airflow, during sleep), is discussed here not because it is considered a psychosomatic disorder, but because it has potentially important health implications and its consequences often seem to have a psychophysiological basis. Sleep apnea is characterized by recurrent episodes of cessation of respiratory airflow during sleep, which result from collapse of the upper airway at the level of the pharynx (Hudgel, 1992). Sleep predisposes the upper airways to narrowing and, in susceptible individuals, to collapse, because of a reduction in the tone of the upper airway muscles combined with their reflex response to the subatmospheric airway pressure generated during inspiration (Hudgel, 1992; Wheatly et al., 1993). Complete airway collapse during sleep is usually preceded by years of narrowing that produces snoring. In a study of the incidence of sleep apnea in a random sample of 602 subjects aged 30–60 years, Young et al. (1993) found that 4% of women and 9% of men had 15 or more episodes of apnea or hypopnea per hour of sleep.

By the time adults with obstructive sleep apnea seek medical attention, they have a long history of loud snoring, often beginning in childhood. When outright obstruction of the airway develops, however, the snoring is interrupted by periods of apnea lasting 15 to 90 seconds, coincident with complete cessation of the airflow. During these episodes severe arterial hypoxia may develop, until the apnea is terminated by a brief awakening and the airway patency is restored. These events are usually accompanied by a generalized startle response, snorting, and gasping. After a few breaths the patient returns to sleep, only to have the cycle repeated as many as 200 to 400 times during 6–8 hours of sleep (Phillipson, 1993).

Sleep apnea, which disturbs the nocturnal sleep rhythm, may result in considerable daytime fatigue. The main clinical expression of obstructive sleep apnea is excessive daytime sleepiness, thought to be due to the fragmentation of sleep as well as the loss of deeper levels of sleep by recurrent arousal, and the effects of hypoxemia on cerebral function. There may also be cognitive dysfunction and memory loss, which together with excessive daytime sleepiness may result in employment difficulties, social disharmony, and emotional disturbances. Among the other important pathophysiological consequences are anoxia, systemic hypertension, and the aggravation of cardiac failure. The fatigue and hypertension, in particular, may be ascribed to psychophysiological factors. It is also easy to see from this description how the patient may be diagnosed as suffering from depression and possibly anxiety.

Among the serious consequences of this condition that have been documented is a link with systemic hypertension (Fletcher et al., 1985; Millman et al., 1991). Half or more of all patients with sleep apnea syndrome are hypertensive, and the severity of the sleep apnea syndrome is linked to the risk of hypertension (Lavie et al., 1993; Hla et al., 1994). In a prospective study of sleep-disordered breathing and hypertension, Peppard et al. (2000) found a significant association between sleep-disordered breathing at baseline and the presence of hypertension four years later that was independent of known confounding factors such as habitus, age, sex, and cigarette and alcohol use. Most important, this study documented the fact that even persons with minimal sleep-disordered breathing (as defined by an apnea–hypopnea index of 0.1 to 4.9 events per hour) had higher odds of hypertension (42% greater odds) than those with no episodes of sleep-disordered breathing. Persons with mild sleep-disordered breathing (as defined by an apnea–hypopnea index of 5.0 to 14.9 events per hour) and those with more severe sleep-disordered breathing (as defined by an apnea–hypopnea index of 15.0 or more events per hour) had approximately two and three times, respectively, the odds of having hypertension at follow-up of those having no episodes of apnea or hypopnea. Furthermore, studies suggesting a causal link between the two conditions have shown that successful treatment of sleep apnea may normalize elevated blood pressure (Fletcher et al., 1985; Mayer et al., 1991; Suzuki et al., 1993).

The mechanism of apnea-induced hypertension is thought to be mediated through sympathetic arousal in that a direct relationship has been shown between oxygen desaturation levels—sometimes below 60% (representing an arterial oxygen tension of below 30 mm Hg)—and the level of acute blood pressure elevation. These patients also display an increased pressor response to induced hypoxia (Hedner et al., 1992; Arabi et al., 1999). Increased sympathetic activity in acute hypoxia has been directly recorded by microneurography (Somers et al., 1988). It has been assumed that repeated, long-term hypoxia during obstructive sleep apnea may reset the chemoreceptor reflex drive to a higher level, causing a chronic increase in sympathetic tone and initiating hypertension (Trzebski, 1992; Carlson et al., 1993).

Other serious consequences of sleep apnea are

- A two- to threefold increase in motor accidents compared to the general population, due to falling asleep at the wheel (Findley et al., 1989).
- An increased risk of stroke, angina, and myocardial infarction (Partinen and Palomaki, 1985; Koskenvuo et al., 1987; Hung et al., 1990).
- Aggravation of left ventricular failure (Malone et al., 1991), pulmonary hypertension, and right ventricular failure (Phillipson, 1993).

Work and Occupation History

A work history is an important part of the assessment of fatigue. There are two main areas of interest: work routine and possible agricultural, industrial, or office exposure to chemicals and gases. A work routine characterized by long hours, substantial emotional demands (due perhaps to responsibility or boredom), and few vacations will almost inevitably lead at some point to feelings of fatigue. This can usually be elicited by inquiry.

A more insidious and potentially dangerous occupational cause of fatigue is exposure to organophosphorus cholinesterase inhibitor insecticides or volatile organic chemicals. Individuals who have had long-term exposure to insecticides or solvents may exhibit symptoms of depression, memory impairment, difficulty concentrating, fatigue, personality changes, headache, and irritability (Hane et al., 1977; Harkonen, 1977; Arlien-Soborg et al., 1979). Exposure for more than 10 years to organic solvents and for a variable time to organophosphorus insecticides is now thought to have subclinical neurobehavioral effects (Bleeker et al., 1991). Only a high index of suspicion on the part of the physician will lead to a search for exposure to hydrocarbon solvents, insecticides, or other potentially toxic chemicals in the patient's work or living environments.

CHRONIC FATIGUE SYNDROME

As mentioned, the diagnosis of CFS implies fatigue lasting more than six months in the absence of an identifiable medical condition. In recent years, well-conducted studies of the prevalence of chronic fatigue have been undertaken in the United States because of the growing professional and public interest in the widely publicized condition. One reason for the medical community's concern is that many people with chronic fatigue syndrome claim to have been quite well and energetic up to the time of a "viral" illness. From that time on they appear to have developed lethargy, extreme forms of fatigability, and, as a result, considerable disability that has severe repercussions on their social and professional lives. Komaroff (1993) interviewed 300 sporadic, that is, nonepidemic, patients diagnosed with CFS, and 85% of the patients stated that their illness had begun suddenly, with an acute "flulike" illness characterized by fever, sore throat, cervical adenopathy, cough, abdominal symptoms, myalgia, arthralgia, or other symptoms suggestive of an acute infectious process. This presumed viral etiology initially received considerable support from a series of reports about chronic Epstein-Barr virus (EBV) infection in which fatigue was a prominent clinical feature (Tobi et al., 1982; DuBois et al., 1984; Jones et al., 1985; Straus et al., 1985). Subsequent studies, however, cast doubt on EBV as the cause of chronic fatigue (Buchwald et al., 1987; Holmes et al., 1987). As this "typical" clinical picture is highly reminiscent of a viral infection, efforts have been directed toward identifying a possible causative role of viruses in CFS.

Fatigue Following Viral Infection

Although the data indicate no proven association between past infection with a particular virus and CFS, the prevalence of fatigue syndromes following viral infection as well as their natural history are problematic. White et al. (1998) studied prospectively a cohort of 250 primary care patients who had suffered a viral infection and found 108 (44%) had EBV infection (GF, glandular fever) confirmed by appropriate serology, 83 (34%) had non-EBV glandular fever (i.e., pharyngitis, cervical adenopathy, and fever but negative serology), and 54 (22%)

had ordinary upper respiratory tract infection (URTI), without serological evidence of a recent EBV infection or infectious mononucleosis. There was no significant difference between the groups in the past psychiatric history or in psychiatric treatment during the year before onset. The incidence of an acute fatigue syndrome was 47% in the GF patients, and this lasted a median of 8 weeks (4 to 16 weeks), but only 3 weeks after URTI. A CFS-like illness was present in 9%–22% (depending on whether the definition of CFS used was American or British) 6 months after GF, compared to 0.6% following URTI. White et al. concluded that new EBV infection may be a risk factor for CFS. While episodes of major depressive disorder were apparently triggered by infection, especially EBV, they lasted only three weeks on average. Furthermore, no psychiatric disorder was significantly more prevalent six months after onset than before. This study indicates that post-EBV acute (i.e., new) infection lethargy is prolonged in some people, but it remains important to distinguish between this condition and most cases of CFS, which reveal little or no evidence of a recent EBV infection. Also, the observation that episodes of major depression associated with the acute viral infection lasted only about three weeks contrasted with Blacker's (1998) finding that the median duration of major depressive disorders in general practice patients is eight months. The patients were studied in the same locality, at the same time, using the same criteria as in the study of White et al. These two studies strongly suggest that lethargy or depression triggered by infection, nevertheless, has a much better outcome.

A number of published studies, however, do point to an association of psychiatric states and psychosocial factors with prolonged fatigue following viral illness. In a study designed to evaluate psychological distress and psychiatric disorder during and after acute infectious mononucleosis (GF), 144 patients with GF were evaluated at initial infection and then at both two and six months later (Katon et al., 1999). As in the White et al. (1998) study, transient psychological distress was common during acute infection, but few patients met accepted criteria (DSM-IIIR) for psychiatric illness. Whereas biological factors such as disturbed liver function still appeared to be important in distressed patients at two months, at six months greater distress correlated with an increased number of adverse life events in the six months after developing GF and of days of reduced activity in the two weeks before the onset of GF.

In two studies of other viral illnesses, one reporting chronic fatigue after hepatitis A and B infections up to 30 months postinfection compared with matched controls hospitalized for other infections (Berelowitz et al., 1995) and the other after viral meningitis (Hotopf et al., 1996), both groups emphasized psychiatric morbidity as a predictive factor for prolonged fatigue. Cope et al. (1994) studied 618 patients diagnosed with viral illnesses in primary care clinics and assessed by questionnaire six months later. Of 502 patients (81.2%) who completed the 6-month questionnaire, and 88 (17.5%) met the criteria for chronic fatigue.

Psychiatric morbidity, belief in vulnerability to viruses, and attributional style at initial interview were all associated with self-designated postviral fatigue. Other researchers from the United Kingdom (Sharpe et al., 1992; Chalder et al., 1996), Australia (Wilson et al., 1994), and the Netherlands (1996) have similarly described a correlation between physical (viral) illness beliefs and functional impairment and have identified such beliefs as the strongest predictor of poor outcome. Thus, the burden of evidence would seem to implicate either preexisting psychiatric conditions or certain psychosocial characteristics as major factors in the development of postviral infection fatigue.

Past Experience with Fatigue Syndromes

Throughout the twentieth century there were reports of epidemic illnesses in different parts of the world, where the predominant symptoms in some cases included marked fatigue and emotional lability (Sabin and Dawson, 1993). In the polio epidemic of 1934 in Los Angeles, for instance, such cases differed in many ways from the clinical picture of polio (Gilliam, 1938). Most came from the ranks of graduate and student nurses who had been exposed to polio patients, leading to the reasonable conclusion that "the majority of them resulted from an infection with the virus of poliomyelitis." Nevertheless, differences between these patients and the proven poliomyelitis patients were sufficiently great to elicit the comment that "certain observers were of the privately expressed opinion that hysteria played a large role in this outbreak ." A similar viewpoint was expressed in relation to other epidemics (Ramsay, 1957; McEvedy and Beard, 1970). Waves of cases of a "mystery illness" were seen following polio epidemics in Australia in 1949 (Pellew, 1954; Pellew and Miles, 1955), in New York State in 1950 (White and Burtch, 1954), and in South Africa in 1955 (Hill, 1955). In Iceland in 1948 (Sigurdsson et al., 1950) the disease thought to resemble polio, whereas in London in 1952 and 1955, it appeared distinctive enough to be called "epidemic encephalomyelitis" or the "Royal Free disease," after the hospital with the largest number of cases (Acheson, 1954; Sumner, 1956; Macrae and Galpine, 1954; Ramsay and O'Sullivan, 1956; Medical Staff of the Royal Free Hospital, 1957). An outbreak in Bethesda, Maryland, in 1952 was cautiously termed *Epidemic neuromyasthenia* (Shelokov et al., 1957).

Certain common features emerging from these epidemics indicated that the illness was nonfatal, relapsing, affected especially young females, and often involved hospital personnel, especially nurses and student nurses. Beyond this, the clinical picture was always variable and ill-defined. It is worth noting, however, that most waves occurred at the time of epidemics of poliomyelitis in the community and, at least in the early years, were referred to as "poliolike." This does not so much hint at the possible involvement of the polio virus in the genesis of the syndrome, as was frequently thought, but points to extreme psychological pressure on the nursing staff and indeed on the general population during these periods. Polio was mainly an affliction of young, active people who either were left disabled or died from the disease, and new outbreaks were always widely publicized in the lay press. It was justifiably considered a fearsome disease from which there was no certain protection.

Pathogenesis of Chronic Fatigue Syndrome

Infectious agents

One of the major problems encountered in the search for a viral cause for CFS is that lifelong infection with EBV beginning in adolescence or with human herpes virus 6 (HHV-6) starting early in life is widespread in the population. In separate studies, some patients with CFS exhibit unusually high levels of antibody to EBV (Schooley et al., 1986), while others have an unusual level of HHV-6 viral replication (Buchwald et al., 1992). Rather than primary infection, these findings have been interpreted to indicate secondary reactivation, which may in turn be an epiphenomenon (Komaroff, 1993). The serological associations between the syndrome and cytomegalovirus (CMV), herpes simplex virus types 1 and 2, and measles virus were found to be as strong as or stronger than the association with EBV. The reemergence in some CFS sufferers of increased antibody titers to persistent virus infections such as EBV and other herpes viruses, for example, could be interpreted as the expression of an enhanced state of Th2 type immunity, as seen in conditions of stress (see Chapter 6). The Th2 immune state occurs when the cytokine profile leads to a weakened cellular immunity (Th1 type)—needed to maintain the virus in a quiescent state—in association with enhanced maturation and stimulation of sensitized, antibody-producing B cells (by a Th2 cytokine such as Il-6), with the persistent virus infection providing continuous antigen stimulation. Other surveys of human herpes viruses (HHVs) that tested for HHV-6, HHV-7, EBV, and CMV in CFS patients and age-, race- and sex-matched controls revealed no differences between the patients and control groups (Wallace et al., 1999). Moreover, the prevalence in the general community of fatigue states that strongly resembled CFS was relatively high, whereas "chronic EBV infection" as an active clinical syndrome is considered to be extremely rare.

Other virus types have also been considered as potential etiological agents of CFS. Following reports of the epidemic occurrence of myalgic encephalomyelitis around the time of polio epidemics, polio virus (in a less virulent form) was thought to be the etiological agent. Enteroviruses are now known to cause a persistent infection of the central nervous system (Sharief et al., 1991), making them potential factors in the etiology of CFS. Circulating enteroviral antigens have been found more often in patients with CFS than in control subjects (Yousef et al., 1988), and enterovirus antigens and nucleic acids are present more often in the muscles of patients with CFS than in healthy controls (Archard et al., 1988; Cunningham et al., 1990; Gow et al., 1991). In a study of enterovirus persistence in eight patients with CFS, Galbraith et al. (1997) found that in serum samples taken five months apart and evaluated by polymerase chain reaction (PCR), the samples were identical in four patients, indicating persistence of the virus, but in the remaining four individuals, the lack of shared sequences suggested reinfection. Thus, the role of enteroviruses in CFS is far from clear.

Nonviral infectious agents have also been linked to CFS (Salit, 1985). One of the best documented causes is infection due to *Borrelia burgdorferi*, the agent responsible for Lyme disease. In this condition, a delay in treatment may result in a state with all the clinical characteristics of CFS (Coyle and Krupp, 1990). No serological evidence of *B. burgdorferi* is found, however, in CFS patients (Pollark et al., 1995; Schutzer and Natelson, 1999).

In a study utilizing a sensitive PCR assay for the detection of mycoplasma species in the peripheral blood mononuclear cells of 100 CFS patients (diagnosed according to the criteria of the Centers for Disease Control) and 100 healthy controls, Choppa et al. (1998) found that the percentage of *Mycoplasma* genus infections in the CFS group was 52% as compared to 15% in the controls. The main types were *M. fermentans*, *M. hominis*, and *M. penetrans* detected in 32%, 9%, and 6% of the CFS patients and in 8%, 3%, and 2% of the controls. In a further study by the same group quantitating the number of *M. fermentans* genome copies in 1 microgram (μg) of DNA for control and CFS patients, genome copy numbers ranging from 130 to 880 and from 264 to 2400 were detected in controls and in CFS patients, respectively. With an enzyme immunoassay against p29 surface lipoprotein of *M. fermentans* to determine the relationship between *M. fermentans* copy numbers and antibody levels, Vojdani et al., (1998) showed that individuals with high genome copy numbers exhibited higher IgG and IgM antibodies against *M. fermentans*–specific peptides. While the exquisite sensitivity of these sophisticated techniques of molecular analysis are helping to define the interplay of pathogens with the immune system and their relationship to clinical states, the changes described may be as much a consequence of immune changes (toward a Th2 state) in CFS as a cause of the disorder.

Fibromyalgia, disturbed sleep patterns, and chronic fatigue syndrome

Fibromyalgia is a clinical condition characterized by muscle pain and stiffness, with tender nodules, or "trigger points," in the muscles, especially those of the back and neck, affecting mainly women aged 30–45 years. Like irritable bowel syndrome, fibromyalgia is normally diagnosed by exclusion; that is, it is accepted as the diagnosis only after other conditions have been eliminated by appropriate clinical and laboratory evaluation. Studies in recent years have pointed to a remarkable overlap in the clinical presentations of fibromyalgia and CFS with at least 80% of patients with either diagnosis complaining of fatigue, myalgia and arthralgia, recurrent headache, and sleep disturbances (Buchwald et al., 1987; Goldenberg et al., 1990). In addition, Buchwald et al. found that as with CFS patients, many of their fibromyalgia patients (about 50%) reported that their condition had begun with a flulike illness.

As pointed out by Moldofsky (1993), many of the clinical features of fibromyalgia and CFS may be induced by total or partial sleep deprivation. Sleep deprivation or prolonged wakefulness causes sleepiness, fatigue, negative mood, and impaired intellectual function, all of which may occur in CFS. A home polysomnography study performed of 18 teenagers aged 11 to 17 years suffering from CFS showed significantly higher levels of sleep disruption by both brief and longer awakenings than in healthy controls matched individually for age and sex (Stores et al., 1998). Fischler at al. (1997) similarly observed difficulties in sleep initiation and sleep maintenance in 49 adult CFS patients. In addition, the percentage of stage 4 deep, restorative sleep was significantly lower in the CFS group as compared to 20 matched healthy controls.

The term unrefreshing (nonrestorative) sleep was introduced by Moldofsky et al. (1975), who observed that an anomalous (in that it occurred during a phase of sleep) alpha rhythm (7.5–11.0 Hz) in electroencephalographic (EEG) recordings during non–rapid eye movement (NREM) sleep was associated with unrefreshing sleep and an overnight increase in muscle tenderness. Anch et al. (1991) reported that fibromyalgia patients had more alpha rhythm in their EEGs during sleep, "were more vigilant during sleep," and had more fatigue, sleepiness, and pain than normal healthy controls. The alpha rhythm normally occurs during quiet wakefulness and tends to disappear with the onset of sleep, although in one study it was observed during sleep in approximately 15% of apparently healthy subjects (Scheuler et al., 1983). It is replaced during sleep by the appearance of other EEG frequencies such as theta (3–7 Hz), K complexes, and sleep spindles (12–15 Hz) and subsequently by the delta or slow waves (0.5–2.5 Hz) of stages 3 and 4 NREM sleep. The alpha frequency appears with induced or spontaneous arousals from sleep. The prominent alpha rhythm during sleep has been interpreted as a physiological indicator of a state of partial wakefulness or a type of arousal disorder within sleep and of the subjective experience of light, unrefreshing sleep (Moldofsky, 1993).

Other authors have observed an association between disturbed sleep and muscular pain. Saskin et al. (1986) reported anomalous alpha EEG rhythm during sleep, as well as diffuse myalgia, fatigue, and emotional distress, in patients after an emotionally distressing but not physically injurious industrial or motor accident. Kolar et al. (1989) and Jacobsen and Danneskiold-Samsoe (1989) also reported a correlation between poor sleep quality and muscle tenderness. Agnew et al. (1967) observed that with selective deprivation of stage 4 slow-wave sleep, subjects became "physically uncomfortable, withdrawn, less aggressive, and manifested concern over vague physical complaints and changes in body feelings." Moldofsky et al. (1975) extended these observations by measuring musculoskeletal pain and altered mood in healthy but sedentary subjects following experimental disturbance of slow-wave sleep. The threshold for joint tenderness was measured with a pressure gauge or dolorimeter over the specific anatomical sites found to be sensitive to pressure in patients with fibromyalgia. The subjects displayed increased tenderness during the three nights of stage 4 sleep deprivation induced by noise. They also complained of musculoskeletal aching, stiffness, generalized heaviness, and unusual fatigue. Some also suffered nausea, diarrhea, and loss of appetite, along with depression and irritability. These symptoms were accompanied by the alpha EEG sleep anomaly, which was produced by the repetitive disruption of stage 4 sleep with the noise stimuli. All the symptoms subsided after two nights of undisturbed sleep. Interestingly, Moldofsky and Scarisbrick (1976) were unable to induce somatic or behavioral symptoms by stage 4 sleep disruption in a small group of physically fit long-distance runners.

The potential role of cytokines in chronic fatigue syndrome and fibromyalgia

The importance of cytokines in mediating both inflammatory and immune responses, as well as neuroimmune interactions, was presented in Chapter 6, particularly in relation to stress responses. There are additional actions of cytokines, however, that have a bearing on this discussion in that they may influence sleep physiology as well as producing neuropsychological change (Kronfol and Remick, 2000). Fatigue, myalgia, irritability, sleepiness, difficulty in concentrating, and negative mood are common to many infected states and similarly occur with the therapeutic administration of cytokines such as interferons in diseases like hepatitis C, malignant melanoma, and multiple sclerosis. The therapeutic administration of cytokines in the management of disorders like these can induce a spectrum of clinical symptoms that strongly resemble those of both CFS and fibromyalgia. The amounts administered are greatly in excess of physiological requirements and therefore the side effects are usually much more severe than might occur as a result of endogenous secretion. The neuropsychiatric side effects of the administered cytokine remits with cessation of the treatment. Alpha-interferon given to hepatitis carriers causes fatigue, cognitive dysfunction, and diffuse myalgia and malaise (McDonald et al., 1987). Interleukin 2 (IL-2), which is given to some patients with metastatic malignancy, may produce an influenzalike syndrome with cognitive impairment. Patients complain of lassitude, fatigue, anorexia, malaise, and sleep disturbance (Denicoff et al., 1987), as well as diffuse musculoskeletal symptoms (Wallace et al., 1990).

Certain viral infections, such as coxsackie B (Nash et al., 1989) and parvovirus (Leventhal et al., 1991), are known to cause fibromyalgia. The occurrence of fibromyalgialike syndromes in 20% of patients infected with human immunodeficiency virus (HIV) (Buskila et al., 1990) and 16% of hepatitis C-infected patients (Buskila et al., 1997) indicates that endogenous secretion of cytokines in response to certain conditions of chronic active viral infection (not simply persistent and nonactive, like EBV) may suffice to produce similar syndromes of fatigue and fibromyalgia. Infection with the parvovirus is also accompanied by the alpha EEG sleep anomaly. Similarly, infection with HIV is associated with sleep disturbance characterized by a delayed onset but increased slow-wave sleep, an increase in the total number of REM periods, the alpha EEG sleep anomaly and increased awakenings during sleep (Norman et al., 1990).

In parallel with these observations showing disturbed sleep patterns in viral infections, studies over the last few years have suggested that a number of cytokines may also play a role in the physiology of sleep. Thus, interleukin 1 (IL-1) is known to promote slow-wave sleep in animals and other mediators may also be important in promoting sleep, such as factor S, muramyl dipeptide (a product of bacterial cell walls), vasoactive intestinal polypeptide, prostaglandin D-2, alpha-2-interferon, tumor necrosis factor (TNF) (Krueger and Johannsen, 1989), and interleukin 2 (Nistico and De Sarro, 1991). Plasma levels of IL-1 and IL-2–like activity in humans are at a maximum during nocturnal sleep (Moldofsky et al., 1986). In cats, IL-1 activity in the cerebrospinal fluid is increased during sleep (Lue et al., 1988). Serum IL-1 may be increased in CFS (Cheney et al., 1989; Cannon et al., 1997). The production of alpha interferon by peripheral mononuclear cells is also increased (Lever et al., 1988), as is IL-6 and TNF-alpha (Gupta et al., 1997), but gamma interferon production is not (Morte et al., 1988). Any function these cytokines have in perpetuating CFS is uncertain. Some of the cytokines mentioned, secreted in response to a viral infection, for example, may induce the clinical symptoms of CFS.

Psychiatric evaluation of chronic fatigue syndrome patients: the psychosocial component

Most patients with CFS reject the suggestion that there may be a psychological basis to their illness (Wessely and Powell, 1989; Wessely, 1990; Blakely et al., 1991). In a psychiatric evaluation of 48 patients with CFS, Hickie et al. (1990) reported high scores on disease conviction (an attitude of certainty about the presence of disease and resistance to reassurance). In a case control study of 133 CFS patients making an insurance claim, 75 multiple sclerosis claimants and 162 non-claimant controls, Hall et al. (1998) found that CFS cases recorded significantly more illness than the two control groups. They reported almost all disease categories to be higher. This study parallels others in which CFS patients scored high on hypochondriasis and disease conviction scales (Schweitzer et al., 1994; Trigwell et al., 1995).

Patients are often able to point to lives of unusual industry and productivity right up to the sudden illness which heralded the onset of CFS. Thus, for example, Salit (1985) reported that patients with CFS are achievement-oriented, goal-driven individuals who have been exceptionally active socially, occupationally, and physically. Similarly, Ware (1993) found that a group of 50 CFS patients had typically led remarkably active lives:

> Men and women who were employed devoted up to 80 hours a week to their jobs. Mothers who worked at home matched this pace, beginning their days early and staying up late to bake, sew or clean after the children were in bed . . . Coping with the number and variety of their responsibilities meant moving fast; hence days were spent racing from one activity to another in a constant, frantic effort to "keep up" . . . Self-professed desires for productivity, high standards for personal performance, and a tendency to "do for others" converge as the driving force behind this whirlwind of activity.

It is important and interesting to note that Blumer and Heilbronn (1982), in an analysis of 900 patients suffering from chronic pain syndrome, had described their patients in extremely similar terms: "The juxtaposition of their frantic premorbid activity with their complete fatigue and helplessness is striking." This overlap of chronic pain syndromes (which certainly may include fibromyalgia) with CFS has been noted by others as well (Clauw and Chrousos, 1997).

However, the life histories of these patients also contained evidence of substantial distress (Ware, 1993): " 'Stress' was cited as either a contributing factor or the single probable cause of CFS by almost half the interviewees, who used the term to mean sensations of being overwhelmed by obligations and commitments, experiences of loss, fears of displeasing others, and feelings of loneliness and isolation." This analysis of life history data of 50 CFS sufferers revealed the following experience:

- Negative life events (serious injury, divorce, job loss, death of a family member or close friend) was recorded by 21 (42%).
- Chronic life difficulties (serious illness in immediate family, troubled or failing marriage, persistent work problems) were noted by 20 (40%).
- Evidence of family psychiatric history (depression, anxiety, alcohol or other drug abuse, and/or physical violence in parents or other close family members) was noted in 26 (44%).
- Abuse, low self-esteem, and family tension in childhood were noted in 22 (44%).

Other authors have also pointed to the high level of activity in CFS patients as a more important feature of their self-image and factor in maintaining self-esteem than in other patient populations (Abbey, 1993). Adolescents referred for the evaluation of persistent fatigue are often described as ambitious and athletic and are usually from an intact, upper middle-class family (Verker, 1992). Nonetheless, in comparing the tendency to perfectionism in 40 CFS sufferers (using the Multidimensional Perfectionalism Scale) and in 31 healthy control subjects, Blenkinron et al. (1999) found no correlation between perfectionism scores and fatigue, anxiety, or depression in either group. Abbey and Garfinkel (1991) summarize the predicament of the CFS sufferer in the following manner: "This group would appear to be particularly susceptible to the psychological impact of incapacity secondary to a severe or protracted illness, because it would remove them from the goal-directed activities which are required to stabilize their self-esteem and provide meaning and pleasure."

Summary

The demographic characteristics of CFS patients appear to include any person subjected to sustained pressure or stress. This could be extraneously derived, perhaps by living in deprived neighborhoods or as a consequence of an excessively demanding life-style and a tendency to perfectionism that ultimately overwhelms the person's ability to cope. While the early literature on the subject tended to describing a population of predominantly white, middle-class women, this perception now may be seen as ascertainment bias that resulted from the ability of this particular population of patients to draw attention to their disorder. A telephone survey by Jason et al. (1999) that canvassed 28,673 adults in Chicago found CFS-like symptoms in approximately 1 in 200 respondents (there was a 65% completion rate of the telephone interview). In this study, the highest levels of CFS were consistently found among women, minority groups, and persons with lower levels of education and occupational status. Thus, we should be prepared to diagnose CFS in women or men, adolescents or adults, and in people from economically privileged or deprived sectors of society. A fairly extensive literature does, however, point to personal characteristics such as perfectionism as creating a special vulnerability. It is this particular quality that predisposes, in particular, the professional woman who combines managerial or professional responsibility with her responsibilities as a mother, wife, and housekeeper, to significant stress, which leads to CFS.

Chronic Fatigue Syndrome and Depression

Could CFS be a depressive illness in a primary sense, with a presentation that is largely somatic? Many authors feel that CFS is not a form of primary depression as defined in the DSM (Rogers and Chang, 1993). Some authors have also pointed out that CFS has certain features distinctly different from those of depression, for example, the shortening of REM latency, that is, the time from falling asleep to the onset of dreaming (REM) sleep. In depression this may be reduced to

35–40 minutes, whereas in CFS patients it is within the normal range (70–120 minutes), though it is slightly shorter (i.e., 50–60 minutes) in CFS patients who are also depressed (Morehouse et al., 1998).

In addition, CFS patients display no evidence of abnormalities of the hypothalamic–pituitary–adrenal (HPA) axis, such as hypercortisolism and loss of dexamethasone suppression, which are typical of major depression. The defect of HPA axis function in 30 patients with CFS compared to 72 normal healthy volunteers was defined as hypoadrenalism of central (hypothalamic–pituitary) origin (Demitrack et al., 1991). This contrasts with the hypercortisolism observed in melancholic depression.

Young et al. (1998) evaluated basal HPA activity by measuring cortisol levels in the saliva and a 24-hour urine collection of 22 patients with CFS and could find no difference from a healthy control group. Scott et al. (1998), however, used a sensitive ACTH (adrenocorticotropic hormone) test involving 1 μg (rather than 250 μg) of ACTH as the adrenal stimulus and were able to show a slightly reduced response in 20 CSF patients, when compared to 20 healthy controls, though basal cortisol values did not differ between the patients and controls. Using an incremental cortisol value of >250 nmol/L as an arbitrary cutoff point, two (10%) of the healthy subjects and nine (45%) of the CSF subjects failed the test ($P < 0.05$). Similarly, MacHale et al. (1998) noted that the diurnal change in cortisol was significantly less in 30 CFS patients compared to 15 age-, sex-, and weight-matched healthy controls, although there was no significant difference between the groups in the morning and evening cortisol levels.

The differences in cortisone secretion between depression and CFS have been confirmed by other workers (Cleare et al., 1995). Nonetheless, the issue is not settled. The CDC criteria for the diagnosis of CFS list depression as an exclusion criterion; the likely result is a selected group of CFS sufferers who normally are unable to easily identify and express their true feelings. In addition, not all patients with depression will show changes in cortisol metabolism, so depression may exist as a comorbid condition, as indicated below.

Comorbidity of CFS with psychiatric diagnoses has been documented in a number of studies. Kruesi et al. (1989), using the Diagnostic Interview Schedule, assessed the lifetime prevalence of psychiatric disorders in a group of 28 CFS patients diagnosed according to the CDC criteria and found that 21 (75%) met the diagnostic criteria for psychiatric illness. Chronic fatigue syndrome followed psychiatric illness in 10 (48%) of these patients and preceded it by a year or more in only 2 (10%). The lifetime prevalence of major depression in this sample was 46%. Studies cited in a review by Katon and Walker (1993) confirm that the symptom of fatigue is associated with high psychiatric comorbidity in community, primary care, and tertiary care samples. In these samples, the prevalence of lifetime major depression among patients with significant fatigue was found to be 18%–23%, 32%–43%, and 46%–76%, respectively. The prevalence of current major depression in these patients was 1.2%–2%, 17%, and 15%–64%. In the community samples, people with significant fatigue and comorbid major depressive and anxiety disorders had significantly more unexplained physical complaints and made more frequent use of medical services than patients with fatigue alone. Buchwald et al. (1997) administered the General Health Questionnaire (GHQ), a 28-item self-report instrument that measures psychological and somatic distress on a four-point scale, to 120 chronic fatigue and 161 CFS patients. Overall, 87 (35%) gave evidence of a current psychiatric disorder and 210 (82%) of such a disorder at some point in their lifetime.

Comorbidity of CFS with a broad spectrum of psychiatric disorders has been described. These include, in addition to depression, generalized anxiety disorder and somatization disorder (Fischler et al., 1997), dysthymia (Brunello et al., 1999), and seasonal affective disorder (Terman et al., 1998). In addition, there may be considerable overlap with other functional somatic disorders, such as fibromyalgia and other chronic pain syndromes (Clauw and Chrousos, 1997), sick building syndrome (Chester and Levine, 1997), and multiple chemical sensitivity (Pollet et al., 1998).

Therapeutic strategies

Promising results of cognitive-behavioral therapy in CFS patients have been reported (Sharpe et al., 1996; Deale et al., 1997; Price and Couper, 2000), in contrast to a lack of benefit from drugs such as antidepressants (Vercoulen et al., 1996), antihistamines (Steinberg et al., 1996), and antiviral agents. The presence of coexistent depression should always be kept in mind, however, including the possibility of more subtle presentations such as dysthymia or seasonal affective disorder.

A program of graded exercise is reportedly beneficial in CFS (McCully et al., 1996; Fulcher and White, 1997). In a randomized trial of fluoxetine and graded exercise in 136 CFS patients, 96 (71%) completed the trial, with a greater tendency of the patients receiving exercise to drop out (Wearden et al., 1998). The graded exercise schedule produced improvements in functional work capacity and fatigue; fluoxetine improved only the depression.

Marginal improvement has been reported with low-dose hydrocortisone therapy (5 or 10 mg daily) (Cleare et al., 1999), but a study with fluorocortisone failed to show any benefit (Peterson et al., 1998). The rationale for hydrocortisone therapy was the assumption that CFS is associated with a state of hypoadrenalism causing at least part of the patients' lethargy.

Conclusion

It seems unlikely that the illness diagnosed as CFS represents a pathological condition resulting from persistent (viral) infection in any more than a small percentage of patients. Psychobiological factors that may be important in initiating CFS include

- Immune mediators (cytokines) secreted in response to an infection and their effects on the nervous system, including lassitude, difficulty in concentrating, easy fatigability, and sleep disturbance.
- Interaction of sleep disorder (including the anomalous sleep alpha rhythm) with the resulting emotional state, leading to a heightened sensitivity with more aches and pains, including fibromyalgia.
- Psychological distress resulting in part from the subject's emotional dependency on hard work for self-esteem and in part from other longstanding unresolved personal problems, which leads to anxiety and perhaps to symptom anticipation.
- The superposition of depression, with its social and biological ramifications.

Clinical experience with a host of treatment modalities, of which cognitive behavior therapy has emerged as the most efficacious, the documented occurrence of frequent comorbidity of psychiatric conditions, particularly depression, as well as with other common psychosomatic conditions have strengthened the categorization of CFS as a psychosomatic disorder. Because CFS patients frequently resist accepting this evaluation, management may prove to be extremely problematic unless approached in a special way.

Management of Chronic Fatigue Syndrome

Among physicians, ideas about the origins of CFS vary markedly. A 1995 survey of 2090 Australian general practitioners about CFS documented considerable diversity of opinion: 70% thought that the most likely cause was depression and 31% reported that they did not believe that CFS is a distinct syndrome (Steven et al., 2000). No wonder patients may be confused about the origins and proper management of CFS. The common tendency of patients with CFS, as documented above, to attribute their illness with considerable conviction to a persistent viral infection often is joined with resistance to the idea of the condition being considered psychosomatic.

My first rule, therefore, is, if resistance is encountered, to avoid being stalemated in my dialogue with the patient by a fruitless discussion about diagnostic labels. Management of the problem may still proceed after the patient accepts the fact that all examinations have failed to locate a definite cause for the fatigue, or if there is a marginal finding that it in no way can account for the profound disability the patient is experiencing. While always being truthful about my perception of the problem, I frequently elicit an attitude of cooperation by expressing my willingness to reevaluate the condition by examining the patient physically or undertaking further laboratory evaluation should the need arise because of lack of clinical progress or because of deterioration. I believe this attitude addresses a major concern of most CSF patients, namely, that the negative investigations have missed a serious underlying (organic) process that is causing the fatigue.

The first step in managing CFS may be profitably spent on planning a physical rehabilitation program. As described in Chapter 13, the outcome of situations of extreme limitation of physical activity, whether caused by anxiety or any other mechanism, is a state of reduced fitness such that even normal physical activity creates distressing discomfort. Much like patients who begin to stand and walk after a period of enforced bed rest and inactivity, orthostatic intolerance (dizziness on standing up due to a fall in blood pressure, with tachycardia and weakness) is also commonly found in CSF patients, both adolescent (Stewart et al., 1999) and adult (LaManca et al., 1999; Schondorf et al., 1999). As in other very unfit people, the reduced blood volume and autonomic lability resulting from their physical inactivity is associated too with impaired oxygen delivery to the exercising muscles (McCully and Natelson, 1999). All these physiological factors work to enhance their discomfort on exertion to discourage continued activity. This debilitating cycle needs to be clearly explained to the patient with the reassurance that not only will physical activity do no harm, even if exercised to exhaustion, but that their ability to reap the benefits from a program of graduated activity is similar to that of any healthy individual—that nothing in their condition that will prevent them from regaining complete good health (Mullis et al., 1999). Furthermore, one can emphasize the already proven efficacy of graduated exercise programs in CFS patients (McCully et al., 1996; Fulcher and White, 1997; Wearden et al., 1998).

As with all debilitating psychosomatic conditions, the most seriously affected are also preoccupied with the pain and frustration of their condition for a significant proportion of their free time; indeed, they usually spend more than 20% and very often 60% to 100% of their time preoccupied with their condition. As mentioned in Chapter 4, this almost invariably indicates that they are struggling with the feeling of having lost control over their lives. While a graduated exercise program helps to return the patient to a reasonable level of fitness, insofar as the patient is party to its planning and execution, it will also help restore a feeling of regaining control, an aspect absolutely fundamental to their emotional and physical rehabilitation.

If the patient still resists the idea of psychotherapy, behavioral techniques such as deep relaxation exercises or a program of mindful meditation may be very helpful in moving the patient in the right direction (see Chapter 19). Although recommending deep relaxation exercises may sound like a curious intervention for an excessively lethargic individual, in my experience in patients suffering from CSF, as with all other psychosomatic conditions, it remains a powerful technique for helping reduce anxiety and restore feelings of self-control with a positive effect on energy levels. As the patient begins to demonstrate increased feelings of self-confidence, it becomes possible to return to the subject of psychotherapy. The initial refusal to consider the psychotherapy option often comes from a feeling of not having the energy to deal with threatening or difficult issues. Beginning the program with behavioral techniques allows those trained in cognitive behavior techniques to easily slip into a dialogue with the patient that begins to examine and explore other relevant issues.

The general experience with drugs in CFS is that they should be reserved for the management of depression and/or anxiety when needed. Even seriously debilitated CFS patients will usually deny feeling depressed, but if in doubt a course of antidepressant medication may be tried (see Chapter 17). Depression symptoms often follow the state of fatigue and improve with periods of less fatigue so provided progress is monitored it is not always necessary to immediately treat depression with medication (Wood et al., 1992). The general experience is that medication makes no difference to the fatigue but that it does result in relief of depression (Wearden et al., 1998; Morriss et al., 1999). To that extent, it may also assist in improving social functioning.

REFERENCES

Aaron LA, Burke MM, Buchwald D (2000). Overlapping conditions among patients with chronic fatigue syndrome, fibromyalgia, and temperomandibular disorder. Arch Intern Med 160:221–227.

Abbey SE (1993). Somatization, illness attribution and the sociocultural psychiatry of chronic fatigue syndrome. In: Kleinman A, Straus SE, eds. Chronic Fatigue Syndrome. Chichester: Wiley (Ciba Foundation Symposium 173), pp 238–261.

Abbey SE, Garfinkel PE (1991). Chronic fatigue syndrome and depression: cause, effect or covariate. Rev Infect Dis 13(suppl 1):S73–S83.

Acheson ED (1954). Encephalomyelitis associated with poliomyelitis virus: an outbreak in a nurses' home. Lancet 2:1044–1048.

Agnew HW, Webb WB, Williams RL (1967). Comparison of stage four and 1-REM sleep deprivation. Percept Mot Skills 24:851–858.

Altay HT, Toner BB, Brooker H, et al. (1990). The neuropsychological dimensions of postinfectious neuromyasthenia (chronic fatigue syndrome): a preliminary report. Int J Psychiat Med 20:141–149.

Anch AM, Lue FA, MacLean AW, et al. (1991). Sleep physiology and psychological aspects of fibrositis [fibromyalgia] syndrome. Can J Psychol 45:179–184.

Arabi Y, Morgan BJ, Goodman B, et al. (1999). Day-time blood pressure elevation after nocturnal hypoxia. J Appl Physiol 87:689–698.

Archard LC, Bowles NE, Behan PO, et al. (1988). Postviral fatigue syndrome: persistence of enterovirus RNA in muscle and elevated creatine kinase. J R Soc Med 81:326–329.

Arlien-Soborg P, Bruhn P, Gyldensted C, et al. (1979). Chronic painter's syndrome: chronic toxic encephalopathy in house painters. Acta Neurol Scand 60:149–156.

Bates DW, Buchwald D, Lee J, et al. (1994). A comparison of case definitions of chronic fatigue syndrome. Clin Infect Dis 18(suppl 1):S11–15.

Berelowitz GJ, Burgess AP, Thanabalasingham T, et al. (1995). Post-hepatitis revisited. J Viral Hepat 2:133–138.

Bigland-Ritchie B (1981). EMG/force relations and fatigue of human voluntary contractions. Exerc Sport Sci Rev 9:75–117.

Blacker CVR (1988). Depression in general practice. London: University of London. Thesis. Quoted by: White PD et al. (1998).

Blakely AA, Howard RC, Sosich RM, et al. (1991). Psychiatric symptoms, personality and ways of coping in chronic fatigue syndrome. Psychol Med 21:347–362.

Bleeker ML, Bolla KI, Agnew J, et al. (1991). Dose-related subclinical neurobehavioral effects of chronic exposure to low levels of organic solvents. Am J Indust Med 19:715–728.

Blenkinron P, Edwards R, Lynch S (1999). Associations between perfectionism, mood, and fatigue in chronic fatigue syndrome: a pilot study. J Nerv Ment Dis 187:566–570.

Blumer D, Heilbronn M (1982). Chronic pain as a variant of depressive disease: the pain-prone disorder. J Nerv Ment Dis 170:381–406.

Brunello N, Akiskal H, Boyer P, et al. (1999). Dysthymia: clinical picture, extent of overlap with chronic fatigue syndrome, neuropharmacological considerations, and new therapeutic vistas. J Affect Disord 52:275–290.

Buchwald D, Cheney PR, Peterson DL, et al. (1992). A chronic illness characterized by fatigue, neurologic and immunologic disorders, and active human herpesvirus type 6 infection. Ann Intern Med 116:103–113.

Buchwald D, Goldenberg DL, Sullivan JL, et al. (1987). The "chronic active Epstein-Barr virus infection" syndrome and primary fibromyalgia. Arthritis Rheum 30:1132–1136.

Buchwald D, Pearlman T, Kith P, et al. (1997). Screening for psychiatric disorders in chronic fatigue and chronic fatigue syndrome. J Psychosom Res 42:87–94.

Buchwald D, Sullivan JL, Komaroff AL (1987). Frequency of "chronic active Epstein-Barr virus infection" in a general medical practice. JAMA 257:2303–2308.

Buskila D, Gladman DD, Langevitz P, et al. (1990). Fibromyalgia in human immunodeficiency virus infection. J Rheumatol 17:1202–1206.

Buskila D, Shnaider A, Neumann L, et al. (1997). Fibromyalgia in hepatitis C infection: another infectious disease relationship. Arch Intern Med 157:2497–2500.

Cannon JG, Angel JB, Abad LW, et al. (1997). Interleukin-1 beta, interleukin-1 receptor antagonist, and soluble interleukin-1 receptor type II secretion in chronic fatigue syndrome. J Clin Immunol 17:253–261.

Carlson JT, Hedner J, Elam M, et al. (1993). Augmented resting sympathetic activity in awake patients with obstructive sleep apnea. Chest 103(6):1763–1768.

Cathebras PJ, Robbins JM, Kirmayer LJ, et al. (1992). Fatigue in primary care: prevalence, psychiatric comorbidity, illness behavior, and outcome. J Gen Intern Med 7:276–286.

Cathey MA, Wolfe F, Kleinheksel SM, et al. (1988). Functional ability and work status in patients with fibromyalgia. Arthritis Care Res 1:1–14.

Chalder T, Power M, Wessely S (1996). Chronic fatigue in the community: a question of attribution. Psychol Med 26:791–800.

Cheney PR, Dorman SE, Bell DS (1989). Interleukin-2 and the chronic fatigue syndrome. Ann Intern Med 110:321.

Chester AC, Levine PH (1997). The natural history of concurrent sick building syndrome and chronic fatigue syndrome. J Psychiatr Res 31:51–57.

Choppa PC, Vojdani A, Tagle C, et al. (1998). Multiplex PCR for the detection of *Mycoplasma fermentans*, *M. hominis* and *M. penetrans* in cell cultures and blood samples of patients with chronic fatigue syndrome. Moll Cell Probes 12:301–308.

Clauw DJ, Chrousos GP (1997). Chronic pain and fatigue syndromes: overlapping clinical and neuroendocrine features and potential pathogenic mechanisms. Neuroimmunomodulation 4:134–153.

Cleare AJ, Bearn T, Allain A, et al. (1995). Contrasting neuroendocrine responses in depression and chronic fatigue syndrome. J Affect Dis 35:283–289.

Cleare AJ, Heap E, Malhi GS, et al. (1999). Low-dose hydrocortisone in chronic fatigue syndrome: a randomized crossover trial. Lancet 353:455–458.

Cope H, David A, Pelosi A, et al. (1994). Predictors of chronic "postviral" fatigue. Lancet 344:864–868.

Coyle PK, Krupp LB (1990). B. burgdorferi infection in the chronic fatigue syndrome. Ann Neurol 28:243–244. (Abstract)

Cunningham L, Bowles NE, Lane RJM, et al. (1990). Persistence of enteroviral RNA in chronic fatigue syndrome is associated with the abnormal production of equal amounts of positive and negative strands of enteroviral RNA. J Gen Virol 71:1399–1402.

David A (1991). Psychiatric disorders in general practice attenders with chronic fatigue syndrome. Presented at the Royal College of Psychiatrists Annual Meeting, Brighton, England, July 1991.

Deale A, Chalder T, Marks I, et al. (1997). Cognitive behavior therapy for chronic fatigue syndrome: a randomized controlled trial. Am J Psychiatry 154:408–414.

Demitrack MA, Dale JK, Straus SE, et al. (1991). Evidence for impaired activation of the hypothalamic-pituitary-adrenal axis in patients with chronic fatigue syndrome. J Clin Endocrinol Metab 73:1224–1234.

Denicoff KD, Rubinow DR, Papa MZ, et al. (1987). The neuropsychiatric effects of treatment with interleukin-2 and lymphokine activated killer cells. Ann Intern Med 107:293–300.

DuBois RE, Seeley JK, Brus I, et al. (1984). Chronic mononucleosis syndrome. South Med J 77:1376–1382.

Edwards RH (1978). Physiological analysis of skeletal muscle weakness and fatigue. Clin Sci Mol Med 54:463–470.

Elert JE, Rantapaa-Dahlquist SB, Henriksson-Larsen K, et al. (1989). Increased EMG activity during short pauses in patients with primary fibromyalgia. Scand J Rheumatol 18:321–323.

Findley LJ, Fabrizio M, Thommi G, et al. (1989). Severity of sleep apnea and automobile crashes. N Engl J Med 320:868–869.

Fischler B, Cluydts R, De Gucht Y, et al. (1997). Generalized anxiety disorder in chronic fatigue syndrome. Acta Psychiatr Scand 95:405–413.

Fischler B, Le Bon O, Hoffmann G, et al. (1997). Sleep anomalies in the chronic fatigue syndrome: a comorbidity study. Neuropsychobiology 35:115–122.

Fletcher EC, DeBehnke RD, Lovoi MS, et al. (1985). Undiagnosed sleep apnea in patients with essential hypertension. Ann Intern Med 103:190–195.

Fulcher KY, White PD (1997). Randomized control trial of graded exercise in patients with the chronic fatigue syndrome. Br Med J 314:1647–1652.

Galbraith DN, Nairn C, Clements GB (1997). Evidence for enteroviral persistence in humans. J Gen Virol 78:307–312.

Gilliam AG (1938). Epidemiologic study of an epidemic diagnosed as poliomyelitis occurring among the personnel of the Los Angeles County General Hospital during the summer of 1934. Public Health Bulletin No. 240, U.S.Treasury Dept.

Goldenberg DL, Simms RW, Geiger A, et al. (1990). High frequency of fibromyalgia in patients with chronic fatigue seen in a primary care practice. Arthritis Rheum 33:381–387.

Gomborone JE, Gorard DA, Dewsnap PA, et al. (1996). Prevalence of irritable bowel syndrome in chronic fatigue. J R Coll Physicians Lond 30:512–513.

Gow JW, Behan WM, Clements GB, et al. (1991). Enteroviral RNA sequences detected by polymerase chain reaction in muscle of patients with postviral fatigue syndrome. Br Med J 302:692–696.

Gupta S, Aggarwal S, See D, et al. (1997). Cytokine production by adherent and nonadherent mononuclear cells in chronic fatigue syndrome. J Psychiatr Res 31:149–156.

Hall GH, Hamilton WT, Round AP (1998). Increased illness experience preceding chronic fatigue syndrome: a case control study. J R Coll Physician Lond 32:44–48.

Hane M, Axelson O, Blume J, et al. (1977). Psychological function changes among house painters. Scand J Work Environ Health 3:91–99.

Harkonen H (1977). Relationship of symptoms to occupational styrene exposure and to the findings of electroencephalographic and psychological examinations. Int Arch Occup Environ Health 40:231–239.

Hedner JA, Wilcox I, Laks L, et al. (1992). A specific and potent pressor effect of hypoxia in patients with sleep apnea. Am Rev Respir Dis 146:1240–1245.

Henriksson KG, Bengtsson A (1991). Fibromyalgia—a clinical entity? Can J Physiol Pharmacol 69:672–677.

Hickie I, Lloyd A, Wakefield D, et al. (1990). The psychiatric status of patients with the chronic fatigue syndrome. Br J Psychiatry 156:534–540.

Hill RCJ (1955). The Durban "mystery disease." S Afr Med J 29:997.

Hla KM, Young TB, Bidwell T, et al. (1994). Sleep apnea and hypertension: a population-based study. Ann Intern Med 120:382–388.

Holmes GP, Kaplan JE, Gantz NM, et al. (1988). Chronic fatigue syndrome: a working case definition. Ann Intern Med 108:387–389.

Holmes GP, Kaplan JE, Stewart JA, et al. (1987). A cluster of patients with a chronic mononucleosis-like syndrome: is Epstein-Barr virus the cause? JAMA 257:2297–2302.

Hotopf M, Noah N, Wessely S (1996). Chronic fatigue and minor psychiatric morbidity after viral meningitis: a controlled study. J Neurol Neurosurg Psychiatry 60:504–509.

Hudgel DW (1992). The role of upper airway anatomy and physiology in obstructive sleep apnea. Clin Chest Med 13:383–398.

Hung J, Whitford EG, Parsons RW, et al. (1990). Association of sleep apnea with myocardial infarction in men. Lancet 336:261–264.

Jacobsen S, Danneskiold-Samsoe B (1989). Inter-relations between clinical parameters and muscle function in patients with primary fibromyalgia. Clin Exp Rheumatol 7:493–498.

Jason LA, Richman JA, Rademaker AW, et al. (1999). A community-based study of chronic fatigue syndrome. Arch Intern Med 159:2129–2137.

Jones JF, Ray CG, Minnich LL, et al. (1985). Evidence for active Epstein-Barr virus infection in patients with persistent, unexplained illnesses: elevated anti–early antigen antibodies. Ann Intern Med 102:1–7.

Katon W, Russo J, Ashley RL, et al. (1999). Infectious mononucleosis: psychological symptoms during acute and subacute phases of illness. Gen Hosp Psychiatry 21:21–29.

Katon WJ, Walker EA (1993). The relationship of chronic fatigue to psychiatric illness in community, primary care and tertiary care samples. In: Kleinman A, Straus SE, eds. Chronic Fatigue Syndrome. Chichester: Wiley (Ciba Foundation Symposium 173), pp 193–211.

Kolar E, Hartz A, Roumm A, et al. (1989). Factors associated with severity of symptoms in patients with chronic unexplained muscular aching. Ann Rheum Dis 48:317–321.

Komaroff AL (1993). Experience with sporadic and "epidemic" cases. In: Dawson DM, Sabin TD, eds. Chronic Fatigue Syndrome. Boston: Little, Brown and Company, pp 25–43.

Komaroff AL (2000). The biology of chronic fatigue syndrome. Am J Med 108:169–171.

Koskenvuo M, Kaprio J, Heikkila K, et al. (1987). Snoring as a risk factor for ischemic heart disease and stroke for men. Br Med J 294:643.

Kroenke K, Mangelsdorff AD (1989). Common symptoms in ambulatory care: incidence, evaluation, therapy, and outcome. Am J Med 86:262–266.

Kroenke K, Wood DR, Mangelsdorff AD, et al. (1988). Chronic fatigue in primary care. Prevalence, patient characteristics, and outcome. JAMA 260:929–934.

Kronfol Z, Remick DG (2000). Cytokines and the brain: implications for clinical psychiatry. Am J Psychiatry 157:683–694.

Krueger JM, Johannsen L (1989). Bacterial products, cytokines and sleep. J Rheumatol 19(suppl):52–57.

Kruesi MJ, Dale J, Straus SE (1989). Psychiatric diagnoses in patients who have chronic fatigue syndrome. J Clin Psychiatry 50:53–56.

Lamanca JJ, Peckerman A, Walker J, et al. (1999). Cardiovascular response during head-up tilt in chronic fatigue syndrome. Clin Physiol 19:111–120.

Lavie P, Yoffe N, Berger I, et al. (1993). The relationship between the severity of sleep apnea syndrome and 24-hour blood pressure values in patients with obstructive sleep apnea. Chest 103:717–721.

Leventhal LJ, Naides SJ, Freundlich B (1991). Fibromyalgia and parvovirus infection. Arthritis Rheum 34:1319–1324.

Lever AM, Lewis DM, Bannister BA, et al. (1988). Interferon production in post viral fatigue syndrome. Lancet 2:101.

Lewis G, Wessely S (1992). The epidemiology of fatigue: more questions than answers. J Epidemiol Comm Health 46:92–97.

Lewis SF, Haller RG (1991). Physiologic measurement of exercise and fatigue with special reference to chronic fatigue syndrome. Rev Infect Dis 13(suppl 1):S98–108.

Lue FA, Bail M, Jephthah-Ochola J, et al. (1988). Sleep and cerebrospinal fluid interleukin-1-like activity in the cat. Int J Neurosci 42:179–183.

Machale SM, Cavanagh JT, Bennie J, et al. (1998). Diurnal variation of adrenocortical activity in chronic fatigue syndrome. Neuropsychobiology 38:213–217.

Macrae AD, Galpine JF (1954). An illness resembling poliomyelitis observed in nurses. Lancet 2:350–.

Malone S, Liu PP, Holloway R, et al. (1991). Obstructive sleep apnea in patients with dilated cardiomyopathy: effects of continuous positive airway pressure. Lancet 338:1480–1484.

Manu P (2000). Chronic fatigue syndrome: the fundamentals still apply. Am J Med 108:172–173.

Manu P, Lane TJ, Matthews DA (1988). The frequency of the chronic fatigue syndrome in patients with symptoms of persistent fatigue. Ann Intern Med 109:554–556.

Mayer J, Becker H, Brandenburg U, et al. (1991). Blood pressure and sleep apnea: results of long-term nasal continuous positive airway pressure therapy. Cardiology 79:84–92.

McCully K, Natelson B (1999). Impaired oxygen delivery to muscle in chronic fatigue syndrome. Clin Sci (Colch) 97:603–608; discussion 611–613.

McCully K, Sisto S, Natelson B (1996). Use of exercise for treatment of chronic fatigue syndrome. Sports Med 21:35–48.

McDonald EM, Mann AH, Thomas HC (1987). Interferons as mediators of psychiatric morbidity: an investigation in a trial of recombinant alpha interferon in hepatitis-B carriers. Lancet 2:1175–1178.

McEvedy CP, Beard AW (1970). Royal Free epidemic of 1955: a reconsideration. Br Med J 1:7–11.

Medical Staff of the Royal Free Hospital (1957). An outbreak of encephalomyelitis in the Royal Free Hospital group, London, 1955. Br Med J 2:895–904.

Millman RP, Redline S, Carlisle CC, et al. (1991). Daytime hypertension in obstructive sleep apnea: prevalence and contributing risk factors. Chest 99:861–866.

Moldofsky H (1993). Fibromyalgia, sleep disorder and chronic fatigue syndrome. In: Kleinman A, Straus SE, eds. Chronic Fatigue Syndrome. Chichester: Wiley (Ciba Foundation Symposium 173), pp 262–279.

Moldofsky H, Lue FA, Eisen J, et al. (1986). The relationship of interleukin-1 and immune functions to sleep in humans. Psychosom Med 48:309–318.

Moldofsky H, Scarisbrick P (1976). Induction of neurasthenic muskuloskeletal pain syndrome by selective sleep stage deprivation. Psychosom Med 38:35–44.

Moldofsky H, Scarisbrick P, England R, et al. (1975). Musculoskeletal symptoms and non-REM sleep disturbance in patients with "fibrositis syndrome" and healthy subjects. Psychosom Med 37:341–351.

Morehouse RL, Flanigan M, MacDonald DD, et al. (1998). Depression and short REM latency in subjects with chronic fatigue syndrome. Psychosom Med 60:347–351.

Morriss RK, Ahmed M, Wearden AJ, et al. (1999). The role of depression in pain, psychophysiological syndromes and medically unexplained symptoms associated with chronic fatigue syndrome. J Affect Disord 55:143–148.

Morte S, Castilla A, Civeira MP, et al. (1988). Gamma-interferon and chronic fatigue syndrome. Lancet 2:623–624.

Mullis R, Campbell IT, Wearden AJ, et al. (1999). Prediction of peak oxygen uptake in chronic fatigue syndrome. Br J Sports Med 33:352–356.

Nash P, Chard M, Hazleman B (1989). Chronic coxsackie B infection mimicking primary fibromyalgia. J Rheumatol 16:1506–1508.

Nistico G, De Sarro G (1991). Is interleukin-2 a neuromodulator in the brain? Trends Neurosci 14:146–150.

Norman SE, Chediak A, Kiel M, et al. (1990). HIV infection and sleep: follow up studies. Sleep Res 19A:339. Abstract.

Olson GB, Kanaan MN, Gersuk GM, et al. (1986). Correlation between allergy and persistant Epstein-Barr virus infections in chronic active Epstein-Barr virus infected patients. J Allergy Clin Immunol 78:308–314.

Olson GB, Kanaan MN, Kelley LM, et al. (1986). Specific allergen-induced Epstein-Barr nuclear antigen-positive B cells from patients with chronic-active Epstein-Barr virus infections. J Allergy Clin Immunol 78:315–320.

Partinen M, Palomaki H (1985). Snoring and cerebral infarction. Lancet 2:1325–1326.

Pellew RAA (1951). Clinical description of a disease resembling poliomyelitis. Med J Aust 1:944–946.

Pellew RAA, Miles JAR (1955). Further investigation on a disease resembling poliomyeleitis seen in Adelaide. Med J Aust 22:480–482.

Peppard PE, Young T, Palta M, et al. (2000). Prospective study of the association between sleep-disordered breathing and hypertension. N Engl Med J 342:1378–1384.

Peterson PK, Pheley A, Schroeppel J, et al. (1998). A preliminary placebo-controlled crossover trial of fluorocortisone for chronic fatigue syndrome. Arch Intern Med 158:908–914.

Phillipson EA (1993). Sleep apnea—a major public health problem. N Engl J Med 328:1271–1273.

Piper BF (1989). Fatigue: current bases for practice. In: Funk SG, Tornquist EM, Champagne MT, Copp LA, Wiese RA, eds. Key Aspects of Comfort: Management of Pain, Fatigue, and Nausea. New York: Springer Publishing Co, pp 187–198.

Pollark RJ, Komaroff AL, Telford SR 3rd, et al. (1995). *Borrelia burgdorferi* infection is rarely found in patients with chronic fatigue syndrome. Clin Infect Dis 20:467–468.

Pollet C, Natelson BH, Lange G, et al. (1998). Medical evaluation of Persian Gulf veterans with fatigue and/or chemical sensitivity. J Med 29:101–113.

Price JR, Couper J (2000). Cognitive behaviour therapy for adults with chronic fatigue syndrome. Cochrane Database Syst Rev 2:CD001027.

Ramsay AM (1957). Encephalomyelitis in northwest London: an epidemic infection simulating poliomyelitis and hysteria. Lancet. 2:1196–1200.

Ramsay AM, O'Sullivan E (1956). Encephalomyelitis simulating poliomyelitis. Lancet 1:761–.

Riley MS, O'Brein CJ, McCluskey DR, et al. (1990). Aerobic work capacity in patients with chronic fatigue syndrome. Br Med J 301:953–956.

Rogers MP, Chang G (1993). Psychiatric aspects. In: Dawson DM, Sabin TD, eds. Chronic Fatigue Syndrome. Boston: Little, Brown and Company, pp 45–68.

Sabin TD, Dawson DM (1993). History and epidemiology. In: Dawson DM, Sabin TD, eds. Chronic Fatigue Syndrome. Boston, Little, Brown and Company.

Sacco P, Hope PA, Thickbroom GW, et al. (1999). Corticomotor excitability and perception of effort during sustained exercise in the chronic fatigue syndrome. Clin Neurophysiol 110:1883–1891.

Salit IE (1985). Sporadic postinfectious neuromyasthenia. Can Med Assoc J 133:659–663.

Saskin P, Moldofsky H, Lue FA (1986). Sleep and posttraumatic rheumatic pain modulation disorder (fibrositis syndrome). Psychosom Med 48:319–323.

Scheuler W, Stinshoff D, Kubicki S (1983). The alpha-sleep pattern: differentiation from other sleep patterns and effect of hypnotics. Neuropsychobiology 10:183–189.

Schondorf R, Benoit J, Wein T, et al. (1999). Orthostatic intolerance in the chronic fatigue syndrome. J Auton Nerv Syst 75:192–201.

Schooley RT, Carey RW, Miller G. et al. (1986). Chronic Epstein-Barr virus infection associated with fever and interstitial pneumonitis: clinical and serologic features and response to antiviral chemotherapy. Ann Intern Med 104:636–643.

Schutzer SE, Natelson BH (1999). Absence of *Borrelia burgdorferi*-specific immune complexes in chronic fatigue syndrome. Neurology 53:1340–1341.

Schweitzer R, Robertson DL, Kelly B, et al. (1994). Illness behaviour of patients with chronic fatigue syndrome. J Psychosom Res 38:41–49.

Scott LV, Medbak S, Dinan TG (1998). The low dose ACTH test in chronic fatigue syndrome and in health. Clin Endocrinol (Oxf) 48:733–737.

Sharief MK, Hentges R, Ciardi M (1991). Intrathecal immune response in patients with the post-polio syndrome. N Engl J Med 325:749–755.

Sharpe MC, Archard LC, Banatvala JC, et al. (1991). A report—chronic fatigue syndrome: guidelines for research. J R Soc Med 84:118–121.

Sharpe M, Hawton K, Seagroatt V, et al. (1992). Follow up of patients presenting with fatigue to an infectious disease clinic. Br Med J 305:147–152.

Sharpe M, Hawton K, Simkin S, et al. (1996). Cognitive behavioural therapy for the chronic fatigue syndrome: a randomised control trial. Br Med J 312:22–26.

Shelokov A, Habel K, Verder E, et al. (1957). Epidemic neuromyasthenia: an outbreak of poliomyelitis-like illness in student nurses. N Engl Med J 257:345–355.

Sigurdsson B, Sigurjonsson J, Sigurdsson JHJ, et al. (1950). A disease epidemic in Iceland simulating poliomyelitis. Am J Hyg 52:222–238.

Somers VK, Mark AL, Abboud FM (1988). Potentiation of sympathetic nerve responses to hypoxia in borderline hypertensive subjects. Hypertension 11:608–612.

Steinberg P, McNutt BE, Marshall P, et al. (1996). Double-blind placebo-controlled study of the efficacy of oral terfenadine in the treatment of chromic fatigue syndrome. J Allergy Clin Immunol 97:119–126.

Steven ID, McGrath B, Qureshi F, et al. (2000). General practitioners' beliefs, attitudes and reported actions towards chronic fatigue syndrome. Aust Fam Physician 29:80–85.

Stewart JM, Gewitz MH, Weldon A, et al. (1999). Patterns of orthostatic intolerance: the orthostatic tachycardia syndrome and adolescent chronic fatigue. J Pediatr 135:218–225.

Stores G, Fry A, Crawford C (1998). Sleep abnormalities demonstrated by home plethysmography in teenagers with chronic fatigue syndrome. J Psychosom Res 45:85–91.

Straus SE, Tosato G, Armstrong G, et al. (1985). Persistent illness and fatigue in adults with evidence of Epstein-Barr virus infection. Ann Intern Med 102:7–16.

Sumner DW (1956). Further outbreak of disease resembling poliomyelitis. Lancet 764–767.

Suzuki M, Otsuka K, Guilleminault C (1993). Long-term nasal continuous positive airway pressure administration can normalize hypertension in obstructive sleep apnea patients. Sleep 16(6):545–549.

Terman M, Levine SM, Terman JS, et al. (1998). Chronic fatigue syndrome and seasonal affective disorder: comorbidity, diagnostic overlap, and implications for treatment. Am J Med 105(3A):115S–124S.

Tobi M, Morag A, Ravid Z, et al. (1982). Prolonged atypical illness associated with serological evidence of persistent Epstein-Barr virus infection. Lancet 1:61–64.

Trigwell P, Hatcher S, Johnson M, et al. (1995). "Abnormal" illness behaviour in chronic fatigue syndrome and multiple sclerosis. Br Med J 311:15–18.

Trzebski A (1992). Arterial chemoreceptor reflex and hypertension. Hypertension 19:562–566.

Vercoulen J, Swanink C, Fennis J, et al. (1996). Prognosis in chronic fatigue syndrome (CFS): a prospective study. J Neurol Neurosurg Psychiatry 60:489–494.

Vercoulen JH, Swanink CM, Zitman FG, et al. (1996). Randomized, double-blind, placebo-controlled study of fluoxetine in chronic fatigue syndrome. Lancet 347:858–861.

Verker MI (1992). Chronic fatigue syndrome: a joint paediatric–psychiatric approach. Arch Dis Child 67:550–557.

Vojdani A, Choppa PC, Tagle C, et al. (1998). Detection of *Mycoplasma* genus and *Mycoplasma fermentans* by PCR in patients with chronic fatigue syndrome. FEMS Immunol Med Microbiol 22:355–365.

Vollestad NK, Sejersted OM (1988). Biochemical correlates of fatigue: a brief review. Eur J Appl Physiol 57:336–347.

Wallace DJ, Peter JB, Bowman RL, et al. (1990). Fibromyalgia, cytokines, fatigue syndromes and immune regulation. Adv Pain Res Ther 17:227–287.

Wallace HL, Natelson B, Gause W, et al. (1999). Human herpesviruses in chronic fatigue syndrome. Clin Diagn Lab Immunol 6:216–223.

Ware NC (1993). Society, mind and body in chronic fatigue syndrome: an anthropological view. In: Kleinman A, Straus SE, eds. Chronic Fatigue Syndrome. Chichester: Wiley (Ciba Foundation Symposium 173), pp 62–82.

Wearden AJ, Morriss RK, Mullis R, et al. (1998). Randomised, double-blind, placebo-controlled treatment trial of fluoxetine and graded exercise for chronic fatigue syndrome. Br J Psychiatry 172:485–490.

Wessely S (1990). "Old wine in new bottles": neurasthenia and "ME." Psychol Med 20:35–53.

Wessely S, Powell R (1989). Fatigue syndromes: a comparison of chronic "postviral" fatigue with neuromuscular and affective disorders. J Neurol Neurosurg Psychiatry 52:940–948.

Wheatly JR, Mezzanotte WS, Tangel DJ, et al. (1993). Influence of sleep on genioglossus muscle activation by negative pressure in normal men. Am Rev Resp Dis 148:597–605.

White DN, Burtch RB (1954). Iceland disease: a new infection simulating acute anterior poliomyelitis. Neurology 4:506–516.

White KP, Speechly M, Harth M, et al. (2000). Co-existence of chronic fatigue syndrome with fibromyalgia syndrome in the general population: a controlled study. Scand J Rheumatol 29:44–51.

White PD, Thomas JM, Amess J, et al. (1998). Incidence, risk and prognosis of acute chronic fatigue syndromes and psychiatric disorders after glandular fever. Br J Psychiatry 173:475–481.

Wilson A, Hickie I, Lloyd A, et al. (1994). Longitudinal study of outcome of chronic fatigue syndrome. Br Med J 308:756–759.

Wood C, Magnello ME, Sharpe MC (1992). Fluctuations in perceived energy and mood among patients with chronic fatigue syndrome. J R Soc Med 85:195–198.

Woods JJ, Furbush F, Bigland-Ritchie B (1987). Evidence for a fatigue-induced reflex inhibition of motorneuron firing rates. J Neurophysiol 58:125–137.

Young AH, Sharpe M, Clements A, et al. (1998). Basal activity of the hypothalamic-pituitary-adrenal axis in patients with the chronic fatigue syndrome (neurasthenia). Biol Psychiatry 43:236–237.

Young T, Palta M, Dempsey J, et al. (1993). The occurrence of sleep-disordered breathing among middle-aged adults. N Engl J Med 328:1230–1235.

Yousef GE, Bell EJ, Mann GF, et al. (1988). Chronic enterovirus infection in patients with postviral fatigue syndrome. Lancet 1:146–150.

Chapter
16

DEPRESSION IN THE MEDICAL CLINIC

> Instead of the myriad sub-divisions of minor illness to be found in
> the ICD or the DSM . . . classifications, we assert that there are
> only a very limited number of ways that the human frame responds
> to psychological stress, and that these are defined by two under-
> lying dimensions of symptomatology: anxious symptoms on one
> hand, and depressive symptoms on the other. These two dimen-
> sions are themselves correlated, and combinations of the two sets
> of symptoms are more common than either set on its own.
>
> (Goldberg and Huxley, "Common Mental Disorders," 1992)

The great majority of individuals with emotional disorders are treated by primary care physicians rather than by mental health professionals (Regier et al., 1978). In fact, depression is more common in primary care than any condition except hypertension (Ballenger et al., 1999). The prevalence, however, varies accord-ing to setting, diagnostic criteria, and method of detection. In five studies using structured interviews with research or clinical diagnostic criteria of depression, its incidence varied from 5.8% (Hoeper et al., 1979) to 20% (Olfson et al., 2000), but most studies of primary care patients put it around 10% (Schulberg et al., 1985; Von Korff et al., 1987; Barrett et al., 1988). Studies employing self-report symptom scales have revealed significant depressive symptomatology in

12%–38% of patients (Rosenthal et al., 1978; Nielsen and Williams, 1980; Linn and Yager, 1984).

To determine whether culture influences the clinical expression of depression, especially with regard to somatization, Simon et al. (1999) screened 25,916 primary care patients from 14 countries on five continents. A total of 1146 patients met the criteria for major depression. The range of patients with depression who reported only somatic symptoms was 45%–95%. Half the depressed patients reported multiple unexplained somatic symptoms, and 11% denied psychological symptoms of depression on direct questioning. Neither of these proportions varied significantly between the centers. The experience of this study suggests, however, that although the symptomatic experience of depression seems to vary little from one country to another, the interaction between doctors and depressed patients may vary considerably and that this influences the patient's presentation of the problem. Thus, a somatic presentation of depression was more common at centers where patients lacked an ongoing relationship with a primary care physician than at centers where most patients had a personal physician. Not surprisingly, it seems an almost universal experience that for patients to speak about their feelings they require a relationship of trust with their physician.

Although most patients with depression are managed in primary care settings, there is thought to be a lack of knowledge and skills in diagnosing and treating the disorder (Thompson and Thompson, 1989; Eisenberg, 1992; Mynors-Wallis et al., 1995). General internists and family practitioners apparently failed to recognize major depression in up to 60% of affected outpatients (Rosenthal et al., 1978; Nielsen and Williams, 1980; Thompson et al., 1983; Zung et al., 1983). In addition, Gerber et al. (1989) and Perez-Stable et al. (1990) found that in 12%–13.6% of cases depression was mistakenly diagnosed when it was absent. This observation, coupled with the problem of underdiagnosis of depression in the clinic, reflects many physicians' uncertainty about the accepted diagnostic criteria for depression. It also indicates a lack of awareness of the clinical implications of demographic and social risk factors predisposing patients to depression, such as poverty, excessive drug use, unemployment, being unmarried, or suffering chronic illness. By contrast, few physicians today would ignore the likelihood that ischemic heart disease might develop or be present in a patient with a history of high blood cholesterol, hypertension, heavy smoking, or diabetes mellitus. When confronted with any of the latter risk factors, most physicians would almost certainly ask a number of probing questions with the intention of including or excluding ischemic heart disease, even if such a patient had presented with a complaint obviously unrelated to the cardiovascular system. In the case of the depression risk factors listed above, asking simple questions such as "Have you lost interest and pleasure in most things you usually enjoy?" "Have you lost energy or do you suffer from unexplained fatigue?" or "Are you feeling sad, blue or depressed?" may help uncover depression (Ballenger et al., 1999).

DIAGNOSTIC CRITERIA OF DEPRESSION

It is important for physicians to be familiar with the diagnostic criteria listed in the *Diagnostic and Statistical Manual of Mental Disorders* (DSM-IV) of the American Psychiatric Association. Interviewing patients in order to include or exclude these criteria is certain to allow a more comprehensive evaluation of their emotional state. The following section outlines the main conditions that need to be considered.

Major Depressive Episode

1. At least five of the following symptoms must be present simultaneously for a period of two weeks or more. The patient's condition represents a change from previous levels of functioning, and one symptom must be either depressed mood or anhedonia (loss of pleasure or interest in all activities).
   - Depressed mood or, in children or adolescents, irritable mood.
   - Anhedonia.
   - Significant weight loss (not due to intentional dieting), weight gain, or chronic increase or decrease in appetite.
   - Insomnia or hypersomnia almost every day.
   - Observable psychomotor agitation or retardation almost every day.
   - Loss of energy or fatigue almost every day.
   - Feeling of worthlessness or of excessive or inappropriate guilt almost every day.
   - Indecisiveness or decreased ability to concentrate almost every day.
   - Recurrent thoughts of death or recurrent suicidal ideation.
2. The disturbance is not caused or maintained by an organic factor or uncomplicated bereavement or by a drug or substance. It should be noted that bereavement can be complicated by a major depressive episode. This is suggested when the bereaved reports morbid preoccupation with worthlessness, suicidal ideation, marked functional impairment, psychomotor retardation (marked slowing down of cerebration and of physical movements).
3. At no time have delusions or hallucinations been present for two weeks in the absence of prominent mood symptoms.
4. The condition is not superimposed on schizophrenia or other psychotic state.

There are two clinical subtypes of major depressive episode, chronic and melancholic.

Chronic. The current episode is defined as chronic if it has lasted for two years or more with no more than a two-month period of symptom remission during that time.

Melancholic. This is a severe form of major depressive episode that seems to be quite responsive to somatic treatments. The diagnostic criteria include at least five of the following depressive symptoms:

- Anhedonia.
- Lack of response to pleasurable stimuli.
- Depression is worse in the morning.
- Early morning awakening, at least two hours before usual time.
- Observable psychomotor agitation or retardation.
- Significant anorexia or weight loss (for example, more than 5% of body weight in a month).
- No significant personality disturbance prior to the first major depressive episode.
- One or more previous major depressive episodes followed by complete or almost complete remissions.
- Previous good response to specific somatic therapy.

If a patient with depression, or a history of depression, has had one or more manic or hypomanic episodes, the condition is regarded as a bipolar disorder. In unipolar depression there are recurrent episodes of depression only. Melancholic depression occurs as part of both unipolar and bipolar illness and accounts for 40%–60% of all hospitalizations for depressive disorder (Klerman, 1984). Despite the depressive features, however, Gold et al. (1988) have pointed out that "the clinical picture of melancholia best illustrates the concept that major depression need not reflect a state of emotional and cognitive inactivation. On the contrary, the hallmark of melancholic depression is an intensely painful arousal and an obsessional preoccupation with personal inadequacy and the inevitability of loss."

Dysthymic Disorder

Today dysthymic disorder is viewed as a common but subtle form of mood disorder in which patients usually continue to function in most spheres of daily activity. However, they are characteristically in a state of chronic dissatisfaction and "down in the dumps." The DSM-IV criteria for diagnosis include the following.

1. A chronically depressed mood that occurs for most of the day for more days than not for at least two years (one year for children or adolescents).
2. During periods of depressed mood, at least two of the following additional symptoms are present:
   - Poor appetite or overeating.

- Insomnia or hypersomnia.
- Low energy or fatigue.
- Low self-esteem
- Poor concentration or difficulty making decisions.
- Feelings of hopelessness.

Because the symptoms are integral to an individual's day-to-day existence, they may not be directly reported unless asked for by the interviewer.

3. During the two-year period (one year for children or adolescents), any symptom-free period lasts no longer than two months.

4. If the chronic depressive symptoms include a major depressive disorder during the initial two years, then the diagnosis is major depressive disorder.

SYMPTOMS OF DEPRESSION

Depression may be expressed as somatic complaints that reflect the depressed state (e.g., disturbed sleep, appetite, or energy level), as symptoms that appear to represent a systemic disorder (such as abdominal pain, headaches, or incapacitating lower back pain), or as a disturbance of affect or cognition (such as depressed mood, gloomy outlook, or poor concentration). The frequency of the symptoms of depression provide a clue to its possible clinical presentation.

Hamilton (1989) evaluated the frequency of 17 symptoms of depression in 239 men and 260 women, all of whom would have satisfied the DSM-IIIR criteria (almost identical to those of DSM-IV) for major depressive illness. In none of the patients did the symptoms appear in the course of schizophrenia or hysterical or obsessional states, and patients diagnosed as suffering from schizoaffective disorders were excluded. The 12 most frequent symptoms in order of frequency are listed in Table 16-1. The three most frequent symptoms, for both men and women, were depressed mood (100%), loss of interest and working capacity (99% or over), and (psychic) anxiety (97%–98%). It is important to note the prominence of physical symptoms as an expression of the depressed state. This was true for both sexes but especially for women, in whom fatigue and loss of energy occurred in 94%, frequently dominating the clinical picture, while somatic symptoms of anxiety were observed in 87% and gastrointestinal symptoms (especially loss of appetite) in 84%. Fatigue was the only symptom in which the difference between the sexes was statistically significant. (Loss of libido was found significantly more often in men, but since many of the women in the study group were widowed or single, assessment of libido among the women was imprecise.) This analysis represents a selected group of patients, those seen in a psychiatric clinic. Had they entered a medical clinic, they would probably have emphasized the somatic expressions of their condition even more.

TABLE 16-1. Frequency of Symptoms in Depression*

MALE		FEMALE	
SYMPTOM	%	SYMPTOM	%
Depressed mood	100	Depressed mood	100
Loss of interest	99.6	Loss of interest	98.8
Anxiety (psychic)	97.1	Anxiety (psychic)	97.7
Anxiety (somatic)	87.4	*Fatigue*	94.2
Insomnia initial	83.7	*Anxiety (somatic)*	87.3
Suicide	82.0	*Gastrointestinal*	83.5
Fatigue	82.0	Suicidal thoughts	80.4
Gastrointestinal	80.3	*Insomnia initial*	77.7
Insomnia delayed	74.1	Guilt	72.7
Weight loss	69.0	*Insomnia delayed*	71.9
Agitation	68.1	*Weight loss*	68.8
Libido reduced	59.8	Agitation	68.1

*Somatic symptoms are italicized.
Source: After Hamilton, 1989.

In a study of 140 patients of different ages suffering from depression, Hopkinson (1963, 1965) found that as many as 26% had an extended prodromal phase (mean duration of 30 months) in which they complained of lack of energy and general feelings of ill health but without the typical mood changes. The length of the prodromal period was unrelated to the age of onset. Sensations of burning and pressure were common. Anxiety was universal, in line with the experience reported in Table 16-1. Hyperphagia and hypersomnia may be expressions of atypical depression (Caspar et al., 1985). This syndrome accounts for approximately 15% of major depressive episodes and is considered to be more common in bipolar than in unipolar illness.

Thus, with depression, as with many conditions, a distinction should be made between "common" and "characteristic" symptoms. Because of the high frequency of somatic symptoms (the "common"), a physician who looks only for the typical mood symptoms of depression (the "characteristic") is likely to miss the diagnosis.

The Course of Depressive Illness

In both unipolar and bipolar forms of illness the frequency of affective episodes increases as a function of the number of previous episodes (Zis and Goodwin, 1979; Post et al., 1981; Cutler and Post, 1982). Episodes in later life, when they are most frequent, tend to have a more precipitous onset and to be more severe than earlier episodes (Post et al., 1981). Clinical observations indicate that the first episode is often preceded by psychosocial stresses, which play a role as precipitating factors. With successive attacks, however, recognizable stressors are less evident as precipitators (Zis and Goodwin, 1979; Lloyd, 1980). Thus, the role of stress in precipitating affective illness seems to depend on the phase of the illness. The mechanism for this facilitated progression of the depression may be analogous to the process of kindling in epilepsy (Chapter 8).

Aside from the disabling effects of depression on patients' personal, social, and professional functioning, the most serious risk with major depression is suicide. In untreated individuals this may be as high as 15%–30% (Taschev, 1974; Winokur, 1975; Tsuang, 1978). Appropriate treatment significantly reduces the danger of suicide (Avery and Winokur, 1976). Long-term follow-up studies show a significant tendency in chronically depressed subjects to increased mortality from all causes, including cancer, pneumonia, and suicide (Brodaty et al., 1997; Takeida et al., 1997).

The Variability of Symptoms

While the discussion thus far has implied that the diagnosis of depression should be made on specific criteria, and that the physician needs to be familiar with the varied psychological (emotional and cognitive) and somatic expressions of depression, there is another aspect of the anxiety–depression problem that should always be kept in mind. That is, variations in mood are fundamental to human nature, and similar fluctuations of mood may also occur among states regarded as specific diagnostic entities. In a study of individuals categorized by psychiatrists as suffering from a "neurotic disorder," fewer than 40% retained their original diagnosis over five years (Kendell, 1974). Among the most obvious of the numerous factors influencing mood are the life experiences of every individual, which may improve or worsen their mood and increase or decrease their feelings of anxiety. The quotation at the start of this chapter emphasizes the frequent comorbidity of depression with anxiety states, as does Table 16-1. To quote Tyrer (1985), "The separation of anxiety and depressive states is particularly difficult and there is frequent 'crossing-over' from one to the other" (with time).

It is another sign of emotional variability that patients with minor depression have an excellent short-term outcome. In one study of depression in primary care, only one-third of patients still have more than one depressive symptom four months after diagnosis, and adequate dosage and duration of treatment were not significant predictors of recovery (Katon et al., 1994). These observations lend support to the assertion that "it is more profitable to look at the circumstances under which symptoms arise than draw a far-reaching conclusion about the management and course of the disorder on the basis of current symptoms. For example, there is evidence that anxiety symptoms arise in the setting of threatening life events and depressive ones in the setting of loss, with mixed symptoms associated with a similar mixture of loss and threatening life events" (Finlay-

Jones and Brown, 1981). The logical implication is that in attempting to account for different depression or anxiety symptoms at different times in the same patient, there is no point in changing one's diagnostic viewpoint; it can create confusion and divert attention from other, more relevant factors such as understanding the circumstances of how the problem came about. There may, in addition, be a major difference in the way the experience is interpreted by the patient and conveyed to the doctor, depending either on the relationship existing with the doctor (as described above) or on the doctor's specialty. To the psychiatrist the patient may talk about tension, depression, or fear; to the nonpsychiatric physician the symptoms are more likely to be expressed in somatic terms such as lethargy, abdominal pain, or weight loss.

DEPRESSION, DISABILITY, AND MEDICAL ILLNESS

There is a general tendency among medical practitioners to regard the disabilities associated with depression as being of a subjective kind and therefore of less clinical significance than those associated with serious medical conditions. This is important because, as mentioned earlier, in the United States at least half of the patients who receive any mental health care obtain it only from general practitioners (Regier et al., 1978; Wells et al., 1986). This pattern of health care is probably representative of other Western countries as well.

In the general medical sector—the non–mental health services—depression is usually recognized in general terms of depressive symptoms rather than as the specific disorders defined by DSM-IV. The Medical Outcomes Study (MOS) was designed to evaluate and compare the morbidity associated with depression as defined by these two paradigms (Wells et al., 1989). In addition, functional impairment resulting from depression was compared to that resulting from eight common categories of chronic medical diseases. A total of 11,242 outpatients from three locations in the United States completed questionnaires dealing with well-being, daily functioning, and the presence of chronic medical conditions. Depression was assessed in two stages:

1. Patients recorded their subjective scores on an eight-item depression symptom scale that elicited information on the intensity of symptoms (e.g., feeling sad, crying) over the previous week and during periods of depression over the preceding year.
2. Those whose scores were indicative, on the basis of predetermined criteria, of a depressive disorder (major depression, dysthymia [see below], or a combination of the two) were interviewed using the National Institute of Mental Health's Diagnostic Interview Schedule (DIS).

The DIS is a highly structured diagnostic tool that identifies psychiatric disorders according to DSM-III criteria (Robins et al., 1981). Among the medical conditions surveyed were a history of hypertension or diabetes mellitus; the presence of advanced coronary artery disease (defined as myocardial infarction during the last year or the presence of heart failure or a large heart, with or without angina); current angina pectoris only; current arthritis; current back problems; current lung problems (asthma or other severe lung problem such as chronic bronchitis or emphysema); and current gastrointestinal disorder (peptic ulcer or chronic inflammatory disease such as enteritis or colitis). The findings of the MOS study were summarized as follows:

> Patients with either current depressive disorder or depressive symptoms, in the absence of a medical disorder, tended to have worse physical, social, and role functioning, worse perceived current health, and greater bodily pain than did patients with no chronic conditions. The poor functioning . . . associated with depressive symptoms, with or without depressive disorder, was comparable with or worse than that . . . associated with eight major chronic medical conditions. For example, the . . . association of days in bed with depressive symptoms was significantly greater than the comparable association with hypertension, diabetes and arthritis. Depression and chronic medical conditions had unique and additive effects on patient functioning. (Wells et al., 1989)

Diagnosing Depression in the Medically Ill

Approximately 20%–33% of medically ill patients in hospitals are suffering from depression (Schwab et al., 1967; Moffic and Pakel, 1975). Cavanaugh (1983) reported mild depression in 18% of medical patients and moderate or severe depression in 14%. Severity was not influenced by age, sex, or race. In approximately 25% of depressed, medically ill patients, the onset of depression had preceded the diagnosis of the medical illness, while in 75% it appeared to follow it (Moffic and Pakel, 1975).

Diagnosing major depression in the medically ill may be problematic. For one thing, it is common for a patient to react with at least transient unhappiness to ill health. This may be a normal response and only a small subset of these patients may be suffering from major depressive illness (Cavanaugh et al., 1983; Rodin and Voshart, 1986). A second difficulty arises out of uncertainty in determining whether a symptom originates in depression or in the underlying medical condition. The DSM-IV, while requiring the presence of certain somatic changes for the diagnosis of major depression, excludes as diagnostic criteria symptoms caused by a medical condition. Physicians who focus on affective and cognitive symptoms in an attempt to circumvent this difficulty, however, will tend to underdiagnose major depression in those medically ill, depressive patients who initially emphasize their somatic symptoms and do not mention cognitive or affective symptoms (Cavanaugh et al., 1983; Rodin and Voshart, 1986). This situation has been studied in patients suffering from an established, well-defined medical disorder (Burkberg et al., 1984; Endicott, 1984; Smith et al., 1985; Minden et al., 1987) and from psychosomatic disorders. In the latter group there is a high incidence of major depression observed, for example, in the irritable bowel and chronic fatigue syndromes (Krupp et al., 1994; Masand et al., 1995; Addolorato et al., 1998). Similarly, 35%–40% of patients with eating disorders such as anorexia nervosa and bulimia are reported to suffer as well from major depression (Piran et al., 1985).

If depression is suspected, in spite of the patient's inclination to initially emphasize somatic symptoms it is important to try to obtain evidence of cognitive–affective symptoms. Cavanaugh et al. (1983) administered the Beck Depression Inventory (BDI), a widely used self-report measure in studies of depression, to 335 medically ill inpatients as well as to depressed and normal controls. They found that although none of the somatic items was a good indicator of severity of depression, the following seven cognitive–affective items were:

- Feeling like a failure.
- Loss of interest in people.
- Feeling punished.
- Suicidal ideation.
- Dissatisfaction.
- Difficulty with decisions.
- Crying.

They further pointed out that since the first four of these items occurred only in more severe degrees of depression, their presence should alert the clinician to the possibility of marked depression. Furthermore, although the last three items, at mild levels, are common in the medically ill population, when pronounced they are good indicators of severe depression. These findings are supported by studies showing that loss of self-esteem (sense of failure) is an important indicator of depression in cancer patients (Plumb and Holland, 1977).

Abbey et al. (1990) used the BDI to study of 271 patients, 92% of whom were outpatients with end-stage renal disease, irritable bowel syndrome, chronic fatigue syndrome, or eating disorders. Analysis of their responses yielded four items, self-hate, indecisiveness, loss of appetite and suicidal thoughts, that best discriminated between patients with and without a current major depressive episode and correctly classified 75% of subjects.

Psychobiological Basis of Depression

Nature and Nuture

Clinical studies are lending credence to the longstanding thesis that traumatic early life events play a major role in predisposing individuals to the subsequent development of affective disorders in particular (Plotsky et al., 1998; Arborelius et al., 1999). For example, Agid et al. (1999) showed that loss of a parent during childhood significantly increased the likelihood of developing major depression during adult life. The increasing sophistication of clinical and experimental studies is providing a stronger basis for the idea that life stressors predispose individuals to the later development of psychiatric disorders.

Nevertheless, not everyone suffering significant stress in early life becomes depressed. The impact of stressful experience in any person thus depends on an interplay of environmental (stress) and constitutional (genetic) factors. In a study of 3790 twin pairs, Kendler and Prescott (1999) found that the heritability of liability to major depression was the same in men and women and equal to 39%, while the remaining 61% of the variance in liability was due to specific environmental factors. That those who develop major depression may inherit genes which influence them to favor high-risk environments is a remarkable idea suggested by Kendler and Karkowski-Shuman (1997) on the basis of a study of 2164 female twins. In this study the authors found that genetic liability to major depression was associated with a significantly increased risk for six stressful "personal" life events (assault, serious marital problems, divorce/breakup, job loss, serious illness, and major financial problems) and one stressful "network" life event, trouble getting along with relatives/friends. This effect was not due to the events occurring during depressive episodes. In a study of 270 twin pairs aged 8 to 17 years, Thapar et al. (1998) similarly found that depressive symptoms and some life events share a common genetic influence, a conclusion also reached by Silberg et al. (1999) in a study of life stress and depression in adolescent girls. The data from the Kendler and Karkowski-Shuman (1997) study showing a significant correlation between personal stressful life events and depression tend to reduce the likelihood that shared environmental factors alone influence the development of the depression (as could easily occur with twins). In some patients and families, evidence may be found for a genetic predisposition to bipolar illness (Egeland et al., 1987; Berrettini et al., 1994; Freimer et al., 1996).

Biological changes in depression

We next consider biological changes associated with depression. With certain effects such as the activation of the HPA axis, the endocrine changes are assumed to be a consequence of the depression. However, whether this and other biological effects to be discussed are associated changes, in the sense of reflecting biophysical processes of which the depression itself is also an additional expression, or result secondarily from the depression may be difficult to determine.

Activation of the hypothalamic–pituitary–adrenocortical axis. A distinctive abnormality in the regulation of HPA function observed in melancholic depression is the pathological activation of the HPA axis coupled with a loss of feedback inhibition of adrenocorticotropic hormone (ACTH) secretion by glucocorticoids (Butler and Besser, 1968; Carroll, 1976; Carroll, 1982; Gwirtsman et al., 1982). The ACTH release mechanism is sensitive to the circulating blood level of glucocorticoids. In the dexamethasone suppression test, following the oral administration of 1 mg of dexamethasone (a very potent glucocorticoid) the previous midnight, the 8 A.M. value for plasma cortisol in normal subjects should be less than 140 nmol/L (normal 8 A.M. values are between 140 to 690 nmol/L). The administration of dexamethasone is normally followed by a measurable reduction in cortisol levels in the peripheral blood because of the inhibition of corticotropin-releasing hormone (CRH) and ACTH secretion. In a number of clinical states, but particularly in major depression (especially of the melancholic type), a significant proportion (40%–50%) of patients show an increased rate of escape of cortisol following dexamethasone administration.

This increased HPA axis activity is also manifested by an augmented total cortisol output, increased ACTH concentration (Pfohl et al., 1985), and adrenal gland hypertrophy as shown by computed tomography (Amsterdam et al., 1987; Nemeroff et al., 1992; Rubin et al., 1995). Rubin et al. (1995) noted that about 70% of depressed patients exhibit adrenal gland enlargement of approximately 1.7-fold compared to matched controls, and that this enlargement normalizes with successful treatment. The circadian rhythm of cortisol secretion is, however, preserved in depression (Sacher et al., 1973).

The frequent occurrence of mood disorders in Cushing's syndrome (Kelly et al., 1983; Haskett, 1985; Hudson et al., 1987; Loosen et al., 1992) and in patients receiving exogenous glucocorticoids (Ling et al., 1981; Perry et al., 1984) indicates that the increased cortisol levels may contribute to the affective state. The strongest evidence that it does is provided by the observation that a reduction of circulating cortisol by a variety of treatment measures, including metyrapone, adrenalectomy, and pituitary radiation or resection, leads to an improvement in mood or a resolution of the affective condition (Kelly et al., 1983; Sonino et al., 1993).

The increase in activity of the HPA axis has been attributed to an increased secretion of the corticotropin-releasing factor from the hypothalamus (Holsboer et al., 1984; Gold et al., 1988). The observed increase in CRF concentration in the cerebrospinal fluid of patients with depression strengthens this hypothesis (Nemeroff et al., 1984; Kling et al., 1991). The importance of CRF secretion as a primary event in the HPA axis changes observed in depressed patients is further supported by the significant increase in pituitary volume in these patients, as determined by magnetic resonance imaging (Krishnan et al., 1991). The blunted ACTH responses to exogenous human (Holsboer et al., 1984) or ovine (Gold et al., 1986) CRF in depressed patients may reflect a potent corticosteroid feedback inhibition of ACTH secretion in response to an intense CRF drive. Elimination of this feedback mechanism with metyrapone, an 11-hydroxylase inhibitor of cortisol synthesis, reveals the intensity of the overdrive (von Bardeleben et al., 1988; Lisansky et al., 1989), especially in dexamethasone nonsuppressors (Ur et al., 1990). Metyrapone inhibition of cortisol synthesis restores the normal hypothalamic–pituitary sensitivity to corticosterone (dexamethasone) inhibition of ACTH secretion, confirming the central role of CRF secretion in driving this process.

The localization of CRF to extrahypothalamic neurons, particularly in the central nucleus of the amygdala and the bed nucleus of the stria terminalis, incriminates it in the mediation of fear and anxiety responses as well (see Chapter 12) (Copland and Lydiard, 1998). For example, posttraumatic stress disorder (PTSD) patients, who suffer intense anxiety and autonomic arousal, show significantly increased concentrations of CRF in CSF (Bremner et al., 1997) and they also exhibit a blunted ACTH response to CRF (Smith et al., 1989). In contrast to depression patients, those with PTSD show hypercortisolism but considerable sensitivity to dexamethasone challenge (Yehuda, 1997).

Activation of central adrenergic and cholinergic mechanisms. The ability to influence brain amine levels by pharmacological means led Janowsky et al. (1972) to postulate a balance between central cholinergic and adrenergic neurotransmitter activity in those areas of the brain that regulate affect, with depression being an expression of cholinergic dominance and mania of central adrenergic (or serotonergic) dominance. In humans, physostigmine and other centrally acting cholinomimetic agents that increase central acetylcholine levels counteract mania and in some individuals may cause depressive symptoms (Davis et al., 1976; Risch et al., 1981; Janowsky and Risch, 1984). Furthermore, reserpine, a drug that induces depression, has central cholinomimetic properties. Acetylcholine stimulates the locus ceruleus through muscarinic receptors. In addition, nondepressed subjects with a history of depression have augmented responses to muscarinic agonists (Sitaram et al., 1980).

The activation of CRF in major depression is associated with the concomitant activation of the locus ceruleus–norepinephrine system (LC-NE) system. Depressed patients show normal or increased levels of norepinephrine in the cerebrospinal fluid, as well as increased levels of urinary 3-methoxy-4-hydroxyphenylglycol (MHPG), a principal metabolite of norepinephrine. Furthermore, cerebrospinal fluid CRF and norepinephrine levels and plasma MHPG levels are positively correlated in patients with melancholic depression (Gold et al., 1988).

Successful response to antidepressant medication is associated with a quietening of the LC-NE system, as indicated by a consistent decrease in cerebrospinal fluid and plasma MHPG (Linnoila et al., 1982). Experimentally, monoamine oxidase inhibitors and tricyclic antidepressants decrease the firing rate of the locus ceruleus, probably through central anticholinergic effects (Nyback et al., 1975).

Serotonergic mechanisms. The therapeutic revolution following the introduction of selective serotonin reuptake inhibitors (SSRIs) such as fluoxetine, paroxetine, fluvoxamine, and sertraline for the management of depression points to the central role of serotonin metabolism in mood regulation. Since most of these drugs belong to different chemical families and their only common property is their capacity to inhibit the 5-HT reuptake carrier, it is clear that they exert their therapeutic effect primarily via the 5-HT system (Blier and de Montigny, 1994). It is clear too from this experience as well as from the effective use of other pharmacological agents, however, that there is an intimate and complex interplay between higher cortical centers, principally frontal lobe, and limbic and hypothalamic regulators of mood that involves adrenergic, cholinergic, and serotinergic mediators. The varying loci of effect of the drugs influencing brain amine metabolism—the tricyclic and SSRI antidepressants and monoamine oxidase A inhibitors, as well as the newer agents with varying degrees of serotonin and norepinephrine reuptake inhibition, as well as central 2-alpha adrenergic autoreceptor antagonism (Kent, 2000), all of which act as antidepressants—underlie the complexity of the relevant pharmacology. These drugs to varying degrees appear to exert their therapeutic influence by increasing noradrenergic and especially specific serotonergic (5-HT$_1$) transmission. These antidepressant drugs are classified by their ability to inhibit reuptake of amines, but it is not this action that directly produces the antidepressant effects. The SSRIs inhibit the 5-HT transporter within minutes, but the antidepressant effects, which take two to three weeks to develop, must be dependent on adaptive changes that result from this action (Blier and de Montigny, 1994) (see also Chapter 17).

Blier and de Montigny (1994) offer the following explanation for this peculiar time sequence of effects: serotonin-containing neurons have serotonin transporters (inhibited by SSRIs) as well as a 5-HT$_{1A}$ autoreceptor on the cell body and dendritic processes (the "somatodendritic 5-HT$_{1A}$ autoreceptor"), which, by binding serotonin, inhibit the neuronal activity. Thus, as confirmed in experimental studies in mice, the immediate effect of SSRI administration, by increasing the extracellular serotonin concentrations—because of the inhibition of transporter—is to produce inhibition of the neuronal firing activity because of serotonin binding to the somatodendritic autoreceptor. This effect is, however, progressively attenuated in the face of continued SSRI administration, where the autoreceptor is downregulated. The effect then is that of enhanced neurotransmission by the released serotonin due to the continued administration of the

SSRIs unopposed by the much reduced autoreceptor influence. As a similar time sequence of events is true too for the antidepressant, predominantly noradrenaline reuptake inhibitors, it seems likely that comparable mechanisms are involved, though it should be noted that some of the newer drugs such as venlafaxine (see below) appear to produce satisfactory therapeutic effects within a shorter period of time (five to ten days as opposed to two to three weeks for the SSRIs and tricyclic antidepressants).

Sleep disturbance in depression

Electroencephalographic sleep patterns in depression are characterized by (Reynolds and Kupfer, 1987)

- Short rapid eye movement (REM) latency (i.e., a decrease in the time taken from falling asleep to the onset of the first REM period).
- Increased REM density (a measure of ocular activity during REM sleep).
- Increased duration of the first REM period.
- Reduced total sleep time, sleep efficiency (i.e., the proportion of time in bed spent asleep), and delta sleep (stage 3 and 4).

The characteristic sleep disturbance that occurs with depression may also be consistent with the cholinergic–aminergic imbalance hypothesis. Thus, REM latency may be shortened in normal volunteers by the systemic administration of cholinergic agonists, such as the cholinesterase inhibitor physostigmine and muscarinic receptor agonists like arecoline and pilocarpine (Sitaram and Gillin, 1980; Berkowitz et al., 1990).

Considerable evidence implicates cholinergic neurons (the pedunculopontine group and the lateral dorsal tegmental nucleus in the pontine tegmentum) in the induction and maintenance of REM sleep and its individual components (electroencephalographic activation, REMs, atonia of the major antigravity muscles, and pontine-geniculate-occipital spikes), probably in inverse proportion to activity in adrenergic and serotoninergic neurons (Shiromani et al., 1987).

Gillin et al. (1979) induced "upregulation" of the muscarinic receptor in normal volunteers by administering a cholinergic muscarinic inhibitor, scopolamine, over three consecutive days. With subsequent scopolamine withdrawal, the sleep pattern in these subjects with heightened muscarinic receptor sensitivity changed in character from normal to a "depressed" pattern, with short REM latency, increased REM density, increased sleep latency, and reduced total sleep time and sleep efficiency. Furthermore, compared to normal controls, patients suffering from depression entered REM sleep more rapidly after the intravenous administration of arecoline (a muscarinic agonist), supporting the assumption of functional supersensitivity of the muscarinic receptor in this condition (Gillin et al, 1991).

Depression, allergy, and autonomic responses

Studies of the concordance of atopic and affective disorders in the last two decades suggest a relationship between them (Gauci et al., 1993; Hashiro and Okumura, 1997; Hurwitz and Morgenstern, 1999). The prevalence of some form of allergy in the general population, as determined by skin tests, is approximately 30% in adults (Freidhoff et al., 1984) and 24% in children (Arbeiter, 1967). Bell et al. (1991) studied the association between type 1 (IgE-mediated) allergies (atopy) and depression in a nonclinical sample of 379 college students. Of those individuals in the survey who were assessed to be depressed, 71% (12/17) had self-reported allergic disorders and 64% (9/14) had professionally diagnosed allergic disorders. In contrast, among those not considered to be depressed, 43% (151/355) had self-reported allergic disorders and 35% (110/315) had professionally diagnosed allergic disorders. In this study, nonallergic and type 1 allergic subjects did not differ in self-rated frequency of depression. These studies suggest that there is an unusually high prevalence of atopic skin reactions in depressed persons, though this is often not expressed as a clinical allergy syndrome.

Ossofsky (1974, 1976) carried out skin tests in an attempt to detect allergies in children and adults referred for psychiatric evaluation because of depression, regardless of whether their complaints included allergic symptoms. Of the 96 patients tested, about half had few or no allergic symptoms but 95 were found to be atopic by skin test. This prevalence of atopy far exceeds the rate in the general population. Impressive as these results are, the study suffered from two defects: there was no control group and the criteria of depression were not specified. This tendency of a high frequency of atopic or allergic states has been similarly noted in patients suffering from the chronic fatigue syndrome (CFS) (Olson et al., 1986; Olson et al., 1986; Straus et al., 1988). Patients suffering from CFS, as with patients suffering from depression, have higher rates of skin test reactivity to allergens (50%) and/or histories of atopy (83%) than in the general population (20%–30%) (Straus et al., 1988).

Sugerman et al. (1982) examined IgE reactivity in the blood of alcoholic, depressive, and schizophrenic patients as well as control subjects. Each person's blood was tested against 12 inhalants and 21 foods. The 10 depressed subjects tested positively on 42%, the alcoholics on 35%, and the schizophrenics on 28% of the tests. In contrast, the 11 controls showed positive IgE reactivity to only 9% of the tests. As the authors had specifically excluded any individual—control or patient—with high levels of total IgE or a history of allergic disease, it seems probable that they underestimated a large number within the psychiatric population with allergen-specific IgE tests.

Of the immune changes that occur in depression, a meta-analysis of the literature reveals a characteristic pattern of change, primarily a decrease in circulating T and B lymphocytes, helper and suppressor/cytotoxic T cells, and natural killer (NK) cells, and a reduced lymphoproliferative response to mitogenic stimulation (Herbert and Cohen, 1993). Changes in B-cell function in depressed patients are manifested, for example, in an increased antibody titer to herpes simplex virus (HSV-1) and cytomegalovirus compared with other hospitalized or healthy controls (Lycke et al., 1974). One may speculate that in depression, as with the immune changes in stress (see Chapter 6), impaired cell-mediated immune response of the Th1 type with enhanced Th2 type responses associated with increased antibody production by sensitized B cells could explain the changes described of enhanced IgE-mediated immune reactions.

A number of studies have addressed the interplay of immune factors such as IgE secretion and tissue cholinergic mechanisms. Endoh et al. (1998) correlated blood IgE levels in healthy subjects and allergic rhinitis patients with the bronchial dilator response to the inhalation of submaximal doses of the anticholinergic agent oxitropium bromide. Oxitropium bromide inhalation induced an increase in FEV_1 (forced expiratory volume in one second) that was significantly greater in allergic rhinitis patients with high serum IgE (155 ± 20 mL) than in healthy subjects (64 ± 21 mL) or those with allergic rhinitis but low serum IgE (82 ± 21 mL). This study raises the question of whether the IgE level has a role in influencing tissue cholinergic metabolism. That IgE may influence tissue acetylcholine metabolism is also suggested by a study of sweat secretion induced by subcutaneous injection of the cholinergic agent pilocarpine in patients with atopic dermatitis and in normal controls (Kato et al., 1999). In both patient and control groups, the time taken from the beginning of sweat secretion to the maximal sweat rate was comparable, but in the patients with atopic dermatitis, the time taken for the sweat rate to fall to half maximal was significantly longer than in controls. These results suggest that the deactivation of pilocarpine-induced sweat secretion is impaired in atopic dermatitis patients. In the Endoh et al. (1998) study it appears that IgE may have enhanced the effects of an administered anticholinergic agent, and in the Kato et al. (1999) study it may have enhanced the effects of an administered cholinergic agent. The mechanism common to both these studies would be through IgE interference with acetylcholinesterase action in the tissues, in the first case enhancing the effect of the anticholinergic and in the second study (Kato et al., 1999) reducing the rate of pilocarpine degredation.

There is no good scientific evidence that food allergies trigger depression, although some patients believe they do (Marshall, 1993). Studies of "total allergy syndrome" or "twentieth-century disease," in which patients claim that food allergies play a role in their depression, indicate that these individuals are suffering mainly from psychiatric disorders such as somatization disorder, hypochondriasis, and depression (Brodsky, 1983; Stewart and Raskin, 1985; Terr, 1986; Seggev and Eckert, 1988). Significantly, this group of patients had a low prevalence of atopic symptoms such as rhinitis, urticaria (hives), bronchitis, asthma, eczema, and gastrointestinal symptoms.

Autonomic function in atopic conditions

Patients suffering from allergic conditions tend to show changes in autonomic responsiveness that are characteristically observed in depression, namely, cholinergic hyperresponsiveness and beta-adrenergic hyporesponsiveness. The latter has been extensively evaluated and confirmed both *in vivo* and *in vitro* in asthmatic subjects (Cookson and Reed, 1963; Inoue, 1967; Lockey et al., 1967; Middleton and Finke, 1968; Logsdon et al., 1972; Parker and Smith, 1973). A detailed review of the literature on this subject by Sventivanyi (1968) led to the suggestion that an unknown mechanism blocking the activation of adenylate cyclase by catecholamines was fundamental to the pathophysiology of asthma in that it impaired mechanisms of endogenous bronchodilatation. This idea was supported by the observed tendency of administered beta-adrenergic antagonists to precipitate asthma in predisposed subjects (Grieco and Pierson, 1971) as well as to enhance the bronchoconstrictive response to histamine and methacholine (Ploy-Song-Sand et al., 1978).

Kaliner et al. (1982) showed that the amount of intravenously infused isoproterenol needed to raise the blood pressure by 22 mm Hg was significantly smaller in normal controls than in asthmatics or patients suffering from allergic rhinitis. Assessment of pupillary cholinergic responsiveness by measuring the concentration of carbamylcholine chloride needed to constrict the pupils showed that it was significantly lower in the allergic subjects than in the controls. Pupillary responses were determined by using an infrared-sensitive television camera focused on the subject's eyes under standard lighting conditions (Smith et al., 1980). In addition, allergic subjects with either rhinitis or asthma produced significantly more sweat in response to intradermal cholinergic stimulation of eccrine sweat glands than did normal controls (Kaliner, 1976). These studies were conducted at a time when the atopic subjects tested were not being exposed to allergens to which they were sensitive. This suggests that allergy-induced changes in cholinergic system sensitivity persist for at least some weeks or months.

The generalized enhancement of cholinergic mechanisms in both depression and allergic conditions requires much more study to be fully understood. Numerous clinical and experimental observations support the proposal of Janowsky et al. (1972) that central adrenergic and cholinergic influences are antagonistic, with adrenergic influences producing behavioral activation and cholinergic influences producing behavioral inhibition. The apparently increased tendency to atopic reactions on skin testing in depressed patients, as well as the demonstration of systemic cholinergic hyperresponsiveness and beta-adrenergic hyposensitivity in persons with allergies, reflects an intriguing overlap of pathophysiological processes. It is probable that a number of mechanisms operate to produce the changes in autonomic function common to depression and atopic states. This could include a shift in the balance of immune function from the Th1 to Th2 type, with impaired cellular suppressor mechanisms and enhanced IgE antibody production, with an influence of the IgE on tissue cholinergic mechanisms that work to potentiate the autonomic changes.

The documented common association in clinical practice of depression and anxiety states with allergic disorders may suggest as well that in the more intractable allergy problems, a comprehensive approach to management, which includes proper attention to the emotional aspects of the patient's condition, will offer the best chance of achieving satisfactory therapeutic results. This association suggests that like the present-day pain clinic (see Chapters 10 and 11), the modern allergy clinic should be staffed too with its resident clinical psychologist.

MANAGEMENT

The management of patients with depression will depend on the symptom severity, the availability of treatment options, and the patient's preferences. In line with the Consensus Statement on the Primary Care Management of Depression (Ballenger et al., 1999), physicians need to educate patients about depressive illness, explain how their symptoms can be managed, explore background problems, define treatment goals, and dispel negative perceptions, such as the belief that antidepressant therapy is addictive (Paykel et al., 1998). This form of psychosocial education and support is an essential component of the management strategy of depression.

The majority of depressed patients seen and managed by primary care physicians will be categorized as mild to moderate. The decision of whether to refer the depressed patient for psychiatric care at the time of diagnosis will in general depend on the following factors:

1. If the patient admits to feeling suicidal, it is important to involve a psychiatrist in assessing the patient's condition and to either transfer the patient or work collaboratively with the psychiatrist in the management of the depression. Thoughts of committing suicide may be associated with depression that does not appear to be clinically severe, and only by systematically questioning every patient who admits to feeling depressed is it possible to determine whether this thought content exists.

2. Patients with depression of sufficient severity to significantly impair their routine function, or with chronic or recurrent depression attacks, should be referred for psychiatric assessment. Combinations of antidepressants or other interventions such as electroconvulsive therapy (ECT) may be indicated.

3. Depressed patients resistant to conventional treatment or with complicating comorbid psychiatric diagnoses such as personality disorder or drug addiction are better referred to a psychiatrist. This is also desirable if the de-

pression is assessed to be part of a bipolar disorder (because of a family history of bipolar disorder or a previous history of hypomanic behavior), to avoid the danger of inducing rapid cycling (i.e., from the depression into the manic phase) through administration of SSRIs or tricyclic antidepressants. These patients require more experience in management from the treating physician.

4. The practitioner's feeling of competence is of overriding importance in determining whether to undertake the treatment of depression in any particular patient. If we were to exclude the specific categories of patient listed above, the majority of depressed patients are mild to moderate in severity and well within the average medical practitioner's competence to treat. Furthermore, the indications for referral for psychiatric management are relative in that a doctor who is very familiar with a particular patient may well feel comfortable managing that patient through a bout of depression, even if the patient admits to having suicidal thoughts. This may be done after having reached an agreement with the patient that he or she will immediately inform the doctor in the event of the suicidal thinking intensifying.

The treatment is influenced by the severity of the depression as well as by the patient's willingness to follow the therapeutic program. Some patients may resist taking drugs, others, the suggestion of psychotherapy—even if offered a short-term program. In the many cases it is beneficial to discuss and analyze with the patient life-style factors that may be contributing negatively to the mood change as well as possible feelings of stress. These might include better time organization, taking an overdue vacation, and planning a more systematized program of recreation and exercise (see Chapter 13). In others, just the opportunity to talk candidly about the feelings of depression may be of considerable benefit.

In patients with mild or moderately severe episodes of major depression, treatment with antidepressant drugs and brief psychotherapies are equally effective; in those with severe episodes, medication is usually recommended (Depression Guideline Panel, 1993). The efficacy of cognitive therapy for the treatment of depression has been confirmed in randomized controlled clinical trials. Fava et al. (1998) reported the six-year outcome in 40 patients, whereas Paykel et al. (1999) assessed 158 patients during 20 weeks of treatment and for a year afterwards. Both studies demonstrated that the benefit of the psychotherapy was sustained and that risk of relapse or persistent symptoms was reduced by 45%–50%. In a collaborative study of depression in 250 outpatients by the National Institute of Mental Health, the number of imipramine (a tricyclic antidepressant) responders was greater than that in patients receiving either cognitive behavioral therapy or interpersonal psychotherapy. Either the medication or psychotherapy was superior to placebo (Elkin et al., 1989). The principles of cognitive therapy are described in Chapter 18.

The treatment of chronic depression is more problematic, however, and these patients have poor responses to single therapies, a very high rate of use of health care resources, and marked impairments in psychosocial function (Keller et al., 1984). The risk of relapse with partial remission to therapies may be as high as 50%–80% (Cornwall and Scott, 1997). Keller et al. (2000) showed, in 681 adults with chronic nonpsychotic major depression, that the combined treatment with an antidepressant (nefazodone over 12 weeks) and cognitive-behavioral therapy (about 16 sessions) produces a greater remission rate (42%) than among patients who receive either nefazodone alone (22%) or psychotherapy alone (24%). These results essentially confirm the outcome of previously reported studies that among patients suffering from a major depressive episode there is a greater overall reduction in the severity of symptoms (by about 25%) in those who receive combined treatment than among those who receive single therapies (Hollon et al., 1993; Thase et al., 1997; Paykel et al., 1999). The pharmacological profile of the major classes of medication used in the treatment of depression is presented in Chapter 17.

REFERENCES

Abbey SE, Toner BB, Garfinkel PE, et al. (1990). Self-report symptoms that predict major depression in patients with prominent physical symptoms. Intl J Psychiat Med 20:247–258.

Addolorato G, Marsigli L, Capristo E, et al. (1998). Anxiety and depression: a common feature of health care seeking patients with irritable bowel syndrome and food allergy. Hepatogastroenterology 45:1559–1564.

Agid O, Shapira B, Zislin J, et al. (1999). Environment and vulnerability to major psychiatric illness: a case control study of early parental loss in major depression, bipolar disorder and schizophrenia. Mol Psychiatry 4:163–172.

American Psychiatric Association (1994). Diagnostic and Statistical Manual of Mental Disorders, 4th ed. Washington, DC: Author.

Amsterdam JD, Martinelli DL, Arger P, et al. (1987). Assessment of adrenal gland volume by computed tomography in depressed patients and healthy volunteers: a pilot study. Psychiatry Res 21:189–197.

Arbeiter HI (1967). How prevalent is allergy among United States school children? A survey of findings in the Munster (Indiana) school system. Clin Pediatr (Phila) 6:140–142.

Arborelius L, Owens MJ, Plotsky PM, et al. (1999). The role of corticotrophin-releasing factor in depression and anxiety disorders. J Endocrinol 160:1–12.

Avery D, Winokur G (1976). Mortality in depressed patients treated with electroconvulsive therapy and antidepressants. Arch Gen Psychiatry 33:1029–1037.

Ballenger JC, Davidson JRT, Lecrubier Y, et al. (1999). Consensus statement on the primary care group management of depression from the International Consensus Group on Depression and Anxiety. J Clin Psychiatry 60 (suppl 7):54–61.

Barrett JE, Barrett JA, Oxman TE, et al. (1988). The prevalence of psychiatric disorders in a primary care practice. Arch Gen Psychiatry 45:1100–1106.

Bell IR, Jasnoski ML, Kagan J, et al. (1991). Depression and allergies: survey of a non-clinical population. Psychother Psychosom 55:24–31.

Berkowitz A, Sutton L, Janowsky DS, et al. (1990). Pilocarpine, an orally active muscarinic cholinergic agonist, induces REM sleep and reduces delta sleep in normal volunteers. Psychiatry Res 33:113–119.

Berrettini WH, Ferraro TN, Goldin LR, et al. (1994). Chromosome 18 DNA markers and manic depressive illness: evidence for a susceptibility gene. Proc Natl Acad Sci USA 91:5918–5921.

Blier P, De Montigny C (1994). Current advances and trends in the treatment of depression. Trends Pharmacol Sci 15:220–226.

Bremner JD, Licinio J, Darnell A, et al. (1997). Elevated CSF corticotropin-releasing factor concentrations in posttraumatic stress disorder. Am J Psychiatry 154:624–629.

Brodaty H, Maccuspie-Moore CM, Tickle L, et al. (1997). Depression, diagnostic subtype and death: a 25 year follow-up study. J Affect Disord 46:233–242.

Brodsky CM (1983). "Allergic to everything": a medical subculture. Psychosomatics 24:731–742.

Burkberg J, Penman D, Holland JC (1984). Depression in hospitalized cancer patients. Psychosom Med 46:199–212.

Butler PW, Besser GM 1968). Pituitary-adrenal function in severe depressive illness. Lancet 1:1234–1236.

Carroll BJ (1976). Limbic-system-adrenal cortex regulation in depression and schizophrenia. Psychosom Med 38:106–121.

Carroll BJ (1982). The dexamethasone suppression test for melancholia. Br J Psychiatry 140:292–304.

Caspar RC, Redmond DE, Katz MN, et al. (1985). Somatic symptoms in primary affective disorder: presence and relationship to the classification of depression. Arch Gen Psychiatry 42:1098–1104.

Cavanaugh S (1983). The prevalence of cognitive and emotional dysfunction in a general medical population: using the MMSE, GHA, and BDI. Gen Hosp Psychiatry 5:15–24.

Cavanaugh S, Clark DC, Gibbons RD (1983). Diagnosing depression in the hospitalized medically ill. Psychosomatics 24:809–815.

Cookson DU, Reed CE (1963). A comparison of the effects of isoproterenol in the normal and asthmatic subject. Am Rev Respir Dis 88:636–643.

Copland JD, Lydiard RB (1998). Brain circuits in panic disorder. Biol Psychiatry 44:1264–1276.

Cornwall PL, Scott J (1997). Partial remission in depressive disorders. Acta Psychiatr Scand 95:265–271.

Cutler NR, Post RM (1982). Life course of illness in untreated manic depressive patients. Compr Psychiatry 23:101–115.

Davis KL, Hollister E, Overall J, et al. (1976). Physostigmine: effects on cognition and affect in normal subjects. Psychopharmacology (Berlin) 51:23–27.

Depression Guideline Panel (1993). Depression in Primary Care. Vol 2. Treatment of Major Depression. Clinical Practice Guideline, number 5. Rockville, MD: Agency for Health Care Policy and Research. (AHCPR publication no. 93–0551).

Egeland JA, Gerhard DS, Pauls DL, et al. (1987). Bipolar affective disorders linked to DNA markers on chromosome 11. Nature 325:783–787.

Eisenberg L (1992). Treating depression and anxiety in primary care: closing the gap between knowledge and practice. N Engl J Med 326:1080–1084.

Elkin I, Shea MT, Watkins JT, et al. (1989). National Institute of Mental Health Treatment of Depression Collaborative Research Program: general effectiveness of treatments. Arch Gen Psychiatry 46:971–982.

Endicott J (1984). Measurement of depression in patients with cancer. Cancer 53:2243–2248.

Endoh N, Ichinose M, Takahashi T, et al. (1998). Relationship between cholinergic airway tone and serum immunoglobulin E in human subjects. Eur Respir J 12:71–74.

Fava GA, Rafanelli C, Grandi S, et al. (1998). Six-year outcome for cognitive behavioral treatment of residual symptoms in major depression. Am J Psychiatry 155:1443–1445.

Finlay-Jones R, Brown GW (1981). Types of stressful life events and the onset of anxiety and depressive disorders. Psychol Med 11:803–815.

Freidhoff LR, Meyers DA, Marsh DG (1984). A genetic–epidemiological study of human immune resposponsiveness to allergens in an industrial population. II. The association among skin sensitivity, total serum IgE, age, sex, and the reporting of allergies in a stratified random sample. J Allergy Clin Immunol 73:490–499.

Freimer NB, Reus VI, Escamilla MA, et al. (1996). Genetic mapping using haplotype, association and linkage methods suggest a locus for severe bipolar disorder (BPI) at 18q22–q23. Nature Genet 12:436–441.

Gauci M, King MG, Saxarra H, et al. (1993). A Minnesota Multiphasic Personality Inventory profile of women with allergic rhinitis. Psychosom Med 55:533–540.

Gerber PD, Barrett JE, Barrett JA, et al. (1989). Recognition of depression by internists in primary care: a comparison of internists and "gold standard" psychiatric assessment. J Gen Intern Med 4:7–13.

Gillin JC, Sitaram N, Duncan WC (1979). Muscarinic supersensitivity: a possible model for the sleep disturbance of primary depression? Psychiatry Res 1:17–22.

Gillin JC, Sutton L, Ruiz C. et al. (1991). The cholinergic rapid eye movement induction test with arecoline in depression. Arch Gen Psychiatry 48:264–270.

Gold PW, Goodwin FK, Chrousos GP (1988). Clinical and biochemical manifestations of depression: relation to the neurobiology of stress (2 parts). N Engl J Med 319:348–353;413–420.

Gold PW, Loriaux DL, Roy A, et al. (1986). Responses to corticotropin-releasing hormone in the hypercortisolism of depression and Cushing's disease: pathophysiology and diagnostic implications. N Engl J Med 314:1329–1335.

Goldberg D, Huxley P (1992). Common mental disorders: a bio-social model. London: Routledge, p 139.

Grieco MH, Pierson RN ((1971). Mechanism of bronchoconstriction due to beta adrenergic blockade: studies with practolol, propranolol, and atropine. J Allergy Clin Immunol 48:143–152.

Gwirtsman HE, Gerner RH, Sternbach H (1982). The overnight dexamethasone suppression test: clinical and theoretical review. J Clin Psychiatry 43:321–327.

Hamilton M (1989). Frequency of symptoms in melancholia (depressive illness). Br J Psychiatry 154:201–206.

Hashiro M, Okumura M (1997). Anxiety, depression and psychosomatic symptoms in patients with atopic dermatitis: comparison with normal controls and among groups of different degrees of severity. J Dermatol Sci 14:63–67.

Haskett RF (1985). Diagnostic categorization of psychiatric disturbance in Cushing's syndrome. Am J Psychiatry 142:911–916.

Herbert TB, Cohen S (1993). Depression and immunity: a meta-analytic review. Psychol Bull 113:472–486.

Hoeper EW, Nycz GR, Cleary PD, et al. (1979). Estimated prevalence of RDC mental disorder in primary medical care. Int J Ment Health 8:6–15.

Hollon SD, Shelton RC, Davies DD (1993). Cognitive therapy for depression: conceptual issues and clinical efficacy. J Consult Clin Psychol 61:270–275.

Holsboer F, von Bardeleben U, Gerken A, et al. (1984). Blunted corticotropin and normal cortisol response to human corticotropin-releasing factor in depression. N Engl J Med 311:1127.

Hopkinson G (1963). The onset of affective illness. Psychiatr Neurol Basel 146:133–144.

Hopkinson G (1965). The prodromal phase of the depressive psychosis. Psychiatr Neurol Basel 149:1–6.

Hudson JI, Hudson MS, Griffing GT, et al. (1987). Phenomenology and family history of affective disorder in Cushing's disease. Am J Psychiatry 144:951–953.

Hurwitz EL, Morgenstern H (1999). Cross-sectional associations of asthma, hay fever, and other allergies with major depression and low-back pain among adults aged 20–39 years in the United States. Am J Epidemiol 150:1107–1116.

Inoue S (1967). Effects of epinephrine on asthmatic children: effects of epinephrine on blood glucose, pulmonary function, and heart rate of children with asthma of varying severity. J Allergy 40:337–348.

Janowsky DS, El-Yousef MK, Davis JM, et al. (1972). A cholinergic–adrenergic hypothesis of mania and depression. Lancet 2:632–635.

Janowsky DS, Risch SC (1984). Cholinomimetic and anticholinergic drugs used to investigate an acetylcholine hypothesis of affective disorder and stress. Drug Dev Res 4:125–142.

Janowsky DS, Risch SC, Parker D, et al. (1980). Increased vulnerability to cholinergic stimulation in affective-disorder patients. Psychopharmacol Bull 16:29–31.

Kaliner M (1976). The cholinergic nervous system and immediate hypersensitivity. I. Eccrine sweat responses in allergic patients. J Allergy Clin Immunol 58:308–315.

Kaliner M, Shelhamer JH, Davis PB, et al. (1982). Autonomic nervous system abnormalities and allergy. Ann Intern Med 96:349–357.

Kato F, Saga K, Morimoto Y, et al. (1999). Pilocarpine-induced cholinergic sweat secretion compared with emotional sweat secretion in atopic dermatitis. Br J Dermatol 140:1110–1113.

Katon W, Lin E, Von Korff M, et al. (1994). The predictors of persistence of depression in primary care. J Affect Disord 31:81–90.

Keller MB, Klerman GL, Lavori PW, et al. (1984). Long-term outcome of episodes of major depression: clinical and public health significance. JAMA 252:788–792.

Keller MB, McCullough JP, Klein DN, et al. (2000). A comparison of nefazodone, a cognitive behavioral-analysis system of psychotherapy, and their combination for the treatment of chronic depression. N Engl J Med 342:1462–1470.

Kelly WF, Checkley SA, Bender DA, et al. (1983). Cushing's syndrome and depression: a prospective study of 26 patients. Br J Psychiatry 142:16–19.

Kendell RE (1974). The stability of psychiatric diagnosis. Br J Psychiatry 124:352–356.

Kendler KS, Karkowski-Shuman L (1997). Stressful life events and genetic liability to major depression: genetic control of exposure to the environment. Psychol Med 27:539–547.

Kendler KS, Prescott CA (1999). A population-based twin study of lifetime major depression in men and women. Arch Gen Psychiatry 56:39–44.

Klerman GL (1984). History and development of modern concepts of affective illness. In: Post RM, Ballenger JC, eds. Neurobiology of Mood Disorders. Baltimore: Williams and Wilkins, pp 1–19.

Kling MA, Roy A, Doran AR, et al. (1991). Cerebrospinal fluid immunoreactive corticotropin-releasing hormone and adrenocorticotropin secretion in Cushing's disease and major depression: potential clinical implications. J Clin Endocrinol Metab 72:260–271.

Krishnan KR, Doraiswamy PM, Lurie SN, et al. (1991). Pituitary size in depression. J Clin Endocrinol Metab 72:256–259.

Krupp LB, Sliwinski M, Masur DM, et al. (1994). Cognitive functioning and depression in patients with chronic fatigue syndrome and multiple sclerosis. Arch Neurol 51:705–710.

Ling MH, Perry PJ, Tsuang MT, et al. (1981). Side effects of corticosteroid therapy: psychiatric aspects 38:471–477.

Linn LS, Yager J (1984). Recognition of depression and anxiety by primary physicians. Psychosomatics 25:593–595, 599–600.

Linnoila M, Karoum F, Calil HM, et al. (1982). Alterations of norepinephrine metabolism with desipramine and zimelidine in depressed patients. Arch Gen Psychiatry 39:1025–1028.

Lisansky J, Peake GT, Strassman J, et al. (1989). Augmented pituitary corticotropin response to threshold dosage of human corticotropin-releasing hormone in depressives pretreated with metyrapone. Arch Gen Psychiatry 46:641–649.

Lloyd C (1980). Life events and depressive disorder reviewed. II. Events as precipitating factors. Arch Gen Psychiatry 37:541–548.

Lockey SD, Glennon JA, Reed CE (1967). Comparison of some metabolic responses in normal and asthmatic subjects to epinephrine and glucagon. J Allergy 40:349–354.

Logsdon PJ, Middleton E, Coffey RG (1972). Stimulation of leukocyte adenyl cyclase by hydrocortisone and isoproterenol in asthmatic and nonasthmatic subjects. J Allergy Clin Immunol 50:45–56.

Loosen PT, Chambliss R, Debold CR, et al. (1992). Psychiatric phenomenology in Cushing's disease. Pharmacopsychiatry 25:192–198.

Lycke E, Norrby R, Roos B-E (1974). A serological study on mentally ill patients with special reference to the prevalence of herpes virus infections. Br J Psychiatry 124:273–279.

Marshall PS (1993). Allergy and depression: a neurochemical threshold model of the relation between the illnesses. Psychol Bull 113:23–43.

Masand PS, Kaplan DS, Gupta S, et al. (1995). Major depression and irritable bowel syndrome: is there a relationship? J Clin Psychiatry 56:363–367.

Middleton E, Finke SR (1968). Metabolic response to epinephrine in bronchial asthma. J Allergy 42:288–299.

Minden SL, Orav J, Reich P (1987). Depression in multiple sclerosis. Gen Hosp Psychiatry 9:426–434.

Moffic HS, Paykel ES (1975). Depression in medical in-patients. Br J Psychiatry 126:346–353.

Mynors-Wallis LM, Gath DH, Lloyd-Thomas AR, et al. (1995). Randomised control trial comparing problem solving treatment with amitriptyline and placebo for major depression in primary care. Br Med J 310:441–445.

Nemeroff CB, Krishnan KKR, Reed D, et al. (1992). Adrenal gland enlargement in major depression: a computed tomography study. Arch Gen Psychiatry 49:384–387.

Nemeroff CB, Widerlov E, Bissette G, et al. (1984). Elevated concentrations of CSF corticotropin-releasing factor-like immunoreactivity in depressed patients. Science 226:1342–1344.

Nielsen AC, Williams TA (1980). Depression in ambulatory medical patients. Arch Gen Psychiatry 37:999–1004.

Nyback HV, Walters JR, Aghajanian GK, et al. (1975). Tricyclic antidepressants: effects on the firing rate of brain noradrenergic neurons. Eur J Pharmacol 32:302–312.

Olfson M, Shea S, Feder A, et al. (2000). Prevalence of anxiety, depression, and substance use disorders in an urban general medicine practice. Arch Fam Med 9:876–883.

Olson GB, Kanaan MN, Gersuk GM, et al. (1986). Correlation between allergy and persistent Epstein-Barr virus infections in chronic active Epstein-Barr virus infected patients. J Allergy Clin Immunol 78:308–314.

Olson GB, Kanaan MN, Kelley LM, et al. (1986). Specific allergen-induced Epstein-Barr nuclear antigen-positive B cells from patients with chronic-active Epstein-Barr virus infections. J Allergy Clin Immunol 78:315–.

Ossofsky HJ (1974). Endogenous depression in infancy and childhood. Compr Psychiatry 15:19–25.

Ossofsky HJ (1976). Affective and atopic disorders and cyclic AMP. Compr Psychiatry 17:335–346.

Parker CW, Smith JW (1973). Alterations in cyclic adenosine monophosphate metabolism in human bronchial asthma. 1. Leucocyte responsiveness to beta-adrenergic agents. J Clin Invest 52:48–59.

Paykel ES, Hart D, Priest RG (1998). Changes in public attitudes to depression during the Defeat Depression Campaign. Br J Psychiatry 173:519–522.

Paykel ES, Scott J, Teasdale JD, et al. (1999). Prevention of relapse in residual depression by cognitive therapy: a controlled trial. Arch Gen Psychiatry 56:829–835.

Perez-Stable EJ, Miranda J, Munoz RF, et al. (1990). Depression in medical outpatients: underrecognition and misdiagnosis. Arch Intern Med 150:1083–1088.

Perry PJ, Tsuang MT, Hwang MH, et al. (1984). Prednisolone psychosis: clinical observations. Drug Intell Clin Pharm 18:603–609.

Pfohl B, Sherman B, Schlecte J, et al. (1985). Pituitary-adrenal axis rhythm disturbances in psychiatric depression. Arch Gen Psychiatry 42:897–903.

Piran N, Kennedy S, Garfinkel PE, et al. (1985). Affective disturbances in eating disorders. J Nerv Ment Dis 173:395–400.

Plotsky PM, Owens MJ, Nemeroff CB (1998). Psychoneuroendocrinology of depression: hypothalamic-pituitary-adrenal axis. Psychiatr Clin North Amer 21:293–307.

Ploy-Song-Sand Y, Corbin RP, Engel LA (1978). Effects of intravenous histamine on lung mechanics in man after beta-blockade. J Appl Physiol 44:690–695.

Plumb MM, Holland J (1977). Comparative studies of psychological function in patients with advanced cancer: 1. Self-reported depressive symptoms. Psychosom Med 39: 264– 276.

Post RM, Ballenger JC, Rey AC, et al. (1981). Slow and rapid onset of manic episodes: implications for underlying biology. Psychatry Res 4:229–237.

Post RM, Kopanda RT (1975). Cocaine, kindling and reverse tolerance. Lancet 1:409–410.

Regier DA, Goldberg ID, Taube CA (1978). The de facto US mental health services system: a public health perspective. Arch Gen Psychiatry 35:685–693.

Reynolds CF, Kupfer DJ (1987). Sleep research in affective illness: state of the art circa 1987. Sleep 10:199–215.

Risch SC, Cohen RM, Janowsky DS, et al. (1981). Physostigmine induction of depressive symptomatology in normal human subjects. Psychiatry Res 4:89–94.

Robins LN, Helzer JE, Croughan J, et al. (1981). National Institute of Mental Health Diagnostic Interview Schedule: its history, characteristics and validity. Arch Gen Psychiatry 38:381–389.

Rodin G, Voshart K (1986). Depression in the medically ill: an overview. Am J Psychiatry 143:696–705.

Rosenthal MP, Goldfarb NI, Carlson BL, et al. (1978). Assessment of depression in a family practice center. J Fam Pract 25:143–149.

Rubin RT, Phillips JJ, Sadow TF, et al. (1995). Adrenal gland volume in major depression: increase during the dperessive episode and decrease with successful treatment. Arch Gen Psychiatry 52:213–218.

Sacher EJ, Hellman L, Roffwarg HP, et al. (1973). Disrupted 24-hour patterns of cortisol secretion in psychotic depression. Arch Gen Psychiatry 28:19–26.

Schulberg HC, Saul M, McClelland M (1985). Assessing depression in primary medical and psychiatric practices. Arch Gen Psychiatry 42:1164–1170.

Schwab JJ, Bialow M, Brown JM, et al. (1967). Diagnosing depression in medical inpatients. Ann Intern Med 67:695–707.

Seggev JS, Eckert RC (1988). Psychopathology masquerading as food allergy. J Fam Pract 26:161–164.

Shiromani PJ, Gillin JC, Henriksen SJ (1987). Acetylcholine and the regulation of REM sleep: basic mechanisms and clinical implications for affective illness and narcolepsy. Annu Rev Pharmacol Toxicol 27:137–156.

Silberg J, Pickles A, Rutter M, et al. (1999). The influence of genetic factors and life stress on depression among adolescent girls. Arch Gen Psychiatry 56:225–232.

Simon GE, Vonkorff M, Piccinelli M, et al. (1999). An international study of the relation between somatic symptoms and depression. N Engl J Med 341:1329–1335.

Sitaram N, Gillin JC (1980). Development and use of pharmacological probes of the CNS in man: evidence of cholinergic abnormality in primary affective illness. Biol Psychiatry 15:925–955.

Sitaram N, Nurnberger JI Jr, Gershon ES, et al. (1980). Faster cholinergic REM sleep induction in euthymic patients with primary affective illness. Science 208:200–202.

Smith LJ, Shelhamer JH, Kaliner M (1980). Cholinergic nervous system and immediate hypersensitivity. II. An analysis of pupillary responses. J Allergy Clin Immunol 66:374–378.

Smith MA, Davidson J, Ritchie JC, et al. (1989). The corticotropin-releasing hormone test in patients with posttraumatic stress disorder. Biol Psychiatry 26:349–355.

Smith MD, Hong BA, Robson AM. (1985). Diagnosis of depression in patients with endstage renal disease. Am J Med 79:160–166.

Sonino N, Fava G, Belluardo P, et al. (1993). Course of depression in Cushing's syndrome: response to treatment and comparison with Grave's disease. Horm Res 39:202–206.

Stewart DE, Raskin J (1985). Psychiatric assessment of patients with "20th century disease" ("total allergy syndrome"). Can Med Assoc J 133:1001–1006.

Straus SE, Dale JK, Wright R, et al. (1988). Allergy and the chronic fatigue syndrome. J Allergy Clin Immunol 81:791–795.

Sugerman AA, Southern DL, Curran JF (1982). A study of antibody levels in alcoholic, depressive, and schizophrenic patients. Ann Allergy 48:166–171.

Sventivanyi A (1968). The beta adrenergic theory of the atopic abnormality in bronchial asthma. J Allergy 42:203–232.

Takeida K, Nishi M, Miyake H (1997). Mental depression and death in elderly persons. J Epidemiol 7:210–213.

Taschev T (1974). The course and prognosis of depression on the basis of 642 patients deceased. In: Angst J, ed. Classification and Prediction of Outcome of Depression. Stuttgart: Schattauer Verlag, pp 157–172.

Terr AI (1986). Environmental illness: a clinical review of 50 cases. Arch Intern Med 146:145–149.

Thapar A, Harold G, McGuffin P (1998). Life events and depressive symptoms in childhood—shared genes or shared adversity? A research note. J Child Psychol Psychiatry 39:1153–1158.

Thase ME, Greenhouse JB, Frank E, et al. (1997). Treatment of major depression with psychotherapy or psychotherapy–pharmacotherapy combinations. Arch Gen Psychiatry 54:1009–1015.

Thompson C, Thompson CM (1989). The prescription of antidepressants in general practice: 1. A critical review. Hum Psychopharmacol 4:91–102.

Thompson TL, Stoudemire A, Mitchell WD, et al. (1983). Underrecognition of patients' psychosocial distress in a university hospital medical clinic. Am J Psychiatr 140:158–161.

Tsuang MT (1978). Suicide in schizophrenics, manics, depressives, and surgical controls: a comparison with general population suicide mortality. Arch Gen Psychiatry 35:153–155.

Tyrer P (1985). Neurosis divisible? Lancet 1:685–688.

Ur E, Turner TH, Clare AW, et al. (1990). The effect of metyrapone on the hypercortisolaemia of depression. J Endocrinol 124(suppl):272.

Von Bardeleben U, Stalla GK, Muller OA, et al. (1988). Blunting of ACTH response to human CRF in depressed patients is avoided by metyrapone pretreatment. Biol Psychiatry 24:782–786.

Von Korff M, Shapiro S, Burke JD, et al. (1987). Anxiety and depression in a primary care clinic: comparison of Diagnostic Interview Schedule, General Health Questionnaire, and practitioner assessment. Arch Gen Psychiatry 44:152–156.

Wells KB, Manning WG Jr, Duan N, et al. (1986). Use of outpatient mental health services by a general population with health insurance coverage. Hosp Comm Psychiatry 37:1119–1125.

Wells KB, Stewart A, Hays RD, et al. (1989). The functioning and well-being of depressed patients: results from the Medical Outcomes Study (MOS). JAMA 262:914–919.

Winokur G (1975). The Iowa 500: heterogeneity and course in manic depressive illness (bipolar). Comp Psychiatry 16:125–131.

Yehuda R (1997). Sensitization of the hypothalamic-pituitary-adrenal axis in posttraumatic stress disorder. Ann NY Acad Sci 821:57–75.

Zis AP, Goodwin FK (1979). Major affective disorders as a recurrent illness: a critical review. Arch Gen Psychiatry 36:835–839.

Zung WW, Magill M, Moore JT, et al. (1983). Recognition and treatment of depression in a family medicine practice. J Clin Psychiatry 44:3–6.

Chapter 17

DRUG TREATMENT OF AFFECTIVE DISORDERS

Any physician interested in the treatment of psychosomatic problems should be aware of the principles of drug therapy. When managing troublesome psychophysiological processes, we are mainly interested in helping patients, through cognitive and behavioral techniques, regain a sense of mastery and self-confidence when relating to their physical predicament, whatever it is. The need to take a drug to improve or control a situation tends to reinforce feelings of dependency on factors not under one's own control. For this reason, many patients are not enthusiastic about the suggestion and often refuse to cooperate, despite their suffering. But in some situations drug treatment may be necessary or desirable. The most acceptable approach is to present the need for drug therapy in the context of a broader program aimed at restoring feelings of control and self-confidence. The simple act of taking a pill is of no educational value to the patient, even if it brings symptomatic relief, unless the rationale for the medication is properly presented. One or another of the reasons enumerated in the next section usually succeeds in eliciting the patient's cooperation.

INDICATIONS FOR THE USE OF PSYCHOACTIVE DRUGS

The main reason for using medication is to treat distressing symptoms. Some patients suffer from symptoms that impair their ability to function. It may therefore be necessary to use medication to help control anxiety or panic disorder, depression or pain. With medication, patients may be less distracted by their symptoms and better able to relate to a program of cognitive and behavioral therapy.

Another important reason for prescribing medication is to help educate the patient about the essentially psychophysiological origin of the clinical state. It often happens that a patient, initially at least, remains extremely skeptical of the doctor's assessment that the physical symptoms have an emotional origin. Administering a psychoactive drug that alleviates the patient's symptoms helps him or her understand the link between emotional distress and physical symptoms. Important as this insight can be to patients' regaining a fuller sense of control over their lives, it still does not provide them with the skills they will need to confront stress in the future. This truism finds expression in almost all studies that compare the outcome of treatment of anxiety disorders by drugs alone with the combination of drug therapy and psychotherapy or cognitive-behavioral therapy. The results usually significantly favor the latter.

Depression too must often be treated with medication, although this is not a universal requirement if the condition is judged to be mild, meeting no more than minimal criteria for a major depressive episode. But all cases diagnosed as moderate to severe should be treated with drugs, usually for at least a year. Any patient who has suffered two bouts of major depression, especially within a five-year period, may have to consider prophylactic drug therapy for life. Among the factors influencing the decision are the severity of previous attacks and a family history of depression.

The most critical issue in managing depression centers on the possibility of suicide. It is advisable to refer any patient expressing suicidal thoughts to a psychiatrist. Furthermore, once the diagnosis of depression is contemplated, and particularly if the patient admits to feeling depressed, the subject of suicidal thoughts should be explored no matter how mild the depression seems to be. It should never be assumed that the patient will volunteer this information. Other affective disorders that may lead to suicidal thinking are panic disorder and posttraumatic stress disorder. In all cases it should be the physician's practice to insist that patients agree to inform the doctor immediately should they contemplate suicide. I accept the responsibility of managing such a problem, assuming I believe that I am able to, only if given this assurance.

THE CHOICE OF A PSYCHOACTIVE AGENT

This section focuses on the medications most widely used for the treatment of anxiety and depression, particularly in general medical practice. In general, the drug categories in this section are very few, and the time-honored practice of knowing well the actions and side effects of a limited selection of the most widely used drugs for each diagnostic category that we are considering is appropriate here. While all the drug types listed are in use, the tendency toward drug dependency especially and sometimes impairment of memory with the benzodiazepines as well as the dryness of mouth, postural hypotension, impotence, and potentially serious cardiac arrythmias with the tricyclic antidepressants have made newer drugs such as buspirol and the selective serotonin reuptake inhibitors (SSRIs) very welcome additions to the list. In situations where price may be of considerable importance, however, the older benzodiazepines and tricyclics are still used, and cost often remains the main reason for choosing one of these older drugs in preference to a newer agent.

Benzodiazepines

Benzodiazepines are most widely used clinically as anxiolytics, sedatives, or hypnotics, though they are also used for their antiepileptic and muscle relaxant effects. Certain benzodiazepine analogues such as alprazolam are considered to be effective in panic disorder as well as depression, though we now have other agents that are much better suited to this role. The extensive use of intravenous benzodiazepines such as diazepam as antiepileptic agents is facilitated by the wide margin of safety between therapeutic efficacy and the danger of respiratory depression in the absence of clinically significant respiratory disease.

Mechanism of action

Benzodiazepines exert their action by potentiating the effect of the inhibitory neurotransmitter γ-aminobutyric acid (GABA), through the $GABA_A$ receptor, on the permeability of the chloride channel. Benzodiazepines and GABA potentiate each other in ability to open the chloride channel and hyperpolarize the postsynaptic cell (Tallman et al., 1980). GABAmodulin, a protein localized in the postsynaptic membrane whose activity is determined by its degree of phosphorylation, can produce changes in the affinity of GABA receptors for GABA. The benzodiazepine binding site may also serve to modulate GABAmodulin activity and the GABA receptor complex allosterically. The $GABA_B$ receptor is not influenced by benzodiazepines. GABA is widely distributed in the mammalian nervous system with high concentrations in the hypothalamus, hippocampus, and basal ganglia of the brain, in the substantia gelatinosa of the dorsal horn of the spinal cord, and in the retina.

Clinical use

The choice of benzodiazepine tends to be somewhat empirical because at the right dose most members of this group will exhibit the full spectrum of clinical effects. However, large differences in metabolic rate and in the production of biologically active metabolites determine the duration of action of the particular agent chosen. Diazepam, the most frequently used benzodiazepine, has a plasma half-life of 1–2 days. In addition, both of its principal metabolites, desmethyl-diazepam and oxazepam, have similar biological activity with half lives respectively of 2–4 days and 12 hours. On the other hand, oxazepam, lorazepam, and alprazolam all have short half-lives around 9–24 hours. These drugs may therefore be more useful in the presence of liver disease, where drug metabolism may be impaired, and in old people, where the continuous presence of a drug with a long plasma life is undesirable, and in this way avoiding the tendency to oversedation and confusion. Chlordiazepoxide, another widely used antianxiety agent, has a half-life of 10–29 hours. Brotizolam, because of its short duration of action (half-life of around 5 hours), has found a place as a nocturnal sedative with little tendency to cause daytime sleepiness or other side effects (Langley and Clissold, 1988).

Undesirable effects of benzodiazepines are mostly related to feelings of light-headedness, lassitude, motor incoordination, confusion, and anterograde amnesia. These symptoms tend to be more pronounced with increasing age and are potentiated by alcohol. In addition, some patients say that they do not feel well after taking benzodiazepines. While they may not be able to describe their feelings precisely, they are insistent that they do not like the experience.

Prolonged use of benzodiazepines leads to dependency. For this reason continuous use, as far as possible, should be restricted to intervals of two to four weeks. Withdrawal symptoms may include a return and intensification of symptoms that prompted their use in the first place, such as anxiety or insomnia. For this reason, too, benzodiazepines are not favored for the management of panic disorder, since more effective medications are available.

Buspirone

The continuing search for antianxiety drugs has produced this agent, which is clinically effective and has additional favorable characteristics for clinical use.

Mechanism of action

Buspirone, an azapirone, differs chemically and pharmacologically from the benzodiazepines. It has a strong affinity for the 5-HT_{1A} (5-hydroxytryptamine[serotonin] type 1A) receptor and consequently alters serotinergic transmission (Peroutka, 1985). While buspirone binds with moderate affinity as well to presynaptic dopamine-2 (D2) receptors as a mixed agonist–antagonist, its main clinical effects are thought to be mediated by its binding to the serotonin receptor. Buspirone does not interact with the benzodiazepine receptor complex or with adrenergic, cholinergic, imipramine, or opiate receptors.

In the serotonergic system, buspirone has varying agonistic activity, acting as a full agonist in the dorsal raphe (presynaptic) and as a partial agonist in the hippocampal formation and cortex (postsynaptic) (Yocca, 1990). This complex interaction with presynaptic and postsynaptic serotonin receptors may explain the dual nature of buspirone's effects in promoting normal neurotransmission in situations of both serotonin excess and deficiency.

When a neurotoxin is used to selectively impair the serotonergic system, this blocks the antiaggression effects of buspirone in the rhesus monkey (Eison et al., 1986). A meta-analysis of six double-blind clinical trials (427 patients) comparing the short-term effectiveness of buspirone to placebo showed significant improvement in patients suffering from anxiety disorders (Feighner and Cohn, 1989). Buspirone also acts as an antidepressant, a useful dual role in view of the frequent coexistence of depression with anxiety symptoms (Gammans et al., 1992). There have also been reports that buspirone can improve successful treatment with standard antidepressants (Jacobsen, 1991).

Clinical use

Unlike the benzodiazepines, which are immediately effective, buspirone appears to have a gradual onset of action. Although some improvement may be expected in the first week, optimal therapeutic effects generally take from two to six weeks to develop (average about three weeks). The usual antianxiety dose is 10 mg three times a day. While the gradual onset of action may be considered a disadvantage in relation to the benzodiazepines, other characteristics of the drug are extremely favorable. Buspirone has almost no sedative effects and may therefore be comfortably taken during the day. There are no disturbing effects on motor coordination or cognition, and so buspirone usually does not disrupt activities requiring alertness and manual dexterity such as driving a car or working a machine. Buspirone does not seem to produce habituation with continued use, as do the benzodiazepines, and alcohol does not potentiate its effects. These characteristics form a remarkable set, making buspirone an almost ideal anxiolytic.

Nevertheless, a word of caution is in order. Many new medications begin their clinical careers as "superior" because they appear to have the advantages of purer clinical effect and fewer undesirable side effects. With continuing use, however, it becomes clear that either the advantages have been exaggerated or there are unanticipated side effects. The key variables are always time and usage. In relation to buspirone, only after a few years will we be able to determine whether the drug is as good as it seems to be or whether there are, in fact, problems with its extended clinical use. Now, after about 10 years in use, the drug shows encouraging signs.

Conditions other than generalized anxiety disorder in which buspirone may prove effective include the aggressive agitation associated with various organic brain syndromes, as well as the augmentation of antidepressive treatment (Schweizer et al., 1986). In higher doses (40–60 mg/day) it may be the sole antidepressant used in some cases. In a psychiatric practice, it is most effective in patients plagued with worry, irritability, and obsessive rumination (Sussman,

1994). Buspirone is considered ineffective for panic disorder and for anxious patients who have been using benzodiazepines a long time.

Selective Serotonin Reuptake Inhibitors

Like buspirone, the selective serotonin reuptake inhibitors (SSRIs) represent an important advance in psychiatry and are widely used to treat depression and panic disorder because of their therapeutic efficacy coupled with a substantial freedom from serious side effects.

Mechanism of action

The SSRIs are relatively specific blockers of serotonin reuptake into presynaptic nerve terminals. Thus, they enhance serotonergic transmission and induce downregulation of postsynaptic receptors. We have some knowledge about the central effects of all the standard antidepressants (e.g., tricyclics, SSRIs, and monoamine oxidase inhibitors) on amine metabolism (e.g., norepinephrine, serotonin, and dopamine) in particular, but the mechanisms explaining their common antidepressive effects are not understood. Significantly, though, every effective antidepressant, including monoamine oxidase inhibitors, tricyclic antidepressants, and SSRIs, as well as electroconvulsant therapy, increases the efficacy of serotonergic neurotransmission (Blier et al., 1987). In addition, some studies have shown that reducing brain serotonin levels is associated with the development of depression (Shopsin et al., 1976; Delgado et al., 1990; Smith et al., 1997). A more detailed account of the neuronal effects of SSRIs in combating depression is given in Chapter 16.

The SSRIs have little or no effect on cholinergic, adrenergic, or histaminergic receptors, which explains why the troublesome side effects associated with blockade of these receptors is rarely a problem with the SSRIs (see TCA side effects below). The SSRIs do have such side effects as anorexia, insomnia, nausea and diarrhea, nervousness, anxiety, and sexual dysfunction. Sildenafil may be helpful in men and women with sexual dysfunction due to SSRIs (Fava et al., 1998). While cardiac side effects are unusual and seldom if ever fatal, there are reports of atrial fibrillation and bradycardia with syncope associated with fluoxetine and other SSRI treatment or overdose (Pacher et al., 1999). Lengthening of the corrected QT interval (QT_c) on the electrocardiogram, an ominous change that may presage fatal ventricular arrythmia and that occurs with tricyclic antidepressants as well as certain neuroleptic drugs such as thioridazine and droperidol, does not appear to occur with SSRIs (Reilly et al., 2000). With the SSRIs, the side effects can often be overcome either by reducing the dosage and building it up gradually or by changing the time of day that the medication is taken (in the morning rather than the evening if the problem is insomnia, or the late evening rather than the morning if the main side effects are gastrointestinal). In any event, side effects caused by SSRIs often diminish with continued use of the drug. Thus, it is often worth trying one of these maneuvers if the side effects are really troublesome; if the side effects are tolerable, encourage the patient to continue taking the medication in the expectation that they will diminish or disappear.

Clinical use

The main use of SSRIs is in the treatment of depression and panic disorder, though in recent years they have been prescribed with increasing frequency for conditions in which anxiety is prominent such as generalized anxiety disorder, social phobia, and simple phobia (Uhlenhuth et al., 1999). The SSRIs have been shown to be efficacious in obsessive-compulsive disorder (OCD). While these patients are usually managed by psychiatrists, occasional patients with psychosomatic disorders show such a pervasive preoccupation with their symptoms that neither a proper conversation nor behavioral interventions such as relaxation techniques are possible; that is, the patient's thinking has a definite obsessional quality. The intrusivity of the repeated symptoms and physical complaints in the conversation makes it impossible to progress with any kind of therapy. In such situations SSRIs to be of value.

The SSRIs are of comparable efficacy to the much older tricyclic antidepressants (TCAs) in the treatment of both depression and panic disorder, and they are now often preferred because they are less likely to produce troublesome side effects and they have a much larger margin of safety for an overdose. The former is of considerable importance in ensuring patient compliance, particularly as these drugs may need to be taken for an extended period. About twice as many patients discontinue treatment with TCAs (30%) due to side effects as discontinue treatment with the SSRI fluoxetine (15%) for the same reason (Montgomery, 1989).

It has been established that fluoxetine taken during pregnancy does not have teratogenic effects (Chambers et al., 1996; Kulin et al., 1998), though there have been assertions that exposure to fluoxetine in the third trimester may be associated with a greater tendency to perinatal complications such as premature delivery and more frequent admission of the newborn to special care nurseries because of respiratory difficulty, cyanosis on feeding, and jitteriness (Chambers et al., 1996). Most important, the neurodevelopment of children whose mothers were exposed to either a tricyclic antidepressant or fluoxetine in the first trimester or throughout pregnancy, tested up to the age of nine years, was found to be normal (Nulman et al., 1997). The assessments included evaluation of global IQ, language development, and behavioral development of preschool children.

These drugs take up to two to three weeks to begin producing relief of any significant kind, but it may be three to four weeks before one is able to decide whether the dose of medication is adequate or should be raised. Better sleep and decreased anxiety are not sufficient indications of improvement in a depressed patient, and care must be taken not to assume that he or she is adequately treated when these symptoms improve (Stokes, 1993). The patient may still be depressed, functioning poorly, and at risk for suicide. The dosage of medication may have to be raised in graduated steps in order to achieve a complete remission of the depression, which should be the goal of therapy. For this reason the drug management of depression and panic disorder requires that the dosage of medication be suited to the individual.

Patients with panic disorder often feel that the symptoms are aggravated in the first five to seven days, and unless they are warned that this could happen, they will stop taking the drug. Because this period may be so difficult for them, however, I routinely warn them of the possibility while also reassuring them that the symptoms mostly subside rapidly (usually within a few days) with continued taking of the medication. In addition, I invariably provide them with my phone numbers and with instructions to call me at any time if they are feeling very worried. It is important that medication be continued both at adequate dosage and for a sufficient time. In practice this means that the medication must be continued at the full therapeutic dosage needed to treat the acute depression. In a bout of major depression, this should be for at least a year. Patients with their first episode of major depression after the age of 50 years or those with more than two episodes in the past five years are at high risk for recurrence and should be encouraged to stay on prophylactic therapy probably for life (Greden, 1993). Average daily doses for the different SSRIs are fluoxetine 20 mg, sertraline 100 mg, paroxetine 20 mg, and fluvoxamine 100 mg.

Tricyclic Antidepressants

For many years the tricyclic antidepressants (TCAs) were the mainstay of treatment for major depression and panic disorder. Historically, imipramine and amitriptyline were the first successful antidepressants. Attempts to minimize side effects while retaining therapeutic efficacy resulted in the development of a series of related compounds, some of which (e.g., clomipramine, doxepin, and nortriptyline) also found widespread clinical use. Because the SSRIs proved similarly effective in the treatment of depression and panic disorder as well as a number of other conditions, however, the TCAs have been largely superseded by the newer drugs.

Mechanism of action

The tricyclic antidepressants block the reuptake of biogenic amines. Their effects, both therapeutic and toxic, result largely from inhibition of presynaptic uptake of norepinephrine and serotonin, and to a much lesser extent dopamine, or from blockade of postsynaptic receptors. While the antidepressant action of these drugs seems to be intimately linked to the blockade of norepinephrine and serotonin uptake, the consistently observed delay between the onset of drug action in blocking amine uptake and the full development of the antidepressant effects (two to three weeks) is probably due to a mechanism similar to that of the SSRIs (Blier and de Montigny, 1994), as described in Chapter 16. Significantly, as mentioned above, a similar delay in reaching therapeutic efficacy is also observed with the buspirone.

The spectrum of TCA side effects is also mostly receptor-mediated and their diversity attests to the relative lack of receptor specificity of this class of drugs. Inhibition of the α_1-adrenergic receptor mediates orthostatic hypotension and reflex tachycardia; inhibition of the H_1 histamine receptor is associated with sedation, drowsiness, and weight gain; and inhibition of the M_1 muscarinic cholinergic receptor may cause dry mouth, constipation, urinary retention, blurred vision, and sinus tachycardia (Richelson, 1987). While all these effects may be troublesome, more sinister are the quinidinelike effects of myocardial depression, which may be particularly dangerous in the presence of conduction defects (bundle branch block), underlying ischemic heart disease, or the use of class I sodium channel–blocking antiarrhythmic agents. Problematic cardiac effects are not confined to old people (Reilly et al., 2000). There have been case reports of sudden death in children and adolescents being treated with TCAs (Nemeroff, 1994), although considering the very widespread usage of these drugs, such reports are rare.

Clinical use

To diminish side effects when TCAs are used to treat depression and panic disorder, the medication is often administered initially at a lower than therapeutic dosage and then gradually increased. This will generally also reduce the intensification of symptoms often experienced by patients with panic disorder during the first five to seven days after starting treatment. As with the SSRIs, it is essential to encourage the patient to continue taking the medication despite the discomfort, in order to pass through this phase of treatment successfully. The advent of slow-release formulations has also been helpful in diminishing side effects, and taking the full daily dose as a single dose at night allows the patient to sleep through the main sedative phase of the daily treatment. The convenience of taking medication as a single dose is also thought to facilitate compliance.

Drugs Inhibiting Noradrenaline and Serotonin Uptake

While all the SSRIs and TCAs may influence both norepinephrine and serotonin reuptake to various degrees, the differing receptor affinities permit the categorization of each drug in both groups according to its predominant pharmacological characteristics. In certain cases, however, the agent may have clinical characteristics which are distinctive enough to be atypical of either group.

One such agent, venlafaxine, has a neuropharmacological profile which differs from that of tricyclic antidepressants because its potency in inhibiting serotonin uptake is approximately five times that of its noradrenaline reuptake inhibitory activity (Holliday and Benfield, 1995). Venlafaxine is effective in treating depression in doses of 75–375 mg/day administered in two or three divided doses. It is well tolerated and any side effects (nausea and sweating) usually subside with continued administration of the drug. A transitory increase in blood pressure has been reported, but there have been no reports of negative cardiac effects, presumably because of very poor interaction with the muscarinic cholinergic receptor. In addition to its efficacy in treating depression, some reports suggest that venlafaxine may be able to achieve a more rapid clinical response rate (four days) when the dose is rapidly increased in hospitalized patients (Rudolph et al., 1991). Under outpatient conditions, however, significant clinical improvement may take two or three weeks to develop. The positive clinical impression of venlafaxine's efficacy, and its low toxicity profile, is almost certainly derived from its very poor affinity for other amine receptors, such as the H_1 histamine and α_1-adrenergic, dopamine, and muscarinic cholinergic receptors (Frazer, 1997).

Additional Therapeutic Agents

Quite a few other psychoactive agents are used to treat anxiety and depression. The trend in drug development in this area is toward agents with increasing specificity for particular receptors. Besides being useful as supplementary drugs to help achieve a greater antidepressant effect when that might be needed, they may also be substituted if the conventional medications are not producing an effect or are causing troublesome side effects.

The older tricyclic antidepressants are being replaced by equipotent newer classes of antidepressant medication such as the SSRIs and other amine reuptake inhibitors that may be more rapid in onset of action and less troubled by side effects that interfere with the quality of life. Prominent among this latter group are venlafaxine (a serotonin noradrenergic reuptake inhibitor), nefazodone (a weaker serotonin and norepinephrine reuptake inhibitor, but a potent serotonin 5-HT$_2$ receptor antagonist), mirtazapine (a potent antagonist of central 2-alpha adrenergic autoreceptors and heteroreceptors as well as an antagonist of serotonin 5-HT$_2$ and 5-HT$_3$ receptors), and reboxetine (the first selective noradrenergic reuptake inhibitor) (Kent, 2000).

While the therapeutic efficacy of all these drugs may be very similar, the decision of which to use may need to be made more on the basis of wanting to either avoid or exploit a certain side effect:

- If a medication interferes with normal sexual function in men or women (a potential side effect of all the SSRIs and TCAs), agents such as nefazodone, bupropion, or mirtazapine may be considered (Langer, 1997; Sanchez and Hyttel, 1999). All these drugs are considered effective and well tolerated with little tendency to interfere with sexual function.

- Weight gain, another side effect of frequent concern to women starting an- tidepressant treatment, occurs with both SSRIs and tricyclic antidepressants and is common with mirtazapine. Nefazodone, venlafaxine, and reboxitine have not been associated with significant weight changes. In certain cases, however, the appetite-enhancing properties of mirtazapine may may be ex- ploited to help to counter significant depression-associated weight loss.
- Sleep disturbances and insomnia, common depression-associated symptoms, may be exacerbated by many antidepressants, significantly affecting pa- tients' sense of well-being and overall functioning. Nefazodone probably best relieves depression-associated sleep disturbance, often making the ad- dition of a nocturnal sedative unnecessary (Kent, 2000).
- Tricyclic and SSRI antidepressants tend to lower the seizure threshold in epileptic patients, whereas nefazodone appears to have no effect on seizure threshold. It would therefore seem to be the drug of choice in patients suf- fering from both epilepsy and depression.
- Venlafaxine, mirtazapine, and reboxetine are associated with low frequen- cies of drug–drug interactions compared with the SSRIs, a consideration of some importance when treating patients with comorbid medical conditions (Gill and Hatcher, 2000) who may already be taking a number of drugs for their medical ailment.

The availability of these newer drugs with their varying side effect profiles is thus helping to improve both efficacy and tolerability and significantly broaden the choice of a suitable agent for any particular patient.

In addition, a selective monoamine oxidase A inhibitor, moclobemide, is free of the side effects of the nonspecific, older generation monoamine oxidase in- hibitors such as hypertensive crises after eating tyramine-rich foods like yellow cheese or drinking wine. Moclobemide is prescribed in particular for depression with atypical features, as well as panic disorder and obsessive-compulsive disorder.

A selective norepinephrine reuptake inhibitor, reboxetine, representing a new class of antidepressants, proved to be effective in the treatment of major de- pressive disorder or dysthymia (Burrows et al., 1998). While being generally well tolerated, the most commonly occurring adverse effects—in more than 15% of patients—were increased sweating, blurred vision, insomnia, and dry mouth. Massana (1998) compared reboxetine (8–10 mg/day) to the SSRI fluoxetine (20–40 mg/day) in a double-blind, randomized clinical trial in 549 patients with major depression. The overall efficacy of both drugs was similar and both were superior to placebo. However, reboxetine appeared to have superior efficacy com- pared to fluoxetine in severely ill patients and was associated with greater im- provement in the social functioning of depressed patients, especially in terms of motivation toward action and negative self-perception.

OTHER CLINICAL USES OF ANTIDEPRESSIVE MEDICATION

Premenstrual Dysphoric Disorder (Premenstrual syndrome)

Premenstrual dysphoric disorder is a DSM-IV diagnosis characterized as markedly depressed mood, marked anxiety, marked affective lability, and decreased interest in activities occurring during the last week of the luteal phase in most menstrual cycles during the past year. The symptoms begin to remit within a few days of the onset of menses (the follicular phase) and are always absent in the week following menses. This incapacitating and distressing state may be viewed as the severest expression of the continuum of symptoms labeled the premenstrual syndrome, and because of its impact on a woman's life it has stimulated a search for effective therapy. In the last few years, repeated placebo-controlled trials of SSRIs, particularly fluoxetine (Steiner et al., 1997; Diegoli et al., 1998), sertraline (Yonkers et al., 1997; Young et al., 1998; Freeman et al., 1999; Jermain et al., 1999), citalopram (Wikander et al., 1998), taken in the luteal phase of the cycle, have shown that these drugs help in reducing the emotional symptoms. This condition represents an unusual exception to the rule emphasized above that these drugs need to be taken continuously for optimal effects. In the case of premenstrual dysphoric disorder, where continuous treatment versus luteal phase administration only has been tested, the later style of administration appeared to provide more satisfactory relief from symptoms or at the least was as effective as continuous dosage (Steiner et al., 1997; Wikander et al., 1998; Freeman et al., 1999; Jermain et al., 1999).

The considerable importance of brain serotonin metabolism in the genesis of premenstrual dysphoria gained further support from a randomized controlled study by Steinberg et al. (1999), where 37 patients with premenstrual dysphoric disorder were treated with the serotonin precursor amino acid L-tryptophan (6 g/day) and 34 were given placebo. The treatments were administered under double-blind conditions for 17 days, from the time of ovulation to the third day of menstruation, during three consecutive menstrual cycles. Subjects receiving L-tryptophan had a 34.5% reduction in their symptom intensity ($P = 0.004$) compared to a 10.4% improvement with the placebo.

Smoking Cessation

Although habituation to cigarette smoking is not categorized as an affective disorder, the exceedingly common association between habitual smoking and affective disorders in particular justifies its inclusion here (Farrell et al., 1998), as does the fact that depression reduces the chances of successful smoking discontinuation (Smith et al., 1999). This is especially important as clinical trials have established that the antidepressant bupropion is effective in helping people stop smoking. Jorenby et al. (1999) conducted a double-blind, placebo-controlled comparison of sustained-release bupropion (244 subjects), a nicotine patch (244 subjects), bupropion and a nicotine patch (245 subjects), and placebo (160 subjects) for smoking cessation. The abstinence rates at 12 months were 15.6% in the placebo group, 16.4% in the nicotine patch group, 30.3% in the bupropion group ($P < 0.001$), and 35.5% in the group given bupropion and the nicotine patch ($P < 0.001$). The weight gain with smoking cessation was also significantly less in the treatment groups than in the placebo, but 34.8% discontinued one or both medications because of side effects such as insomnia and headache. The mechanism of these side effects is probably related in some way to the interaction of bupropion with nicotinic acetylcholine receptor subtypes (Fryer and Lukas, 1999). A history of depression or alcoholism, conditions associated with poorer smoking treatment outcomes, does not appear to interfere with the effect of bupropion in smoking cessation (Hayford et al., 1999), though major depression may occasionally appear during treatment with bupropion for smoking cessation (Patten et al., 1999). Similar effects in facilitating smoking cessation have not been demonstrated with other antidepressants.

COMPLIANCE IN DRUG TAKING

One of the curious paradoxes of clinical practice, familiar to most physicians with even a few years of practical experience, is the seemingly anomalous behavior of the suffering but nevertheless noncompliant patient. The physician prescribes medication for the relief of symptoms and the patient fails to take the prescribed medication but continues to complain of the symptoms. This phenomenon is especially commonly encountered in the field of psychosomatic medicine and often relates to the intention of prescribing antidepression or antianxiety medication. The key to understanding it is to appreciate that for many patients suffering from stress-related problems, the taking of a tablet may be yet another symbol of having lost control over their lives—that is, it represents the need to be reliant on a substance foreign to their being in order to help solve the problem.

While patients are not usually able to formulate the problem in quite this way, the difficulty nevertheless expresses itself in one of several characteristic responses. Patients don't take the prescribed medication in spite of their symptoms; or they are unable to tolerate a range of drugs because of a tendency to develop intolerable side effects with almost any medication they take; or they remain unresponsive or partially responsive to what should be adequate therapy for the underlying medical problem. It is important to understand that the underlying medical problem may be organic in etiology. Thus, the patient, who could be suffering from rheumatoid arthritis, may complain that the medication she is receiving is not helping her morning stiffness or her joint pain. The apparent lack of response may give the impression that the underlying disease is not responding to treatment and this may lead the physician to consider using drugs with potentially more serious side effects, such as corticosteroids. However, what needs to be considered in such a case is that the lack of response may have a treatable emotional basis. To a certain extent this may also be articulated as a fear of dependency on drugs. A physician not understanding the process underlying these responses may become impatient and be tempted to label the patient as uncooperative. Relating to the patient's specific fears or concerns in the therapeutic interaction is, however, likely to increase the patient's willingness to take the prescribed medication.

Other patients in a similar clinical predicament may prefer the idea of medication as opposed to psychotherapy or counseling. This may be for reasons of convenience, but not infrequently the preference stems from a reluctance to confront the possibility that the clinical problem has a psychophysiological basis, which behavioral intervention or a program of psychotherapy clearly implies. Here it is important to remember that failure to deal specifically with an underlying cause of the anxiety can condemn any attempt at drug therapy to failure, though drugs may be used as an adjunct to other forms of therapy. As a general rule, with appropriate cognitive and behavioral management, many patients suffering from psychosomatic disorders may find their symptoms alleviated sufficiently to reduce symptom-relieving drug requirements to minimal levels. This is particularly true for many chronic or intermittent pain syndromes.

The presence of disturbing side effects is a formidable obstacle to long-term compliance in drug taking. The introduction of the newer drugs, many of which appear to be more specific in their pharmacological actions, has also extended considerably the likelihood of being able to find a drug with the required therapeutic efficacy but without disturbing side effects. This chapter presented examples of how these agents may be used in response to specific clinical needs.

SUMMARY

Patients are likely to respond most favorably when the use of drugs for anxiety or depression is suggested as a means to regain a measure of the control and self-confidence that have been undermined by their clinical condition. In some patients this may be perceived as the treatment of choice. In others, it may be seen as a means of stabilizing an unstable and stressful clinical state in order to allow a program of psychotherapy to proceed. As with all forms of effective communication with patients, here too specific fears—such as concern about drug dependency—must be explored and directly responded to.

A characteristic of the drugs used for the treatment of depression is the apparent plateau effect of drug efficacy in relation to their therapeutic effect. Of all the antidepressants currently available, no one agent regarded as effective has been shown in properly conducted trials to be clearly superior in alleviating depression (i.e., as being more efficient) compared to any other drug. The selection of a drug in this group will thus be very much determined by other characteristics such as the speed of onset of the therapeutic action and lack of side effects. To this end the newer categories of drugs discussed here promise a therapeutic advantage. The older drugs will, nevertheless, continue to be prescribed in spite of suboptimal characteristics (longer interval to achieve a therapeutic effect and more troublesome side effects), often because of price considerations, although it is reassuring to know that from the point of view of efficacy they may be regarded as similar to the newer drugs.

The tendency of many antidepressants to seemingly accentuate arousal symptoms with the onset of therapy, leading to considerable patient discomfort with increased agitation, and the tendency to stop taking the drug because of this, is common enough to be regarded as a general problem. This may be especially problematic in the treatment of panic disorder because here arousal symptoms are typically associated with intense feelings of distress. Quite naturally, most patients interpret this response as a deterioration in their condition caused by the new drug. All patients should, therefore, be warned that this may happen. However, starting with very low doses that are built up gradually may alleviate or avoid the problem completely. In addition, offering the patient a line of facilitated contact is also reassuring and will allow the physician to encourage continuation of the drug if the patient is agitated by the apparent deterioration. In many cases this intensification of symptoms passes within three to four days and in the majority by five to seven days.

REFERENCES

American Psychiatric Association (1994). Diagnostic and Statistical Manual of Mental Disorders. Washington, DC: Author.

Blier P, de Montigny C (1994). Current advances and trends in the treatment of depression. Trends Pharmacol Sci 15:220–226.

Blier P, de Montigny C, Chaput Y (1987). Modifications of the serotonin system by antidepressant treatments: implications for the therapeutic response in major depression. J Clin Pharmacokinet 7(6, suppl):24S–35S.

Burrows GD, Maguire KP, Norman TR (1998). Antidepressant efficacy and tolerability of the selective norepinephrine reuptake inhibitor reboxitine: a review. J Clin Psychiatry 59 (suppl 14):4–7.

Chambers CD, Johnson KA, Dick LM, et al. (1996). Birth outcomes in pregnant women taking fluoxetine. N Engl J Med 335:1010–1015.

Delgado PL, Charney DS, Price LH, et al. (1990). Serotonin function and the mechanism of antidepressant action: reversal of antidepressant-induced remission by rapid depletion of plasma tryptophan. Arch Gen Psychiatry 47:411–418.

Diegoli MS, da Fonseca AM, Diegoli CA, et al. (1998). A double-blind trial of four medications to treat severe premenstrual syndrome. Int J Gynaecol Obstet 62:63–67.

Eison AS, Eison MS, Stanley MM, et al. (1986). Serotonergic mechanisms in the behavioural effects of buspirone and gepirone. Pharmacol Biochem Behav 24:701–707.

Farrell M, Howes S, Taylor C, et al. (1998). Substance misuse and psychiatric comorbidity: an overview of the OPCS National Psychiatric Morbidity Survey. Addict Behav 23:909–918.

Fava M, Rankin MA, Alpert JE, et al. (1998). An open trial of oral sidemafil antidepressant-induced sexual dysfunction. Psychother Psychosom 67:328–313.

Feighner JP, Cohn JB. (1989). Analysis of individual symptoms in generalized anxiety— a pooled, multistudy, double-blind evaluation of buspirone. Neuropsychobiology 21:124–130.

Frazer A (1997). Pharmacology of Antidepressants. J Clin Psychopharmacol 17:2S–18S.

Freeman EW, Rickels K, Arredondo F, et al. (1999). Full- or half-cycle treatment of severe premenstrual syndrome with a serotinergic antidepressant. J Clin Psychopharmacol 19:3–8.

Fryer JD, Lukas RJ (1999). Noncompetitive functional inhibition at diverse, human nicotinic acetylcholine receptor subtypes by bupropion, phencyclidine and ibogaine. J Pharmacol Exp Ther 288:88–92.

Gammans RE, Stringfellow JC, Hvizdus AJ, et al. (1992). Use of buspirone in patients with generalized anxiety disorder and coexisting depressive symptoms: a meta-analysis of eight randomized, controlled studies. Neuropsychobiology 25:193–201.

Gill D, Hatcher S (2000). Antidepressants for depression in people with physical illness. Cochrane Database Syst Rev 2:CD001312.

Greden JF (1993). Antidepressant maintenance medications: when to discontinue and how to stop. J Clin Psychiatry 54(8, suppl):39–45.

Hayford KE, Patten CA, Rummans TA, et al. (1999). Efficacy of bupropion for smoking cessation in smokers with a former history of major depression or alcoholism. Br J Psychiatry 174:173–178.

Holliday SM, Benfield P (1995). Venlafaxine: a review of its pharmacology and therapeutic potential in depression. Drugs 49:280–294.

Jacobsen FM (1991). Possible augmentation of antidepressant response by buspirone. J Clin Psychiatry 52:217–220.

Jermain DM, Preece CK, Sykes RL, et al. (1999). Luteal phase sertraline treatment for premenstrual dysphoric disorder: results of a double-blind, placebo-controlled, crossover study. Arch Fam Med 8:328–332.

Jorenby DE, Leischow SJ, Nides MA, et al. (1999). A controlled trial of sustained-release bupropion, a nicotine patch, or both for smoking cessation. N Engl J Med 340:685–691.

Kent JM (2000). SnaRIs, NaSSAs, and NaRIs: new agents for the treatment of depression. Lancet 355:911–918.

Kulin NA, Pastuszak A, Sage SR, et al. (1998). Pregnancy outcome following maternal use of the new selective serotonin reuptake inhibitors: a prospective controlled multicenter study. JAMA 279:609–610.

Langer SZ (1997). 25 years since the discovery of presynaptic receptors: present knowledge and future perspectives. Trends Pharmacol Sci 18:95–99.

Langley MS, Clissold SP. (1988). Brotizolam: a review of its pharmocodynamic and pharmacokinetic properties, and therapeutic efficacy as an hypnotic. Drugs 35:104–122.

Massana J (1998). Reboxitine versus fluoxetine: an overview of efficiency and tolerability. J Clin Psychiatry 59(suppl 14):8–10.

Montgomery SA (1989). The efficacy of fluoxetine as an antidepressant in the short and long term. Int Clin Psychopharmacol 4(suppl 1):113–119.

Nemeroff CB (1994). Evolutionary trends in the pharmacotherapeutic management of depression. J Clin Psychiatry 55:(12, suppl):3–15.

Nulman I, Rovet J, Stewart DE, et al. (1997). Neurodevelopment of children exposed in utero to antidepressant drugs. N Engl J Med 336:258–262.

Pacher P, Ungvari Z, Nanasi PP, et al. (1999). Speculations on difference between tricyclic and selective serotonin reuptake inhibitor antidepressants on their cardiac effect: is there any? Curr Med Chem 6:469–480.

Patten CA, Rummans TA, Croghan IT, et al. (1999). Development of depression during placebo-controlled trials of bupropion for smoking cessation: case reports. J Clin Psychiatry 60:436–441.

Peroutka SJ (1985). Sedative interaction of novel anxiolytics with 5-hydroxytryptamine$_{1A}$ receptors. J Biol Psychiatry 20:971–979.

Reilly JG, Ayis SA, Ferrier IN, et al. (2000). QTc-interval abnormalities and psychotropic drug therapy in psychiatric patients. Lancet 355:1048–1052.

Richelson E (1987). Pharmacology of antidepressants. Psychopathology 20(suppl 1):1–12.

Rudolph R, Entsuah R, Derivan A. (1991). Early clinical response in depression to venlafaxine hydrochloride. Biol Psych 29:630S. Abstract P-26-12.

Sanchez C, Hyttel J (1999). Comparison of the effects of antidepressants and their metabolites on reuptake of biogenic amines and on receptor binding. Cell Mol Neurobiol 19:467–489.

Schweizer EE, Amsterdam J, Rickels K, et al. (1986). Open trial of buspirone in the treatment of major depressive disorder. Psychopharmacol Bull 22:183–185.

Shopsin B, Friedman E, Gershon S (1976). Parachlorphenylalanine reversal of tranylcypramine effects in depressed patients. Arch Gen Psychiatry 33:811–819.

Smith KA, Fairburn CG, Cowen PJ (1997). Relapse of depression after rapid depletion of tryptophan. Lancet 349:915–919.

Smith PM, Kraemer HC, Miller NH, et al. (1999). In-hospital smoking cessation programs: who responds, who doesn't? J Consult Clin Psychol 67:19–27.

Steinberg S, Annable L, Young SN, et al. (1999). A placebo-controlled clinical trial of L-tryptophan in premenstrual dysphoria. Biol Psychiatry 45:313–320.

Steiner M, Korzekwa M, Lamont J, et al. (1997). Intermittent fluoxetine dosing in the treatment of women with premenstrual dysphoria. Psychopharmacol Bull 33:771–774.

Stokes PE (1993). A primary care perspective on management of acute and long-term depression. J Clin Psychiatry 54 (8, suppl):74–84.

Sussman N (1994). The uses of buspirone in psychiatry. J Clin Psychiatry 12:3–19.

Tallman JR, Paul SM, Skolnick P, et al. (1980). Receptors for the age of anxiety: pharmacology of the benzodiazepines. Science 207:274–281.

Uhlenhuth EH, Balter MB, Ban TA, et al. (1999). International study of expert judgement on therapeutic use of benzodiazepines and other psychotherapeutic medications: VI. Trends in recommendations for the pharmacotherapy of anxiety disorders, 1992–1997. Depress Anxiety 9:107–116.

Wikander I, Sundblad C, Andersch B, et al. (1998). Citalopram in premenstrual dysphoria: is intermittent treatment during luteal phases more effective than continuous medication throughout the menstrual cycle? J Clin Psychopharmacol 18:390–398.

Yocca FD (1990). Neurochemistry and neurophysiology of buspirone and gepirone: interactions at presynaptic and postsynaptic 5-HT$_{1A}$ receptors. Psychopharmacology 10(suppl):68–125.

Yonkers KA, Halbreich U, Freeman E, et al. (1997). Symptomatic improvement of premenstrual dysphoric disorder with sertraline treatment: a randomized controlled trial. Sertraline Premenstrual Dysphoric Group. JAMA 278:983–988.

Young SA, Hurt PH, Benedek DM, et al. (1998). Treatment of premenstrual dysphoric disorder with sertraline during the luteal phase: a randomized, double-blind, placebo-controlled crossover trial. J Clin Psychiatry 59:76–80.

Chapter

18

General Principles of Stress Management

I do believe that there is a large body of knowledge about behavior that is required before one can be clinically effective, and I believe that knowledge is what is missing from the repertoire of many, if not most physicians.

(Engel "Psychosomatic Medicine," 1986)

Every emotional state has its somatic correlate, which is mediated mostly through autonomic activation. In situations where emotions are intensely felt, the coupling of particular kinds of thoughts and feelings with specific autonomic responses is thought to play a role in maintaining problematic patterns of behavior. It is as if emotionally troublesome thoughts and experiences are "locked in" and experienced in association with often distressing somatic effects of autonomic activation. This type of experience has the quality of a conditioned response in that it cannot be influenced by will.

The somatic component is central to the emotional state. When it is possible to uncouple memory and feelings from the reflex autonomic response, an individual may acquire the ability to reevaluate a situation in cognitive terms that are less disturbing emotionally, with concomitant relief of the symptom. Clinical experience has shown that reduction of the reflex autonomic activation associated with a particular context-related emotion such as anxiety, fear, or anger may help free the individual from the emotion itself. In this way patients may in turn be "released" from the inevitability of the body responses or symptoms which are triggered by the emotional state and which can exacerbate distress. This may be achieved either by cognitively modifying a patient's perception of the symptom so that it ceases to be threatening or by moderating, through some behavioral intervention, the activity of the autonomic nervous system associated with the symptom. Most techniques of behavioral intervention are directed at both the cognitive and the autonomic levels.

Four main categories of intervention can be used to deal with emotions and undesirable autonomic activation:

1. Cognitive modification.
2. Techniques of deep relaxation and meditation.
3. Biofeedback.
4. Miscellaneous techniques of exposure and graduated "desensitization."

Well-controlled clinical studies have shown relaxation and meditation training to be effective in the management of conditions which are classically associated with chronic disability and suffering, including chronic pain syndromes and anxiety states, which are often unresponsive or only partially responsive to all forms of "conventional" medicine (Benson et al., 1978; Kabat-Zinn et al., 1985; Kabat-Zinn et al., 1987; Hellman et al., 1990; Caudill et al., 1991; Kabat-Zinn et al., 1992). Behavioral intervention has been shown to be effective in chronic insomnia (Jacobs et al., 1996). In a reevalaution after three years of 18 of 22 patients with anxiety disorders who initially participated in an eight-week outpatient stress reduction intervention based on mindful meditation (Kabat-Zinn et al., 1992), Miller et al. (1995) found that the gains obtained in the original study were maintained, judged by the Hamilton and Beck anxiety scales as well as their respective depression scales, the Hamilton panic score, and the number and severity of panic attacks were maintained. Ongoing compliance with the meditation practice was also demonstrated in the majority of subjects at three years. A program of mindful meditation–based stress reduction was shown by Kabat-Zinn et al. (1998) to significantly facilitate the rate of skin clearing in 37 patients suffering from moderate to severe psoriasis who underwent ultraviolet light therapy.

Principles of cognitive therapy as well as techniques of deep relaxation and meditation, the approaches with the most general utility to physicians interested in managing the psychosomatic aspects of medical practice, are discussed here in some detail. Biofeedback is also used to considerable effect in the management of stress-related symptoms as well as in rehabilitation programs where patients have to relearn such functions as sphincter control. As the management of most anxiety-inducing experiences involves some exposure to the specific trigger for the emotional response, the fourth point listed above may be an important component of the first two techniques. While in a state of deep relaxation, for example, a patient may imagine the anxiety-inducing experience, or actually be accompanied to the place or shown the object which induces the anxiety. First, however, we consider some of the general principles of patient management.

REDUCING ANXIETY IN ILLNESS BY INFORMING
THE PATIENT: A PREVENTIVE STRATEGY

A growing body of literature supports the contention that educating patients about specific illnesses or clinical states substantially reduces their concerns, enabling more effective management of the clinical condition and leading in turn to a lower rate of utilization of medical services. For patients to be adequately reassured, the physician must provide them with information that is relevant to their clinical condition, in a form they can easily understand (Ley, 1982; Warwick and Salkovskis, 1985). This principle is illustrated by the following studies.

In a Southern California clinic where fever was the most common reason for pediatric visits, accounting for 20%–25% of all pediatric complaints, the local health maintenance organization (HMO) designed a health education program to increase knowledge about fever in children. In a study aimed at evaluating how parents use medical care (Robinson et al., 1989), 500 families who visited the doctor with a feverish child under the age of 13 were divided into two groups, one of which was shown a 10-minute slide presentation on fever. All participants in both groups were seen individually by a physician. All parents were supplied with a pamphlet covering the major points of the slide presentation and were given the opportunity to ask questions. After seven months, the group that watched the slide presentation had made 35% fewer visits for fever than the group that only received a pamphlet. After eight months, the slide group had made 25% fewer visits for all acute illnesses.

A diagnosis of diabetes mellitus imposes a radical change in life-style as patients learn how to manage their condition, and especially how to balance diet and exercise requirements with drug therapy (insulin injections or oral medication). They must also learn to monitor their own blood glucose. At the Los Angeles County–University of Southern California Medical Center, an integrated program of diabetes education and care decreased the rate of hospitalization in a group of 6000 patients by 73% and the average length of stay by 78%, with an estimated saving of $2319 per patient each year (Miller and Goldstein, 1972).

In Atlanta, Georgia, diabetes outpatient education and care reduced the incidence of severe diabetic ketoacidosis by 65% and the number of lower extremity amputations by 49% in a group of 12,950 patients. The total estimated saving was $437,500 per year (Davidson et al., 1979).

In Germany, a five-day intensive outpatient education program attended by 212 patients over three years cut the number of days spent in hospitals from 16.7 to 6.3 days per year (Muhlhauser et al., 1983; Assal et al., 1985).

In 1978, Children's Hospital Medical Center in Cincinnati, Ohio, introduced a program of structured education for children with diabetes. The program was presented by a diabetes nurse-educator and a dietitian, with social and psychiatric support services. Initial interventions were geared to the child's development level and the family's attitudes and health values. Round-the-clock telephone support was made available. Admission records of 798 diabetic children between 1973 and 1987 showed that the program saved the hospital about $342,000 per year. The savings derived mainly from a reduction in the length of hospitalization of children admitted with diabetic ketoacidosis.

A meta-analysis of 191 studies conducted between 1963 and 1989 evaluated the effects of psychoeducational interventions on recovery, postsurgical pain, and psychological distress of adult surgical patients (Devine, 1992). The operations in these studies were both minor and major, and included abdominal (gall bladder, bowel, or gastric) and thoracic (heart and lung) surgery. The psychoeducational interventions were grouped in three broad categories:

1. Health care information about what would be done before and after surgery, timing of the various procedures and activities, and the functional roles of different health care providers.
2. Skill-building exercises for coughing, breathing, and relaxation.
3. Psychosocial support, identifying and attempting to alleviate patient concerns, providing reassurance, encouraging patients to ask questions throughout hospitalization, and shaping specific expectations of recovery.

Between 79% and 84% of the studies indicated beneficial effects from these interventions. The length of hospital stay was decreased by an average of 1.5 days.

Another analysis of 13 studies showed that psychological intervention reduced hospitalization after surgery or after a heart attack by about two days below the control group's average of almost 10 days (Mumford et al., 1982). Significantly, the psychological interventions were modest and in most of the studies were not matched to the emotional needs of particular patients or to their coping styles. The techniques included presentation of specific information about the patient's condition and about any planned surgery and its expected aftermath. This information was delivered by a nurse-practitioner or psychologist, or by audio- or videocassette. Some studies also used relaxation techniques.

Certain chronic conditions, such as asthma, may be associated with significant disability and high rates of health care utilization. In the 1979–1981 National Health Interview Surveys, 27% of individuals with asthma or frequent wheezing reported one or more days in bed in the past year, 21% reported long-term lim-

itations on their usual activities, and 18% reported five or more visits to the doctor in the past year. There is widespread evidence of poor self-management practices among asthmatic patients, including poor compliance with medication
(Klieger and Dirks, 1979; Kinsman et al., 1980), and many physicians believe
that the increasing mortality from asthma in recent years is partly explained on
this basis (Evans et al., 1987; Sly, 1988). The overall death rate from asthma in
1988 was 1.9 per 100,000 population, with much lower rates in persons under
45 years and a dramatic increase with age. Bailey et al. (1990) found a significant improvement in medication compliance and functional status associated with
education, but no decrease in rate of utilization of health care services over a 12-
month follow-up period. George et al. (1999) found, however, that inpatient education at the time of admission with acute asthma produced a markedly higher
follow-up attendance (60% versus 27%) and significantly fewer emergency department visits and hospitalizations in the six months following the intervention.
This was demonstrated to substantially reduce health care costs (O'Dowd et al.,
1997). In a study of 323 patients suffering from moderate to severe asthma, Wilson et al. (1993) reported an education-dependent difference in the time course
over which changes in outcome occurred. With small-group education, there was
an almost immediate improvement in control of asthma symptoms (reduced
"bother" due to asthma and increased symptom-free days) and in the level of
physical activity. But the rate of utilization of medical care for acute attacks took
much longer to show an effect, decreasing gradually over the two-year follow-
up period. It should be noted that 48% of the total group had pets to which they
were known to be allergic, and 34% still allowed these pets into the house. Similarly, approximately 10% of the participants were active smokers.

These latter factors must have militated against a better outcome, and they
serve to emphasize an important point that emerges from the foregoing studies:
education that simply informs can still have a strong impact on the patient. It reinforces feelings of control by eliminating uncertainty and the likelihood of un-
grounded fears. However, education whose primary aim is to bring about behavioral change other than increasing compliance in drug taking (George et al.,
1999) often is much less successful and presents a more formidable challenge.
A good example of this problem is the randomized, controlled trial of an educational program to prevent low back injuries undertaken by Daltroy et al. (1997)
in about 4000 postal workers (described in Chapter 10). The subjects were followed for over five and a half years. Comparison of the intervention and control
groups showed that the education program did not reduce the rate of low back
injury, the median cost per injury, the time off from work per injury, the rate of
related musculoskeletal injuries, or the rate of repeated injury after return to work.
A possible reason for the failure is the fact that these educational programs should
have led to increased practice of safe lifting and handling techniques, a behavioral change that did not take place.

Management Versus Treatment

The word "management" often implies a comprehensive, holistic therapeutic approach to dealing with a particular clinical problem. "Treatment" usually denotes a process which is narrower and more specific, such as prescribing a drug or performing an operation. Patients suffering from psychosomatic problems often require several types of treatment and the physician has to evaluate the appropriateness of each. For this reason, patients with psychosomatic disorders are "managed" rather than "treated."

Who manages the patient?

The first question to consider is whether a particular patient is to be managed by the primary care physician alone or referred for psychiatric evaluation and management. Even if the physician opts for psychiatric referral, it is by no means certain that the patient will acquiesce in this proposal. The physician may have to convince the patient that this would be in his or her best interests, a task that may take time and requires patience. Patients who resist consultation with a psychotherapist may feel threatened by the potential implications, in particular the possibility of being labeled with a psychiatric diagnosis.

As an immediate objective, the physician should work on the patient's sense of control through cognitive intervention and, if necessary, through deep relaxation or meditation. The support provided by these measures often helps patients, over a number of weeks or months, to view the prospect of psychotherapeutic consultation in a more positive light. Patients are further helped by the physician's reassurance of continued interest and expressed desire to remain "in the picture." Because the original complaint was of a physical nature, the physician's continued involvement is reassuring not only to the patient but also to the psychotherapist. If it is decided that the problem is to be managed by the physician, a number of therapeutic options are available.

How is the patient to be managed?

No one therapeutic approach can possibly suit all situations. In all cases, however, the physician must have a clear understanding of the problem as a prerequisite for establishing effective therapeutic rapport with a patient. The various management options may then be presented to the patient and discussed in a spirit of joint planning of the therapeutic program. In this approach, patients feel personally involved from the outset in the management of their problems. Communication in this spirit is itself therapeutic. A discussion then follows on the most suitable way of managing the emotional aspects of the problem, whether it be by referral to a psychotherapist or a stress-management program utilizing techniques such as deep relaxation or meditation, or the teaching of biofeedback, or treatment with antianxiety or antidepressant medication.

The process of doctor–patient communication may seem to create an anomalous situation in which patients are being asked how they feel their problems should be managed. This is not the case, however. What in fact happens is that, depending on the physician's assessment of the problem, a number of therapeutic options are offered with the intention of determining which would be the most appropriate. This will be decided in accordance with patients' responses to the options presented. Some patients strongly resist the suggestion of taking pills, especially tranquilizers or antidepressants, and much prefer to try deep relaxation. Others are not interested in trying deep relaxation and instead opt for drugs. The physician may have to accommodate these personal preferences, especially if patients cannot be persuaded to accept what is recommended first. It should be emphasized that the general physician's style of managing psychosomatic problems is different from the psychotherapist's. The physician, unlike the psychotherapist, must involve patients in a full discussion of therapeutic options and help them make the choices. Moreover, the physician tries to convey not only that the patients are controlling the interaction insofar as they are participating in management decisions, but also that all aspects of the therapeutic interaction will be directed toward strengthening their feelings of control.

Therapeutic Options

The basic elements of comprehensive management should include cognitive aspects of management, which in most cases means effective reassurance.

Principles of cognitive therapy

One of the most important techniques in psychotherapy is a highly effective, directed approach in which the therapist first elicits then challenges and modifies patients' rational understanding of their physical symptoms, particularly when these are manifested as anxiety or depression. Patients' interpretation or understanding of their clinical condition may be distorted or erroneous, so that any anxiety or depression may be sustained and even reinforced by an inappropriate, often illogical, interpretation of their clinical state. Demonstrating the illogicality of their underlying thought processes helps undermine the supposedly "rational" basis for the negative mood, leading to a change in mental image and thus in feeling. Patients are shown that the same information may be differently (and more plausibly) interpreted and that the new interpretation is much less threatening. Clinical experience indicates that emotional states of depression or anxiety may be substantially alleviated in this way (Beck, 1991; Clark, 1999; DeRubeis et al., 1999). Cognitive-behavioral therapy has proven to be effective and to enhance the efficacy of drug treatment in other prevalent affective disorders, such as panic disorder (Bruce et al., 1999), obsessive-compulsive disorder (O'Conner et al., 1999), posttraumatic stress disorder (Devilly and Spence, 1999), and hypochondriasis (Clark et al., 1998).

In the field of medical practice, both the clinical context and the thought sequence that lead to emotional problems in most cases are fairly predictable. As stated by Hollon (1998): "Patients often suffer as a consequence of their misperceptions without having any underlying motivation for doing so or for maintaining those beliefs, other than that they fear they might be true." Information processes tend to be dominated by strategies that are unduly conservative and are structured to maintain existing beliefs, even in the absence of motivation. Patients may react to symptoms (or even to innocuous body sensations) with the thought that they represent serious underlying disease and may become anxious or depressed as a result, regardless of the fact that they come to no harm even over extended periods of time. This sequence is characterized as the A–B–C of cognitive therapy, where A represents a stimulus (activating events, the body sensation or symptom) and C the state that it provokes (consequences, anxiety or depression). The challenge for the physician is to determine the precise content of B, which is the patient's belief about the significance of A (e.g., that the symptom indicates impending death or disability) (Ellis and Grieger, 1977). The physician's understanding of B is vital to the objectives of adequately reassuring patients and helping to change, in a fundamental way, their perception of the problem.

The cognitive aspect of evaluating control

The subject of control and its central importance to the stressed individual was discussed in Chapter 4. Its immediate relevance to the medical context derives from the tendency of symptoms or medical diagnoses to arouse fears of life-threatening illness or of intense suffering, and if indeed true this represents an extreme example of complete loss of control. While an existential threat does represent an unfortunate reality for certain sufferers of serious illnesses, in most stressed patients it is a fear with no or at most little basis in reality. This is particularly true for the sizable group of somatizing patients in whom emotional distress is transduced into a physical symptom. Even with symptoms the patient understands will not endanger life, such as intense vertigo or severe pain, however, the sense of lack of control in being able to influence the attacks substantially amplifies the apprehension felt around the occurrence of the symptom.

Given the obvious relevance of this topic to an understanding of the worried patient, as well as the many years the subject of control has been a major topic in psychology literature, it seems surprising that it has never found its way into medical texts or into discussions of aspects of the doctor–patient interaction. The causal role of cognitive processes in the development of emotional reactions was stressed by Arnold (1960, 1970), Lazarus (1966; Lazarus and Alfert, 1964), and others. It is their different cognitive interpretations that lead different people to react in widely different ways to very similar stimuli. The experience of a specific emotion depends not only on the state of physiological arousal but also on how this state is interpreted (Schachter and Singer, 1962; Nisbett and Schachter, 1966).

For the practitioner, an appreciation of this cognitive component, whether expressed as clinical anxiety or through other symptoms, can be of the utmost importance in the management of the patient's condition. Changing a subject's perception of what a symptom might mean can lead to a substantial change in the emotional reaction and therefore in the intensity of symptoms.

It follows from these considerations that it is very important, in all clinical encounters, to encourage patients to verbalize their specific worries. They should be urged to express their thoughts and feelings about the meaning and implications of their symptoms, particularly in terms of health and survival. Some patients are ashamed to admit to their fears and may be afraid of ridicule, or they may be unable to explain what they are afraid of and may find prompting by the physician helpful. Kleinman (1980) proposed the following series of questions to help determine patients' beliefs about their illness:

1. What do you call your problem? What name does it have?
2. What do you think caused your problem?
3. Why do you think it started when it did?
4. What does your sickness do to you?
5. How severe is it? Will it have a short or long course?
6. What do you fear most about your sickness?
7. What are the chief problems your sickness has caused you?
8. What kind of treatment do you think you should receive? What do you hope to achieve with the treatment?

Patients who show signs of anxiety without verbalizing their specific fears could be asked directly whether they are concerned about dying during an attack, or are fearful of suffering a heart attack or stroke, or believe that the symptoms mean they have an incurable disease. Patients' anxiety is usually found to be centered on one of these possibilities. If patients are not encouraged to articulate the specific fears induced by the symptoms, the reassurance offered them is all but useless. Differences between physicians in their ability to provide patients with adequate reassurance hinges to a large degree on understanding and relating to their patients' specific concerns.

This is well illustrated by the panic disorder patient who complains of chest pain and palpitations. Characteristically, after numerous electrocardiographs, chest radiographs, and physical examinations, she is told that there is nothing to worry about and that she should go away and forget it. The physician attempts to demonstrate to the patient that the complaints have been taken seriously by performing a thorough evaluation. Nevertheless, the patient is left frustrated and dissatisfied because she still has a symptom which provokes intense fear and for which she has received no adequate explanation. As opposed to the well-intended but practically worthless kind of general reassurance described above, panic attack patients in the early phase of their illness are amenable to reassurance when the physician pinpoints their particular fears and concerns, such as having a heart attack at the time of feeling chest pain. Furthermore, because panic attacks mostly occur in young women in good physical health, it is usually easy to reassure the patient (after having excluded significant disease through appropriate examinations) that no matter how disturbing the symptoms, nothing adverse is going to happen.

Analyzing the sequence of symptom-related events together with the patient usually has a reassuring effect, especially when the panic attacks are of recent origin. But since many patients are correctly diagnosed only after some months of experiencing symptoms, it may be necessary at first to repeatedly reassure patients who are easily worried by almost any body sensation. This may be especially necessary at the beginning of drug therapy, when symptoms may be exacerbated.

Symptoms and Anxiety: A Chicken–Egg Predicament

Body sensations or symptoms arouse differing degrees of anxiety in different patients. The tendency in anxious patients is to suppose that the symptom indicates the presence of serious illness. Specific thought content often precedes feelings of anxiety or even panic, but this sequence is usually not recognized by patients. Also, patients often insist that the emotional distress is caused by the symptom. If anxiety follows the symptom, they argue, the symptom cannot be due to the anxiety. This claim may be expressed with conviction, as if in response to the physician's suggestion, even if unspoken, that the problem is anxiety-induced. The discomfort that certain patients feel at the suggestion that they may be suffering from the consequences of an emotional state may also be reflected in their disappointment at the news that routine laboratory test results are normal. Positive laboratory investigations would vindicate their claim that the clinical state is derived from an organic process.

Physicians who lack experience in managing the emotional aspects of clinical disorders are more easily convinced by patients that their anxiety results from the presence of the symptom. The implication is that if the symptom—the physical problem—could only be dealt with, the anxiety would disappear. It is therefore important for the physician to realize that the temporal relationship between anxiety and the onset of symptoms may be quite obscure and is in any case of little relevance in practical terms. Whether anxiety precedes the symptom or vice versa is of no practical consequence in the management of the problem according to the principles described above. What is important, as already emphasized, is *to determine how the symptoms are interpreted by the patient*. Dealing with significant anxiety as efficiently as possible should be a primary objective. If this is successfully accomplished, most other aspects of the clinical problem are likely to become much less important to the patient.

Having just stated that regardless of which came first, it is the anxiety which should be attended to, I must hasten to add that it nevertheless is important for the physician to acquire a deeper understanding of the relationship between anxiety and symptoms in each case. This knowledge serves two main functions. First, it may be extremely difficult to identify anxiety as the main component of certain clinical situations, and the following discussion may aid in the analysis. Second, the physician may need to use this information to help elicit patients' cooperation in the management of the emotional state.

Three processes may complicate evaluation of the order of events in the clinical situation. In many psychosomatic disorders, especially when chronic, there is no obvious temporal relationship between a stressor and the onset of symptoms. A period of stress may be separated by weeks, months, or even years from the onset or exacerbation of a functional disorder such as irritable bowel syndrome or migraine. In this situation patients will emphasize that they were feeling perfectly well and relaxed when the symptom started. Consequently, it is probable that neither the patient nor the physician will think of connecting the two events. Thus, a stress-related illness may begin a substantial period after the stressful experience has passed.

In cases of extreme anxiety, it may be impossible to dissect out the sequence of events. This is often the case with panic attack patients, who may find it impossible to state whether the attack started with physical symptoms (e.g., palpitations, chest pain, or breathing difficulty) that rapidly led to the fear of death or serious illness, which then caused intense anxiety, or the experiencing of anxiety triggered the symptoms, which in turn led to the fear of illness or death. We know from dreams that elaborate thoughts may form in the brain with astounding speed. The process may be illustrated by the following anecdote in which an individual, while sleeping, is stung on the arm by a bee. He awakens suddenly from a dream that he had been riding in a fast-moving train with his arm out of the window, when the arm hit a pole on the side of the track and the pain awakened him. The sequence, therefore, is: sting, dream, awakening. Anyone who has been stung or seen someone being stung by a bee is aware of the fraction of time it takes from the stinging to the sensation of pain. It is during these milliseconds that this highly coherent dream content is formed. By analogy, it seems likely that in a panic attack, from the moment of the first palpitation induced by an extrasystole, or from the earliest awareness of light-headedness induced by hyperventilation, it is a matter of seconds or milliseconds to the thought of death or disabling illness, and a similar time lapse to anxiety or panic. Repeated attacks will have a facilitatory effect on subsequent ones so that the time it takes for the full-blown attack to develop may be extremely short, in conformity with clinical experience. The speed of development also helps explain the difficulty such patients often have in accounting for the sequence of events. Although symptoms may develop as a result of anxiety or tension, patients view the anxiety or tension as resulting from the symptom; in other words, they do not recognize the predisposing emotional basis of the symptom. The sequence is clearly seen, for example, in patients who respond to stress with hyperventilation, which presents as recurrent attacks of dizziness or light-headedness. Usually, these patients do not immediately see the problem as resulting from the stressed condition.

Summary

The protocol for successful management of anxious patients has certain essential elements.

- The physician must create an appropriate context for a discussion of the patient's emotional problems. This requires that the patient's symptoms first be evaluated fully, as with any other physical complaint, even if the physician suspects from an early stage that the disorder is psychosomatic. A complete physical examination and laboratory investigations must be directed at excluding possible organic causes for the symptoms.
- For the reassurance of anxious patients, their specific worries must be determined and directly addressed. General expressions of reassurance, even when based on extensive investigations, are unlikely to calm anxious patients for more than a very limited time.
- Except for certain conditions such as depression or panic disorder, it is generally better to avoid diagnostic labels. Most patients will find the term "stress reaction" nonthreatening and acceptable as a basis for allowing the physician to plan with them a therapeutic strategy, which in any event is the main reason for the consultation.
- A detailed explanation of the patient's condition, whatever the basis, particularly when it is presented in simple terms, can be highly effective in alleviating anxiety. Among patients with chronic or recurrent diseases, it leads to a lower rate of utilization of medical services. But a single interview session may be inadequate for this purpose and repeated explanations, workshops, printed material, and/or group discussions may be needed to enable patients to fully assimilate the relevant information.

PSYCHOTHERAPY

Referral for Psychotherapy

As mentioned, the physician should make it perfectly clear to patients that anyone, not only those with neurotic disorders, may respond to stress or emotional pressure with symptoms that have a psychophysiological basis. It should be pointed out that everyone has a limit when it comes to coping with such pressures. When the limit is exceeded, the resulting emotional state may well affect one or another body system, being expressed as a symptom such as headache, diarrhea, dyspnea, abdominal pain, or palpitations. This is a useful way to explain why a particular set of clinical symptoms should receive the attention of a psychotherapist rather than an internist. A patient, however, may have already undergone some psychotherapy without feeling any benefit, or have consistently refused to agree to such a referral. Such patients may nevertheless gain considerable benefit from a stress-management program, either as preparation for psychotherapy or as a management strategy on its own.

The Psychotherapist as a Clinical Collaborator

Many questions that arise during therapy might best be answered by a trained psychotherapist. For this reason, any physician who uses stress-management techniques is advised to establish a good working relationship with a number of psychotherapists, including psychiatrists. This will facilitate consultation and, if necessary, referral. In some cases patients may best be managed jointly by the psychiatrist and the physician. Under these circumstances it is imperative that a clear definition of roles be established in advance by discussing the issues to be addressed by each party. Furthermore, a physician should not undertake any form of behavioral intervention such as deep relaxation therapy with patients known to be in psychotherapy without the knowledge and approval of the psychotherapist.

One of the aims of this book is to convince medical practitioners, whether primary care physicians or medical specialists, that the great majority of psychophysiological processes may be relatively easily understood and effectively managed, according to the principles set out here. The general rules that govern the clinical evaluation of these disorders are fairly well defined and work well in most cases. However, any practitioner who attempts to work according to these rules should also be prepared to encounter problems that turn out to be much more complicated than originally anticipated. This is especially true for those who choose to apply deep relaxation or meditation techniques in their clinical practice.

For example, an apparently straightforward clinical problem manifested as a particular symptom may, during the course of deep relaxation therapy, turn out to be the tip of the iceberg, in terms of the extent of the emotional involvement that emerges during therapy. Effective psychiatric consultation is never more important than in this situation. However, referring the patient to a psychiatrist may not immediately solve the problem. Because of the special relationship created by the therapy, the physician may have to continue managing the problem at least temporarily, but under psychiatric supervision. The act of suggesting and undertaking stress-management therapy of this kind must be accompanied by responsibility for the welfare of the patient; the physician may not simply drop the patient like the proverbial hot coal when the problem begins to look complicated. The transfer of patients to a psychotherapist, if this becomes necessary, must be done in an orderly way, in consultation with the psychotherapist and with the patient's understanding and consent.

BEHAVIORAL INTERVENTION

While the notion of behavior is extremely broad, the focus here is on certain specific aspects of it, particularly the resources needed by any patient to deal effectively with stress that is proving to be harmful to her or his health, regardless of whether it derives from illness or life events of a stressful kind. The objective in all cases is to provide the individual with an understanding of the processes involved as well as the behavioral techniques needed to effectively regain a sense of both control and of self-confidence in dealing with the disease or symptoms.

In presenting the idea of a stress-management program to patients, it must be emphasized that the technique to be learned, such as deep relaxation or meditation, *forms part of an educational package* designed to teach the individual how best to cope with stress and its consequences. The physician explains that we all possess unexploited resources which we can learn to mobilize to help us deal with stress. While the actual technique of relaxation or meditation is relatively simple, familiarity turns it into a potentially powerful (and proven) tool for helping patients to understand and control their own body responses. A biofeedback program can also enhance feelings of control.

When patients first seek consultation, they may be aware only that the symptoms occur at times of "tension." But over just a few weeks, practice of the deep relaxation technique, for example, can help create a much more sensitive awareness of the development of tension in the body. Patients may become aware of certain muscle groups developing tension well before onset of the symptoms that precipitated the visit to the doctor in the first place. In addition, familiarity with the relaxation or meditation process allows patients to respond to tension by relaxing the tense muscles to some extent, and in this way to abort or modify the development of the symptom. This change in patients' ability to cope with the problem in a more active and independent way represents a substantial achievement and reflects a very real measure of control, the significance of which is usually apparent to symptomatic patients. It is important to present the relaxation or meditation program in the context of these objectives and not simply as an end in itself.

The treating physician must take care not to offer something sounding like a wonder cure, but must emphasize that the symptom or clinical condition is unlikely ever to be completely eliminated. That is, never suggest that complete cure is imminent and that the program will eliminate the problem. The aim is to help patients develop the ability to change the problem from one that dominates their lives, or controls them, to one they may largely control.

Another point to be emphasized is that patients are intended to be active participants in their own management. The apparent passivity inherent in the relaxation or meditation exercises is a necessary step in leading patients to greater involvement in the management of the clinical problem. That patients are expected to participate actively is repeatedly conveyed by encouraging them to become increasingly independent in using the experience gained from the exercises, and giving strong positive reinforcement of any tangible achievements resulting from the program.

The benefits obtained from the program occur gradually and are often subtle. Patients may register in conversation a difference in their clinical condition only after three or four weeks of therapy (one session per week). Often they express awareness that the severity and/or frequency of attacks has changed for the better. A surprising number of patients use the same language in describing their perception of events: "I don't know if what we are doing has anything to do with it, but things are better than they were!"

A patient will occasionally deny feeling any real change in the clinical condition but, when pressed for a more specific evaluation, will concede that the symptom now responds to medication whereas it did not before, or that attacks are shorter-lived or less frequent. It is important to point out this progress, and in discussing it most patients will acknowledge a sense of increased control. Growing independence may also be encouraged by tape-recording an exercise on the third or fourth visit, after patients are familiar with the relaxation exercise. In my experience, however, the use of a commercial relaxation tape, without the necessary introduction, interaction, and dialogue during the process of learning the technique, is not successful in helping to resolve significant clinical problems. As emphasized, this type of intervention must be managed as part of an ongoing educational process designed to teach patients about their own bodily reactions and how they may best interpret and respond to whatever discomfort they feel. During exercises the physician may also need to introduce material of relevance for the particular problem, as well as other techniques (see Chapter 19) that may be useful.

Some patients become overdependent on the physician and claim that they are unable to perform the exercises or to "concentrate" in the physician's absence, or even with the help of the physician's tape, or they may simply return for their appointment without having made any attempt at practice. This attitude may also reflect a high level of anxiety about relaxing deeply when alone, a predicament that requires special consideration and is usually recognizable on appropriate questioning. These patients frequently admit to a fear of being unable to control the situation when deeply relaxed.

Greatest caution is necessary when dealing with patients who have a history of psychosis or a persistently high level of anxiety such as "free-floating" anxiety or the anxiety associated with posttraumatic stress disorder. In such cases, considerable energy may be expended by patients in maintaining a tenuous hold on reality and the deep relaxation exercise could lead to a deterioration of their condition. These patients should be referred to a psychiatrist for management.

The psychophysiology of altered states and the technical aspects of deep relaxation and meditation exercises are discussed in Chapter 19.

REFERENCES

Arnold MB (1960). Emotion and personality. New York: Columbia University Press, 2 vols.

Arnold MB (1970). Perennial problems in the field of emotion. In: Arnold M, ed. The Loyola Symposium: Feelings and Emotion. New York: Academic Press.

Assal JP, Muhlhauser I, Pernet A, et al. (1985). Patient education as the basis for diabetes care in clinical practice and research. Diabetologia 28:602–613.

Bailey WC, Richards JM, Brooks CM, et al. (1990). A randomized trial to improve self-management practices of adults with asthma. Arch Intern Med 150:1664–1668.

Beck AT (1991). Cognitive therapy: a 30 year retrospective. Am Psychol 46:368–375.

Benson H, Frankel FH, Apfel R, et al. (1978). Treatment of anxiety: a comparison of the usefulness of self-hypnosis and a meditational relaxation technique: an overview. Psychother Psychosom 30:229–242.

Bruce TJ, Spiegel DA, Hegel MT (1999). Cognitive-behavioral therapy helps prevent relapse and recurrence of panic disorder following alprazolam discontinuation: a long-term follow-up of the Peoria and Dartmouth studies. J Consult Clin Psychol 67:151–156.

Caudill M, Schnable R, Zuttermeister P, et al. (1991). Decreased clinic utilisation by chronic pain patients after behavioral medicine intervention. Pain 45:334–335.

Clark DM (1999). Anxiety disorders: why they persist and how to treat them. Behav Res Ther 37 (suppl 1):S5–S27.

Clark DM, Salkovskis PM, Hackman A, et al. (1998). Two psychological treatments for hypochondriasis. a randomized controlled trial. Br J Psychiatry 173:218–225.

Daltroy LH, Iversen MD, Larson MG, et al. (1997). A controlled trial of an educational program to prevent lower back injury. N Engl J Med 337:322–328.

Davidson JK, Delcher HK, Englund A (1979). Spin-off cost/benefits of expanded nutritional care. J Am Dietetic Assoc 75:250–257.

DeRubeis RJ, Gelfand LA, Tang TZ, et al. (1999). Medications versus cognitive behavior therapy for severely depressed outpatients: mega-analysis of four randomized comparisons. Am J Psychiatry 156:1007–1013.

Devilly GJ, Spence SH (1999). The relative efficacy and treatment distress of EMDR and a cognitive-behavior trauma protocol in the amelioration of post traumatic stress disorder. J Anxiety Disord 13:131–157.

Devine EC (1992). Effects of psychoeducational care for adult surgical patients: a meta-analysis of 191 studies. Patient Educ Counseling 19:129–142.

Ellis A, Grieger R (1977). Handbook of Rational–Emotive Therapy, Vol 1. New York: Springer Publishing Company.

Engel BT (1986). Psychosomatic medicine, behavioral medicine, just plain medicine. Psychosom Med 48:466–479.

Evans R, Mullally DI, Wilson RW, et al. (1987). National trends in the morbidity and mortality of asthma in the US: prevalence, hospitalization and death from asthma over two decades, 1965–1984. Chest 91:65S–74S.

George MR, O'Dowd LC, Martin I, et al. (1999). A comprehensive educational program improves clinical outcome measures in inner-city patients with asthma. Arch Intern Med 159:1710–1716.

Hellman CJ, Budd M, Borysenko J, et al. (1990). A study of the effectiveness of two group behavioral medicine interventions for patients with psychosomatic complaints. Behav Med 16:165–173.

Hollon SD (1998). What is cognitive behavioral therapy and does it work? Curr Opin Neurobiol 8:289–292.

Jacobs GD, Benson H, Friedman R (1996). Perceived benefits in a behavioral-medicine insomnia program: a clinical report. Am J Med 100:212–216.

Kabat-Zinn J, Lipworth L, Burney R (1985). The clinical use of mindfulness meditation for the self-regulation of chronic pain. J Behav Med 8:163–190.

Kabat-Zinn J, Lipworth L, Burney R, et al. (1987). Four-year follow-up of a meditation-based program for the self-regulation of chronic pain: treatment outcomes and compliance. Clin J Pain 2:159–173.

Kabat-Zinn J, Massion AO, Kristeller J, et al. (1992). Effectiveness of a meditation-based stress reduction program in the treatment of anxiety disorders. Am J Psychiatry 149:936–943

Kabat-Zinn J, Wheeler E, Light T, et al. (1998). Influence of a mindfulness meditation-based stress reduction intervention on rates of skin clearing in patients with moderate to severe psoriasis undergoing phototherapy (UVB) and photochemotherapy (PUVA). Psychosom Med 60:625–632.

Kinsman RA, Dirks JF, Dahlem NW (1980). Noncompliance to prescribed-as-needed (PRN) medication use in asthma: usage patterns and patient characteristics. J Psychosom Res 24:97–107.

Kleinman A (1980). Patients and Healers in the Context of Culture. An Exploration of the Borderland between Anthropology, Medicine, and Psychiatry. Berkeley: University of California Press. p 106.

Klieger JH, Dirks JF (1979). Medication compliance in chronic asthmatic patients. J Asthma Res 16:93–96.

Lazarus R (1966). Psychological Stress and the Coping Process. New York: McGraw-Hill.

Lazarus R, Alfert E (1964). The short-circuiting of threat by experimentally altering cognitive appraisal. J Abnorm Soc Psychol 69:195–205.

Ley P (1982). Satisfaction, compliance and communication. Br J Clin Psychol 21:241–254.

Miller JJ, Fletcher K, Kabat-Zinn J (1995). Three year follow-up and clinical implications of a mindfulness meditation-based stress reduction intervention in the treatment of anxiety disorders. Gen Hosp Psychiatry 17:192–200.

Miller LV, Goldstein J (1972). More efficient care of diabetes in a county hospital setting. N Engl J Med 286:1388–1391.

Muhlhauser I, Jorgens V, Berger M, et al. (1983). Bicentric evaluation of a teaching and treatment program for type 1 (insulin-dependent) diabetes patients: improvement of metabolic control and other measures of diabetes care for up to 22 months. Diabetologia 25:470–476.

Mumford E, Schlesinger HJ, Glass GV (1982). The effects of psychological intervention on recovery from surgery and heart attacks: an analysis of the literature. Am J Publ Health 72(2):141–151.

Nisbett R, Schachter S (1966). Cognitive manipulation of pain. J Exp Soc Psychol 2:227–236.

O'Conner K, Todorov C, Robbilard S, et al. (1999). Cognitive-behaviour therapy and medication in the treatment of obsessive-compulsive disorder: a controlled study. Can J Psychiatry 44:64–71.

O'Dowd LC, George MR, Atkins P, et al. (1997). Does an asthma referral center (ARC) reduce hospital utilization and health care costs in a managed care organization (MCO)? Am J Respir Crit Care Med 155:A891. Abstract.

Robinson JS, Schwarz ML, Magwene KS, et al. (1989). The impact of fever health education on clinic utilization. Am J Dis Child 143:698–704.

Schachter S, Singer J (1962). Cognitive, social, and physiological determinants of emotional state. Physiol Rev 69:379–399.

Sly RM (1988). Mortality from asthma, 1979–1984. J Allergy Clin Immunol 82(5 pt 1): 705–717.

Warwick HM, Salkovskis PM (1985). Reassurance [editorial]. Br Med J 290:1028.

Wilson SR, Scamagas P, German DF, et al. (1993). A controlled trial of two forms of self-management education for adults with asthma. Am J Med 94:564–576.

Chapter
19

BEHAVIORAL INTERVENTION IN STRESSED STATES

This chapter describes the physiological basis and effects of the behavioral techniques commonly used in clinical practice. All of these techniques have the common characteristic of reducing autonomic activity. It must be stressed that they are most effective when used in the context of a dialogue between patient and physician. This is because the cognitive aspects of this interaction are of the utmost importance and may contribute greatly to the impact of the behavioral intervention.

RELAXATION THERAPY AND ALTERED STATES OF CONSCIOUSNESS

Relaxation therapy is one of several technique that employ the principle of the "altered state." This section considers the principles underlying some of the more commonly applied therapeutic techniques that exploit the altered state, with no discussion of the wide variety of altered mental states in sleep, sensory deprivation, and trance-inducing rituals or dances in some cultures. The therapeutic techniques that employ altered states of consciousness include hypnosis, guided imagery, meditation (Kabat-Zinn, 1990), the "relaxation response" (Benson et al., 1975), yogic therapy (Patel, 1984), autogenic training (Schultz and Luthe, 1959), and other types of deep relaxation. Although the various techniques differ in details, there is nevertheless a mix and overlap of key elements common to them all. Because their physiological impact seems to be similar, there seems to be no justification for distinguishing between them on that basis (Benson et al., 1975; Shapiro, 1982).

Definitions of an altered state of consciousness tend to vary, depending on the professional background and interests of the person offering the definition. I will define an altered state of consciousness simply as *a physiological state that develops after attention is focused on a subject which does not specifically require mathematical or critical reasoning.* This usually also means that the focus of attention is on an emotionally neutral image or sensation. This definition is similar to that given by Shapiro (1982) in a review of meditative states. He similarly took the focusing of attention as the basis, and defined meditation as "a family of techniques which have in common a conscious attempt to focus attention in a nonanalytical way and an attempt not to dwell on discursive, ruminating thought."

The act of focusing attention in this manner leads to distinct changes in the physiology of the central nervous system (CNS). These changes are exploited to create the therapeutic effect. Not all attention-requiring tasks, however, produce the same physiological state. Concentrating on internal cognitive operations, such as mental arithmetic, is likely to increase autonomic activity, as reflected in an accelerated heart rate and a rise in blood pressure (Lacy, 1967), a technique that has remained an important exprimental paradigm of mental stress (Moriguchi et al., 1992; Critchley et al., 2000; Willemsen et al., 2000). Furthermore, tasks that demand motor readiness also involve the left hemisphere and may produce an increase in both pulse rate and metabolic activity in anticipation of motor activity (Obrist et al., 1970). It follows that the attentional states most likely to be associated with a reduction in autonomic activity are those that are not involved in analytic or mathematical thinking. Much of the mysticism and even fear surrounding techniques of altered state therapy tend to dissipate when it is understood that the process is essentially a physiological one. We all tend to shift into and out of altered states of consciousness during a normal day's activities as our attention is more or less focused on a specific activity, object, or thought process.

In beginning a stress-management session the patient is encouraged to focus her or his attention on something specific—like the act of breathing, muscle tension, guided imagery, or a mantra. (The mantra in meditation is a word, sound, or brief expression which the subject should retain as the focus of attention by constant, usually silent repetition, usually in synchrony with the breathing rate; a commonly chosen mantra is the sound "ohmmm,"—pronounced as in "rom.") Whatever the method, the aim is to achieve a state of focused (and therefore selective) attention. In many techniques, such as meditation, the level of relaxation is not important. I will attempt to show, through a consideration of the relevant literature and from personal observations, that most of the mental and physiological changes found to occur in altered state therapy result from the primary event of focused attention.

NEUROPHYSIOLOGY OF ALTERED STATES

Both clinical experience and laboratory studies demonstrate that the act of focusing attention is accompanied by well-defined changes in both neuronal and certain complex cerebral activities. A growing body of scientific data relates to the physiology of selective attention.

Selective Attention

Selective attention has a central role in information processing, as we are all compelled constantly to select from moment to moment specific items of information from numerous environmental signals. Most of the literature concerning selective attention is devoted to experimental work on visual and auditory processes. The evidence favors the view that the act of focusing one's thoughts on a recalled or imagined image utilizes a neuroanatomical substrate very similar to that required for actually viewing or hearing it. Mental imagery seems to involve the efferent activation of visual areas in the prestriate occipital cortex, the parietal and the temporal cortex, which represent the same kinds of specialized visual information in imagery as they do in actual perception (Farah, 1989; Kosslyn, 1996). Functional brain imaging studies have shown that asking someone to imagine making a movement activates very much the same areas as asking someone to prepare to make that movement (Stephan et al., 1995). Similarly, imagining the sound of a voice increases activity in the superior temporal cortex (auditory association cortex) in addition to frontal regions, including Broca's area mediating speech production (McGuire et al., 1996).

The parietal lobe is considered one of the main cortical regions involved in selective attention. It mediates both the functions of selective attention (particularly through area 7) and the integration of proprioception with concepts of size, form, and texture in the ability known as stereognosis (posterior parietal cortex). An example is the ability to identify an object in the palm of the hand by feel alone, which presupposes the combined and coordinated contribution of two modalities, cutaneous touch and position sense. Given intact peripheral sensation, this function is thought to be mediated by the posterior parietal lobe (Werner, 1980). Lesions of the posterior parietal lobe (temperoparietal region) result in the patient's ignoring events in the contralateral hemisphere, a disorder called *neglect*. Human parietal cortex is also richly endowed with connections not only from the association cortex but also from the limbic and reticular systems. In humans, lesions of the right hemisphere induce more frequent and severe attentional disorders than do lesions of the left hemisphere (Faglioni et al., 1971; Albert, 1973). Studies utilizing positron emission tomography have similarly demonstrated the right hemisphere's involvement in attention. This asymmetry of hemispheric function will be discussed further, since it may well have repercussions in the therapeutic situation.

Observations of commisurotomized patients, in whom connections between the right and left hemispheres are severed, show that priority is given to left hemisphere operations when task demands are complex, involving, for example, use of both hands or mathematical and other cognitive functions. Situations requiring active attention, such as responding to a question asked during hand activity, will disturb activity of the right hand (left hemisphere) but not of the left hand (right hemisphere). In addition, Dimond and Beaumont (1973) have shown experimentally that the right visual field (left hemisphere) is superior to the left, in maintaining a state of vigilance when subjects must respond to a stimulus without warning. Other attentional tasks that do not require vigilance and motor readiness may also be performed better by the right hemisphere (Tucker and Williamson, 1984).

The ability to focus one's attention on certain memory traces and ignore others is a central act that is independent of sensory input. But as Mountcastle (1978) has written, "the capacity for central attention to recalled images is facilitated by an overall reduction in afferent bombardment." Muscular relaxation reduces afferent input by reducing proprioceptive impulses that are also processed by the parietal cortex, in this way facilitating the mechanisms of selective attention.

The debate concerning hemispheric dominance in relation to different aspects of brain function is today considered virtually meaningless given the complexity of cerebral function (Hellige, 1993), although some psychophysiological studies have favored such a functional asymmetry. Frumkin et al. (1978) used *dichotic* listening tests to demonstrate hypnosis-induced changes in hemispheric lateralization (a reduction of left hemisphere dominance) and concluded that the hypnotic state was associated with greater participation of the right hemisphere than of the left. Dichotic listening tests are used to determine the extent to which performance on tasks using auditory stimuli depends on the ear to which the stimulus is presented. Each ear sends information to both cerebral hemispheres. However, the pathway from each ear to the contralateral hemisphere contains more fibers than does the pathway to the ipsilateral hemisphere. In addition, when two items are presented simultaneously to both ears (called dichotic presentation), the pathway from each ear to the ipsilateral hemisphere is inhibited, especially if the two items are acoustically similar. Thus with dichotic presentation, information presented to one ear projects primarily or exclusively to the contralateral cerebral hemisphere. Accordingly, ear differences in audition are likely to be influenced by hemispheric asymmetries and so have become an important converging technique both in split-brain patients and in neurologically intact individuals.

While some of the answers will undoubtedly come from functional brain imaging untilizing techniques such as positron emission tomography (PET) and functional magnetic resonance imaging (fMRI), we do not yet understand fully the functional role and interrelationship of brain regions subserving the psychological states induced by our behavioral techniques. The anterior cingulate cortex, a midline structure, shows prominent activity on brain imaging, in selective attention to emotional responses (Lane et al., 1997) as well as in clinical paradigms of hypnosis (Rainville et al., 1999) or meditation (Lazar et al., 2000). A complex structure with functional subdivisions, the affect division of the anterior cingulate cortex, modulates autonomic activity and internal emotional responses, while the cognition division is engaged in response selection associated with skeletomotor activity and responses to noxious stimuli (Devinsky et al., 1995). The anterior cingulate cortex is part of a larger matrix of structures engaged in similar functions. These structures form the rostral limbic system and include the amygdala, periaqueductal gray, ventral striatum, orbitofrontal, and anterior insular cortices.

Facilitative and Inhibitory Processes

In the act of focusing attention, neuronal responses to a specific sensory stimulus acquire a coherence of frequency (Gray et al., 1989; Singer, 1993). This process results in particular channels of activity being favored over others, and synchronization of this kind is most evident when individuals are asked to attend selectively to a stimulus (Tiitinen et al., 1993). Neurophysiological studies in primates combining neuronal and behavioral measures have demonstrated that increasing attention to a stimulus enhances the responsiveness and selectivity of the neurons that process that stimulus (Richmond and Sato, 1987; Spitzer et al., 1988) and inhibit the activity of neurons not involved in the attention process (Moran and Desimone, 1985). Similar processes operate in humans, and a series of studies showed that when a subject attends to a location in visual space, information is processed more efficiently at that location and less efficiently at other locations (Posner and Presti, 1987). An analogous process appears to be operative in language processing. When attention is given to a selected word, related words appear to be facilitated and unrelated words are processed more slowly (Neely, 1977). These studies demonstrate not only a potentiation in the processing of sensory or verbal images that are the focus of attention, but also a concomitant reduction in the processing of other stimuli.

These observations provide a physiological basis for explaining what has long been known through clinical experience: being in an altered state of consciousness facilitates the recollection of related experiences and memories, even if long forgotten. Furthermore, recall of an event or thought while in this condition may be much clearer and more detailed than would otherwise be the case. At the same time, the subject ignores other internal and environmental signals not of immediate relevance. It is a common experience in patients suffering from pain, regardless of the cause, that concentrating attention on something else may substantially reduce the pain. The mechanism described above provides a physiological explanation for this experience and suggests that when attention is distracted, the processing of pain signals is correspondingly reduced. This situation is also expressed during therapy by patients' ability, when in a state of deep relaxation or when in a hypnotic trance, to transfer a thought rapidly, at the therapist's suggestion, from an emotionally charged subject to a more neutral one with an appropriate change in emotional response.

The following clinical experience dramatically illustrates this mechanism. One day, while I was working with a deeply relaxed patient, a fire alarm bell began ringing suddenly with deafening intensity outside my door. There was no reaction from the patient, and I knew that the signal was a false alarm so I continued with the session in spite of considerable difficulty caused by the noise. Such was the intensity of the noise, in fact, that I was not even sure that the patient could hear what I was saying. At the end of the exercise I asked the patient whether she had been disturbed by the ringing, which must have continued for two or three minutes. It turned out that she had been only remotely aware of the bell and not in the least disturbed by it! Her attention had been specifically focused on my voice, resulting in almost total exclusion of the intense noise produced by the fire alarm signal.

Suspension of Critical Faculty

The inhibition of associated thought processes during the selective focusing of attention may be demonstrated by the absence of critical responses during the therapeutic exercise. This suspension of critical faculty, also referred to as a reduction or suspension in reality testing, is one of the most striking as well as the most intriguing of the mental processes associated with the altered state. It is particularly pronounced when, as is sometimes necessary during a relaxation exercise, the patient is asked to imagine an incongruous situation which to a normal observer may sound quite ludicrous. As described by Hilgard (1965), the patient's reality distortion "includes acceptance of falsified memories, changes in one's own personality, modification of the rate at which time seems to pass, doubling of persons in the room, absence of heads or feet of people observed to be walking around the room, inappropriate naming, hallucinating the presence of animals that talk and all manner of other unrealistic distortions."

These absurd situations were induced in experimental studies of hypnosis, not during therapy. Suspension of reality testing has a different character when employed in the therapeutic context. The awareness of subject matter that characterizes normal conversation contrasts with the lack of reaction by the patient to a totally incongruous suggestion, which is accepted without even a smile of curiosity or of embarrassment. After the therapy session the patient may ask "What was that about?" More often, if nothing is said by the therapist, the patient will say nothing. A sense of incongruity or embarrassment requires that the therapist's suggestion be compared to the standards and norms of our everyday lives. A discrepancy between what is presented and what we regard as congruent or appropriate will then be further evaluated, generally with an emotional reaction (humor, embarrassment, revulsion, etc.) that reflects the sense of inappropriateness. Clearly, this process involves a substantial amount of additional parallel cortical activity that in a state of deep relaxation and focused attention is at least partially, if not completely, inhibited.

Suggestibility

Suggestibility is another attribute of an altered state of consciousness and the one typically exploited in hypnotherapy, though all forms of altered state therapy utilize it in one way or another. Hypnosis depends on suggestibility because through it the hypnotist establishes a controlling status in the therapeutic interaction. For example, by suggesting (instructing) that the patient respond in a counterintuitive way, such as having the arm drift upward "as if carried by helium balloons," or being unable to open eyelids "as if they are stuck together by glue," the hypnotist demonstrates to the patient the extent of this control.

Suggestibility, however, is not solely an outcome of the altered state. In the initial phases of the therapeutic interaction, it seems to be mainly an expression of a person's ability to relinquish control to the therapist, or a readiness to be controlled. The dynamic of the therapist–patient interaction here is best illustrated by the widespread experience of successful altered state therapy in "unhypnotizable" subjects, through permissive and minimally directive techniques (Barber, 1980; Baker, 1987). The depth of the hypnotic trance is related to the degree of suggestibility, which in some situations also correlates with therapeutic outcome in the management of certain disorders, such as asthma and migraine. In most cases dealt with in the medical clinic, however, depth of trance is not an important criterion for successful therapy. Consequently, clinical tests of hypnotizability are irrelevant when altered state techniques are applied in the management of clinical problems in internal medicine.

Respiration Rate and Autonomic Activity

A striking physical effect of the altered state is the distinct slowing of respiratory activity (Allison, 1970). In certain subjects, especially those practiced in relaxation techniques, meditation, or yoga, respiration slows the moment attention is restricted to a particular focus. In individuals who are learning relaxation techniques the process of respiratory slowing is more gradual but serves as an important indicator of whether they are in an altered state. Studying 36 meditating subjects, Wallace et al. (1971) documented reduced respiratory activity during meditation as manifested by decreased oxygen consumption, CO_2 elimination, respiratory rate, and minute ventilation with no change in respiratory quotient. Skin resistance markedly increased (due to decreased perspiration resulting from lowered sympathetic activity), while systolic, diastolic, and mean arterial blood pressure remained unchanged. Electroencephalograms showed an increased intensity of slow alpha waves and occasional theta wave activity. The close association between respiratory and autonomic activity was discussed in Chapter 14. Here it suffices to emphasize that the slowing of respiration is associated with a reduction in both autonomic activity and responsiveness. This contributes to the release of physical (and therefore emotional) tension and may be exploited during the therapeutic encounter.

Respiratory rate remains an important indicator of the subject's emotional state throughout the exercise. A sudden speeding up of respiration gives a clear indication that the subject is more anxious, for whatever reason. Conversely, a marked slowing of respiration is usually associated with relaxation, regardless of the subject matter being presented by the therapist.

Since reduced respiratory activity is recognized as one of the main physical expressions of altered states such as in yoga and meditation, slow breathing may be used to promote the development of a relaxed state. In a traditional therapeutic context, the physician helps the patient relax via a reduction in respiratory rate by having the subject voluntarily take three or four deep breaths. This has the effect of inducing hypocapnia by blowing off carbon dioxide, with immediate reflex slowing of the respiratory rate.

Neurophysiological studies in cats link the amygdaloid complex to the respiratory changes observed in the attentional states described above (Ursin and Kaada, 1960). Stimulation of the amygdaloid complex by implanted electrodes resulted in an attention response associated initially with respiratory inhibition. In higher animals projections from the frontal cortex may modulate the function of the amygdala, which has a feedback influence on the hypothalamic control of arousal (Pribram and McGuiness, 1975). In order to focus on a particular stimulus an organism must be aroused. In our context, interest has to be stimulated before attention is directed; consequently, arousal precedes or parallels attention.

Muscular Relaxation

A striking physical consequence of being in an altered state of consciousness is the ability to achieve a more profound degree of muscular relaxation than is otherwise possible. Deeper levels of muscular relaxation, especially when the subject is totally immobile, are often associated with a heavy, leaden feeling of the limbs or the whole body. Absence of proprioceptive stimulation as a result of immobility may also lead to a distorted perception of limb position; the subject may feel that his hands are in a different position from the actual one. In very profound states of relaxation, the subject may feel that his body is floating, or he may be unable to feel part (usually the legs) or the whole of the body. But muscular relaxation is not an essential requirement for the development of an altered state. A subject may also be hypnotized while performing physical activity such as riding a stationery bicycle (Banyai and Hilgard, 1976). Relaxation is not necessary for the therapeutic use of meditative states.

THE CLINICAL CONTEXT

In the medical clinic, anxious patients are usually also the most symptomatic. Most of these patients are struggling to maintain a sense of control because things are happening to them (their symptoms) over which they have very little or no control. Clinical experience has shown that a sense of losing control or feeling out of control is a potent and universal anxiety-inducing state. The anxiety serves to accentuate or aggravate the symptoms, leading to more intense feelings of loss of control. It is this confusion of tension, symptoms, and anxiety-inducing feelings of being out of control that the physician must relate to in discussion at the outset, offering both a better understanding and the hope of relief. This requires an explanation of how symptoms work to create a feeling of losing control, which in turn undermines feelings of self-confidence, how the feeling of loss of control and loss of self-confidence increase the anxiety and feelings of stress, how these feelings aggravate and promote the symptom, and how the symptom represents simply the physical expression of the emotional state. The relaxation exercise will work to help regain feelings of control by reducing the symptom intensity while at the same time showing the patient the natural resources she or he has to help deal with the stressor.

The physician may then suggest a program of behavioral therapy as part of an educational package geared toward strengthening feelings of control by the patient through increasing awareness of mind–body interactions. Such a program may be based on one or more techniques, including meditation and yoga, deep relaxation, and biofeedback. Although some patients are able to point to a close association between feeling "stressed" or anxious and an intensification of physical symptoms, most are focused almost exclusively on the physical symptoms as the primary problem. The techniques mentioned here may substantially help a patient develop a much greater sense of association between emotional state and body awareness, which in turn will lead to enhanced feelings of control.

The dialogue with the physician during treatment is of cardinal importance in providing ongoing guidance for the cognitive management of patients' beliefs, which are often inaccurate, about the nature of the problem, and in reinforcing their progress with the technique chosen. Change in this process is usually subtle, and the real significance of a difference in response may not be fully appreciated by the patient. In essence, the task of the practitioner is to enable patients to become aware of processes not previously evident to them, so that they can appreciate how increased control leads to an alleviation of the clinical condition, learn how to achieve that increased control, and in this way turn the crisis of illness into a personal growth experience.

The Importance of Terminology to the Medical Patient

Some psychotherapists refer to all forms of therapy utilizing the altered state as hypnosis, a particularly unfortunate use of the term from the point of view of the average medical patient. This term is likely to be a major deterrent to the introduction of any techniques of behavioral intervention in the management program because being hypnotized means, in effect, transferring control to another person, so that changes in one's reactions and responses may be produced through suggestion, while in a hypnotic trance. The patient who consults a hypnotherapist expects this to happen. In the case of patients who consult a physician, however, being hypnotized is the last thing they expect to do. Behavioral intervention is generally considered for the most anxious and symptomatic patients who, as indicated previously, are also those feeling most out of control. Consequently, for the great majority of medical patients in emotional distress, hypnosis in the popular sense often has negative, even frightening connotations. The "resistance" of many subjects to being hypnotized is probably centered on this problem.

With this caveat in mind, altered states of consciousness are usefully classified according to who *controls* the experience (Figure 19-1). Maneuvers commonly employed in classical hypnotic inductions, such as arm levitation or the demonstration of inability to open the eyelids, are not used in this context, as they are employed to emphasize the extent of the therapist's control over the subject and to facilitate suggestibility. In contrast to the classical hypnotic experience, the objective of the deep relaxation program is to strengthen the patient's own feelings of control, and therefore the exercises employed are totally permissive. Permissive here means that the subject is given no instruction or order in the relaxation exercise. It is emphasized that no part of the exercise is critical to its overall success and that the individual may respond to whatever he or she feels comfortable with. Thus patients are invited in this way to "control" the experience by choosing not to respond if they so wish.

Even those patients with strong though unexpressed reservations about the procedure can thus be reassured that they are not about to be hypnotized (in the clas-

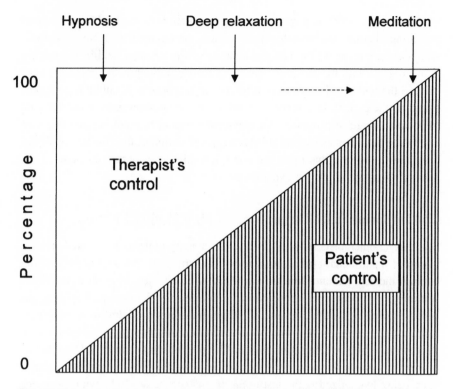

FIGURE 19.1 In the therapeutic context, the altered state is defined by the dynamic of perceived control between therapist and patient. With behavioral interventions such as deep relaxation, the subject is encouraged to greater independence (increased self-control), as indicated by the broken arrow.

sical sense), that they are controlling the experience, and that the exercise is permissive and cannot be impaired should they decide at any stage not to respond. Furthermore, it should be emphasized that the objective is to move them further and further along the path of increasing self-control and independence from medications, doctors, and medical institutions.

From the patient's viewpoint, the important difference between these techniques lies in *the extent to which each is more or less directed (controlled) by the therapist* (Figure 19-1). With hypnosis, the therapist may try to acquire as much control as possible during the therapeutic interaction. At the other end of the altered state spectrum, in meditation and the contemplative Zen states, the entire experience is initiated and controlled by the subject. All intermediate practices fall between these two extremes in relation to the degree of control the subject has, or is expected to exhibit, during the therapeutic encounter.

A physician may propose the relaxation program in an attempt to demonstrate to a skeptical patient that the medical problem has a significant psychophysiological component. A successful course of relaxation exercises in which the patient's feelings of control are strengthened and symptom intensity is reduced will undoubtedly help overcome resistance and make it much easier to convince the patient to seek appropriate psychotherapeutic consultation, if necessary

Contrary to the common perception of symptom management through altered state techniques, a physician may successfully manage a symptomatic patient in this way without ever mentioning the troublesome symptom during the relaxation exercise. Moreover, with minimal investment of time and effort, the relaxation program may provide the patient with the resources to identify tension with more certainty in its earlier phases, and may serve to dissipate the tension before it manifests itself as a troublesome symptom. Such an achievement would unquestionably enhance the patient's control of the situation.

Main Elements of Techniques for Inducing Deep Relaxation

Focusing attention to produce the altered state

A key element of all relaxation techniques is to have the subject focus attention on some specific thought or object. The neurophysiological changes described above that accompany this act are then exploited to develop the therapeutic content of the exercise. When the approach is permissive, as advocated here, the physician may provide the focus by drawing attention to a completely neutral phenomenon such as the feeling of contact or pressure between the patient's body and the chair or bed and/or the feeling of pressure between the soles of the feet and the floor. It is important to be aware of the fact that being directed to do or feel certain things may be disturbing to the patient. Anything in the encounter that is construed as instruction emphasizes the physician's control and hence the patient's lack of it; even in a permissive atmosphere this may arouse negative feelings.

The least directed focus is provided by guided imagery, where in most cases the patients themselves fill in the details from personal experience. Before beginning the exercise it is worth asking patients how they best enjoy relaxing, and then developing the theme they present. Thus, asking the subject to imagine a garden or a beach usually provides a focus that is sufficiently neutral (i.e., without emotional significance) and effective. Sometimes, however, imagery that is assumed to be neutral is of disturbing significance to the subject. I have attempted to treat patients for whom the sea was an object of fear. Similarly, I once encountered a patient who was disturbed by the image of a park because it reminded him of a 12-year-old daughter who had committed suicide. It is therefore worthwhile, before starting the exercise, briefly to elicit a reaction from the patient to the particular imagery you intend to use. An additional advantage of using guided imagery is that it is easy to incorporate suggestion in the imagery by using appropriate adjectives, for example, "a quiet, *tranquil* garden or park" or "a warm, *relaxing* day."

Appropriate suggestion

The suggestions of a general kind, aimed at promoting relaxation and strengthening feelings of control, are the basic structure of all exercises. There are also specific suggestions, which are tailored to the individual and intended to assist in the management of a particular problem. Only the general suggestions are discussed here.

An important principle of the technique being developed here is that all suggestions must have, at least at the beginning of the relaxation program, a coherent and logical structure. As the program progresses and the patient feels more comfortable with the exercises, the physician may introduce more contradictory material, such as a blatant nonsequitur if the situation demands it (see below). If the initial experience is handled sensitively and appropriately, the uncertainty encountered in this new phase is usually resolved with the first exercise.

The basis of all exercises are the suggestions *coupling the state of physical relaxation with feelings of control*. The logic of this juxtaposition is that the individual who feels "out of control" is unable to relax; if you are relaxed, you must be in control. This assumption allows the following generalizations:

- Since a state of relaxation represents being in control, if you are enjoying the relaxation, you may also enjoy the feelings of control.
- You can strengthen the feeling of control by allowing the state of relaxation to deepen.
- You can demonstrate the extent of your control by allowing yourself to relax deeply.
- By being deeply relaxed you are demonstrating the extent of your control.

During an exercise the words "control" and "relaxation" are coupled, emphasizing the link between them. As the exercise progresses they are also interchanged, as if their meaning were identical.

Another important aspect of the exercise is muscular relaxation, which facilitates the altered state of consciousness and helps reduce the intensity of sympathetic responses. Deep relaxation, however, is not a prerequisite for success and an exercise may be satisfactory even if the patient is not very relaxed. The physician can help to promote relaxation at the beginning of the exercise by instructing the patient to relax muscle groups one after the other, as follows:

1. The muscles of the face and neck.
2. The muscles of the shoulders and arms.

3. The muscles of the legs.
4. All the muscles of the body.

As the exercise progresses, the process is facilitated by suggestions like "let go," "release all the tension," "enjoy the feeling of freedom from all physical and emotional tension," as well as "enjoy the feeling of pleasant relaxation." In some techniques, such as in autogenic relaxation, the patient is instructed systematically to contract and relax specific muscle groups. This is done so that the patient can learn to identify a state of muscle relaxation by being able to contrast it with the contracted, tense, state.

As the degree of muscle relaxation achieved during these exercises may be more profound than at other times, the experience may have a considerable impact on anxious or very tense patients. After experiencing the relaxation attained in such an exercise, some patients comment that they have never before been relaxed. With practice, this experience also heightens patients' sensitivity to the development of tension in specific groups of muscles, enabling them to recognize tension (physical and emotional) in themselves more easily than before. Before beginning the program, most subjects first become aware of their problem (i.e., the emotional tension) only through developing a particular symptom such as headache. As the program progresses, their enhanced sensitivity allows them to take immediate remedial action through directed relaxation of the affected muscle groups, say, in the neck or shoulders, with resulting dissipation of the symptom or reduction in intensity of the attack. In this way, the patient is shown the immediate benefit of having a greater degree of control.

Slowing the breathing rate

As discussed in preceding sections and Chapter 14, the rate of breathing and the activity of the sympathetic nervous system are tightly coupled. Under normal circumstances most anxious people tend to breathe rapidly, and slowing the rate of breathing also appears to reduce the intensity of their anxiety. In the early phase of the exercise many therapists encourage the subject to breathe slowly, either by direct instruction or by requesting three or four very deep breaths. In certain practices, such as yoga and mindful meditation, the subject is encouraged to make breathing the primary focus of attention. Although the relaxation exercise recommended here contains little direct reference to breathing, it is certainly relevant and may comfortably be included.

Depth of Relaxation: Is It Important?

The depth of relaxation serves as an indicator of the efficiency of a relaxation exercise. It may seem logical to assume that the more deeply a patient is able to relax during an exercise, the more successful the exercise will be, but this is by no means true.

Whatever the reasons for patients deciding on relaxation therapy, before the program begins they always feel some degree of uncertainty about the experience. Despite the physician's detailed reassurances and explanations about what will or will not be done during the exercise, most patients retain at least some apprehension. To foster positive experience for the patient, who at the end of the exercise should feel that it was easily manageable, unthreatening, and pleasant, it is just as well not to be too successful at inducing relaxation in the initial sessions! The aim should be to proceed gradually so that the patient retains a feeling of reasonable control at all times. For this reason, I always make sure that the first relaxation exercise is performed with the patient sitting in a comfortable but straight-backed chair. Lying down, the patient may relax more deeply than I intend. This deliberate restraint on the part of the physician is of special importance at the start of the program and may considerably increase the patient's willingness to continue with the program. Conversely, improper handling of this issue at the beginning of the program is probably the most effective deterrent to continued cooperation. Once the process is well accepted by the patient, depth of relaxation is not a very important factor in most therapeutic encounters. On occasions I have conducted perfectly satisfactory exercises with the patient sitting in a chair and looking at me. As they acquire self-confidence, however, patients are more inclined to lie back, shut their eyes, and relax deeply.

A BASIC RELAXATION EXERCISE

This section presents a standard relaxation exercise. Successive portions are numbered to permit easy access to the points discussed in the comments.

1. "Make yourself comfortable . . . you can begin the exercise by allowing yourself to concentrate your attention on the feeling of contact between your body and the couch that you are lying on (or the chair you are sitting on) . . . Permit yourself to focus your attention on that feeling of contact . . . or perhaps the feeling of pressure, from the weight of your body pressing on the couch (or chair). When you have done that . . . when you are aware of that feeling of contact or pressure . . ."

Comment: This initial phase is intended to direct the individual attention to a specific focus in order to induce an altered state of consciousness. The focus provided is simple, nonthreatening and neutral for all subjects and is quite sufficient to initiate the exercise. In meditation, focusing one's attention on the breath (or mantra) serves a similar function. The object of attention may be entirely without meaning. In directing a person's attention to a particular focus, an important technical aspect is the rhythm of the therapist's speech and its relationship to the patient's rate of breathing. The rate of speech should be no faster than the patient's rate of breathing (called by some "pacing"). By speaking more slowly, the therapist may also prompt the patient to breath more slowly. Slow, shallow breathing is typical of an altered state.

The breathing pattern will also reflect the patient's emotional state. When specific content is introduced into the relaxation exercise, an increase in the breathing rate will always indicate a rise in tension. Similarly, an unexpected increase in the rate of breathing is likely to mean that the patient has lost concentration. It is usually best to ask what is happening so that if the patient has become anxious for any reason, reassurance can be given and the exercise can continue.

2. "... you can allow yourself to begin releasing all the tension in all the muscles of your body ... you can allow yourself to release the tension in the muscles of your face and of your neck ... to release the tension in the muscles of your shoulders and from your arms ... you may permit yourself to release the tension in the muscles of your legs ... from your whole body ... so that with each comfortable breath, you may allow yourself to feel ... more and more comfortably ... more and more pleasantly, relaxed ..."

Comment: Directed but simple suggestion is aimed at beginning the process of muscular relaxation. It is unnecessary to mention particular muscles or specific muscle groups in greater detail than in the above example.

3. "... remembering all the time that you, and only you, are controlling the experience ... you and only you are allowing it to happen ... you are permitting yourself to unwind ... you are allowing yourself to feel more and more pleasantly, more and more comfortably ... relaxed ..."

Comment: Here suggestion strengthens feelings of control. Slowly enunciated repetition of the main suggestions is an important part of the process.

4. "... then as you do that, as you permit that comfortable feeling of control and pleasant deep relaxation to grow and to deepen ... you may gradually become aware of a pleasant feeling of heaviness in your body ... a feeling of heaviness, that may be greater in the legs than in the arms ... a feeling of heaviness, that could be greater in the arms than in the legs ... of course, it doesn't matter, it really doesn't matter, as you permit yourself to unwind ... as you allow yourself to feel comfortably ... pleasantly ... maybe even heavily ... relaxed ..."

Comment: This additional suggestion of heaviness assists in deepening the relaxation. It may be left out of the first exercise because, as mentioned previously, it is better if the patient is not too deeply relaxed on the first occasion. It may prove useful in subsequent exercises, however, particularly where the intention is to confront painful or feared situations and a deeper state of relaxation is desirable (although not essential). Feelings of heaviness serve the additional purpose of helping to teach patients how to recognize in themselves a state of deep relaxation. Thus, when relaxing on their own, feeling heavy is an indication that they are relaxed. While most subjects feel heaviness in part or the whole of the body, when very deeply relaxed some may experience a sensation of floating or an inability to feel part or the whole of their body.

5. ". . . as you do that, as you allow that comfortable feeling of control and of pleasant relaxation to grow and to deepen . . . you can allow yourself to imagine that you are standing in a tranquil, beautiful park or garden . . . try to picture that . . . try to see yourself there . . . enjoying the tranquillity and the beauty of the place . . . perhaps imagine yourself standing next to a bed of beautiful, brightly colored flowers . . . try to picture that as clearly as you can . . . try to see those flowers at this very minute right in front of you, their shape and their color . . . as you permit yourself to unwind, as you allow yourself to feel comfortably and pleasantly relaxed . . . and then you can imagine yourself walking along a path, enjoying the beauty and the tranquillity of that setting . . . you can see the plants and shrubs, the beautiful beds of brightly colored flowers, perhaps an expanse of green grass . . . and tall, shade-giving trees dotted around . . . you may even find that you can hear the happy sound of birds singing in those trees . . ."

Comment: This part of the exercise employs guided imagery, which is less directed in its structure than the preceding section. Many subjects will find it much easier to relax, particularly in the earlier exercises, at this stage. The object of the detailed description of flowers or trees is to establish an additional focus of attention, which promotes the development of an altered state, and this in turn facilitates the response to the suggestion of relaxation. Notice the indirect suggestion embedded in the text: "the **tranquillity** of that setting . . . the **happy** sounds."

6. ". . . so that everything you see . . . and everything you hear strengthens a growing feeling of optimism and self-confidence in your own ability to control yourself . . . a growing feeling of optimism and self-confidence in permitting yourself to relax . . . remembering all the time that you and only you are controlling the experience . . . you and only you are allowing it to happen . . . you are the only one who can decide where and under what circumstances you wish to activate this very simple technique . . ."

Comment: There is a return to suggestion, reinforcing feelings of control, self-confidence, and optimism.

7. ". . . as you continue relaxing . . . as you permit yourself to relax . . . you can allow yourself to enjoy that comfortable feeling of freedom from tension . . . that comfortable feeling of freedom from all kinds of physical and emotional tension . . . continue relaxing . . . continue permitting yourself to enjoy that pleasant, comfortable feeling of control and of deep . . . comfortable relaxation . . . for as long as you wish to do so . . ."

Comment: References to feelings of control, freedom from tension, and relaxation are juxtaposed and used interchangeably so that they seem to mean the same thing. The suggestion that the subject may maintain this state of control and relaxation "for as long as you wish to do so" also carries the clear message that concluding the exercise does not have to terminate the agreeable state developed during the exercise.

8. ". . . I am going now to conclude the exercise by counting from 5 to 1: 5 . . . 4 . . . 3 . . . 2 . . . 1."

Comment: Although this is an extremely permissive protocol with emphasis on the patient's control throughout, it is important to provide a clear demarcation of the conclusion of the exercise in view of the increased state of suggestibility associated with the deeply relaxed state.

Additional Techniques

The content of the exercise may be influenced by various factors, including of course the patient's personality, attitude, and sensitivities as well as the therapist's own experience and judgment about what is likely to be most effective in a particular situation. The preceding relaxation exercise contains all the basic elements of the content. It may be applied exactly in the form presented, in order to test the patient's response as part of a trial-and-error approach. But it is sometimes clear from the start, or becomes clear during the program, that something more is needed. The techniques described next may be incorporated into the exercise as appropriate, in order to achieve additional therapeutic effects.

Confronting anxiety- or fear-inducing situations

In treating patients suffering from situational anxiety or phobias, there is general agreement that successful management often requires having the patient in some way confront the anxiety-inducing problem (Marks, 1987). Relaxation therapy offers the optimal approach to the problem of symptom-associated anxiety because the relaxed patient may be much more easily encouraged to recreate through imagery the physical and emotional aspects of the experience. This content may be alternated with the suggestion of "feeling comfortably in control and deeply relaxed" as part of the relaxation exercise. On one hand, the patient is being encouraged to recreate an unpleasant and stressful experience while on the other hand receiving the reassuring, albeit contradictory suggestion of control and relaxation. This process corresponds to the technique of reciprocal inhibition developed by Wolpe (1976) for the management of anxiety states. Wolpe observed that

> An anxiety response habit can be weakened by evoking a response incompatible with anxiety in the presence of the anxiety-evoking stimulus. Each time anxiety is inhibited by the evocation of an incompatible response, a measure of conditioned inhibition of the anxiety response habit results, so that eventually the strength of the habit may be reduced to zero.

In this situation, the initial response will be one of increased anxiety, detectable as an increase in breathing rate. However, if reassurance is given at the same time, the exposure (imagined) has the effect of deconditioning the patient to the anxiety-producing situation. It is often convenient to alternate the neutral imagery (garden, beach) of the basic exercise with recall of the threatening experience. This should be done two to three times in each cycle. In most cases, the intensity of reaction will diminish with each repeated cycle. This technique is particularly useful in patients suffering from anticipatory anxiety. Panic disorder patients, for example, may be encouraged to experience any of the distressing symptoms of an attack. Thus, if symptoms (such as palpitations) unexpectedly appear as the patient begins relaxing and the patient becomes restless and agitated, the appropriate response on the part of the therapist is *not* to stop the exercise but to encourage the patient to "allow the symptoms to develop" (see section on paradoxical suggestions below). Asking a patient to imagine the most feared aspect of a panic attack while he or she is in a state of deep relaxation helps in the management of the disorder by reducing the intensity of the anticipatory anxiety.

Symptom anticipation may be difficult to diagnose. In general, the physician should suspect it in any situation where the symptom tends to recur with *consistent associations*, such as under specific weather conditions or with certain foods or environmental conditions not normally thought of as causative. If a patient is convinced that a specific factor always induces an attack, then the mechanism for producing the attack may be symptom anticipation, as described in Chapter 8. Reducing this anxious expectation of the symptom may contribute to its management.

CASE REPORT: UNCONTROLLED RAYNAUD'S PHENOMENON

A 65-year-old woman presented in a highly agitated condition because of repeated attacks of Raynaud's phenomenon over a period of four months, during the winter. Although otherwise well, she was found to have a raised erythrocyte sedimentation rate and a serum antinuclear factor titer of 3+. The patient claimed that the attacks could occur at any time of the day, but closer questioning revealed that she frequently suffered an attack when getting out of bed in the morning. Presumably, the transition from the warm bed to the cooler room air was sufficient to trigger an attack. Adamantly refusing to try medication, the patient showed an interest in the relaxation program. In the course of her six-week treatment, she was taught deep relaxation and was encouraged to practice the basic exercise at home on a regular basis. Part of the exercise was devoted to the guided imagery of getting out of bed in the morning "while feeling comfortably relaxed and in control." No direct reference was made to the distressing attacks of Raynaud's phenomenon that usually occurred at this time. Within three weeks both the intensity and the frequency of attacks had noticeably diminished, and in six weeks attacks were much less frequent. This progressive improvement was sustained until the episodes disappeared completely. The relaxation exercises were performed at longer intervals and were discontinued after about four months. There have been no further attacks through five winter seasons since that time.

Paradoxical suggestions

In some situations, especially where a symptom is extremely persistent, it may be helpful actively to encourage the development of the symptom during the deep relaxation exercise. This approach was developed by Frankl (1960) as part of the psychotherapeutic technique known as "logotherapy." Frankl observed that "fear brings about that which one is afraid of (anticipatory anxiety), and that hyperintention makes impossible what one wishes (paradoxical intention):" In referring to hyperintention, Frankl was referring in particular to problems such as insomnia and impotence. In the clinical context under discussion here, however, where suffering is due to the anxiety associated with a symptom, another mechanism appears to be operative. The apparently inappropriate or paradoxical suggestion effectively puts the patient in the predicament of either suffering the symptom with greater intensity (as suggested by the therapist) or inhibiting its development. This technique is especially valuable in the management of persistent pain syndromes. The usual practice is to emphasize the severity of the symptom by describing it vividly and dwelling on the considerable distress it may be causing. Here is an example:

> I want you to allow the usual discomfort in your lower back to develop in the usual place . . . permitting the pain on this occasion to feel particularly severe . . . much more severe than it may normally be . . . almost as if someone is applying a ball of red-hot steel to the point of maximum tenderness . . . not only touching the skin with this ball of red-hot steel . . . but pressing it with considerable force into the site of maximum tenderness . . . just allow the pain to develop with as much intensity as you can possibly imagine . . .

This may seem like a bizarre way to treat an ailment, but the positive effect at times is quite dramatic. The difficulty for the physician, especially if inexperienced, is to overcome the reluctance to say these things to a suffering patient! As mentioned above, however, in an altered state of consciousness the normal critical faculty is diminished and the reaction of the patient usually differs from that of an unrelaxed observer.

This method is particularly effective when the paradoxical content is embedded in and alternated with the neutral content of the relaxation exercise. Similarly, a patient who suffers from panic disorder and begins to experience palpitations during a relaxation exercise could be encouraged to feel the symptom "in all its intensity" while at the same time feeling "comfortably relaxed and in control." Here too the therapist can exaggerate the intensity of the symptom but encourage the patient to experience all the fears and concerns that it usually provokes.

Undesirable Effects of Deep Relaxation

Relaxation-induced anxiety

Occasionally a patient may suffer an anxiety attack during a relaxation exercise (Heide and Borkovec, 1983). Among 30 chronically anxious patients, 5 (17%) reported increased anxiety during the relaxation exercise (Braith et al., 1988). This is more likely to occur in patients with free-floating or trait anxiety (i.e., anxiety unrelated to specific events or situations or to obvious precipitating stimuli in the environment) who normally spend a considerable amount of energy in dealing with the anxiety on a daily basis. As they begin relaxing, the anxiety breaks through and may make it difficult to continue with the exercise. In most such patients, in my experience, it is possible to continue with the exercise by giving reassurance to encourage them to experience whatever symptoms they may be feeling. Panic disorder patients may also feel typical somatic symptoms as they begin a relaxation exercise. Here too the experience may be exploited to help decondition the patient to the symptoms, as described above.

Unmasking depression

In some patients the presenting symptom may be masking a state of depression. The severity of the symptom demands attention, but as it decreases in intensity with appropriate management, depression becomes increasingly evident clinically and must then be suitably treated. This sequence is illustrated by the following case report.

CASE REPORT: CONCEALED DEPRESSION

The patient, a 38-year-old mother of two, presented with a nine-month history of dyspepsia, nausea and vomiting, and abdominal pain. She was able to eat only very slowly, very small amounts of food, and then tended to vomit after eating. A gastroenterologist could find no physical explanation for the symptoms. A barium meal and abdominal ultrasound were normal. The patient was referred to a psychiatrist who had unsuccessfully treated her for six months with medication including clomipramine and maprotiline, and then she consulted a second psychiatrist over a further three months but without satisfaction. The patient had lost about 8 kg in weight since the start of her illness and reported amenorrhea for two months. Blood tests, including routine blood count, biochemistry, and thyroid function tests were all normal. The husband commented that his wife had eaten very little for about six months and that she slept a lot and had largely neglected her family responsibilities during this period. Although the patient was not herself convinced of the likely emotional causation for her symptoms, she did agree to try a course of relaxation exercises, mainly because of a feeling of desperation. After five meetings twice a week at this stage, she began to admit to feeling anxious and depressed, with periods of weeping, though she enjoyed the relaxation exercises. She was encouraged to return to her normal work routine and to take food as a medicine, that is, not because she was hungry but because the doctor had asked her to. This she did after playing a tape with the relaxation exercise, and within six weeks she had regained about 3 kg in body weight. Reference was made on the tape only to relaxation and reinforcing feelings of control.

At this point a discussion of her feelings about her father's death was initiated. He had died 14 years before and all mention of him was forbidden by the patient's mother, who had also removed pictures of him from the walls, from the moment of this death. The patient admitted never having actually mourned properly for her father, whom she had been very attached to. During the relaxation exercises, the patient was encouraged to remember her interactions with her father. She expressed surprise at the happy memories that returned to her. Dealing with the memories of her father and the sad thoughts of his death became a central subject both in our discussion and in the relaxation exercises over the next few weeks, as the patient reported continuing progress and increasing weight gain. Attention was also given to family problems, especially her attitude toward her mother, who tended to dominate her life, as well as a father-in-law who was very dependent on her and her husband. She mentioned feeling over a few years that she never had time alone for herself or with her husband. It seemed that it had been the buildup of these family pressures, coupled with the patient's inability to confront the frustration and dissatisfaction that they evoked in her, which had initially precipitated this emotional crisis with its attendant somatic expression. However, the unresolved mourning process following her father's death contributed significantly to the development of depression. Intermittent follow-up meetings for 18 months helped to consolidate the progress made as the patient returned to a normal family life and work routine. There has been no tendency to relapse over an 11-year follow-up period.

Exaggerated dependency on the physician

In some dependent personalities there may be a tendency for a therapeutic interaction of the kind being described here to accentuate the patient's dependent tendencies. Both the idea and experience of "being relaxed" by the therapist serve to reinforce the feelings of passivity on the part of the patient. The attitude seems to be "I want you to do it to me . . . you make me better." A fairly obvious expression of this state is the patient's reluctance to do homework such as the practicing of deep relaxation exercises, even with the aid of a tape prepared by the practitioner. In some, this reluctance to act more independently may reflect a serious lack of self-confidence by a person with a poor sense of control. Being aware of the problem helps the practitioner encourage and guide the patient to a greater independence and self-reliance with appropriate support and reassurance.

SUMMARY

The main objective of this chapter is to explain the nature of behavioral intervention by describing in some detail its main elements, using deep relaxation as an example. A number of points emerge from the analysis presented.

- Patients will most easily be persuaded to cooperate with a therapy program when convinced that the intervention being offered is directed specifically at helping to restore their sense of personal control and with that their self-confidence. While this in effect means that a successful therapy program will unquestionably lead to diminution in the intensity of symptoms, and perhaps even to their eradication, it is important to note that aside from exceptional cases, the symptoms themselves are generally not even referred to in the relaxation exercise.
- The text of a typical relaxation exercise should always retain the internal logic given by the suggestions that if you are in control, you can allow yourself to relax, or that if you are relaxed, you must be in control.
- The relaxation exercise utilizes the physiological changes in brain function that result from directing attention in a nonanalytical way on a specific focus, which in itself is invariably totally unimportant. The technique exploits specifically three consequences of this state. The first, increased suggestibility, is selectively used to emphasize the points mentioned above. Second, in this condition of focused attention the ability to relax is facilitated to a considerable degree. Third, reflex autonomic activity, which normally reinforces the emotional texture of a traumatic memory or experience, is substantially reduced. This enables uncoupling of the stressful experience from the reflex autonomic responses and with that a diminution in the intensity of the anxiety associated with the symptom.

Understanding the physiological principles underlying this therapeutic intervention, as well as the relevant cognitive content, is the basis for its successful application to a very wide range of stress problems encountered to clinical practice. Restoring through this intervention even a very modest degree of control in situations of stress or suffering where the feeling of loss of control may be overwhelming usually goes a long way in helping to alleviate the problem.

REFERENCES

Albert ML (1973). A simple test of visual neglect. Neurology 23:658–664.

Allison J (1970). Respiratory changes during transcendental meditation. Lancet 1:833–834.

Baker EL (1987). The state of the art of clinical hypnosis. Int J Clin Exp Hypnosis 35:203–214.

Banyai EI, Hilgard ER (1976). A comparison of active–alert hypnotic induction with traditional relaxation induction. J Abnorm Psychol 85:218–224.

Barber J (1980). Hypnosis and the unhypnotizable. Am J Clin Hypnosis 23:4–9.

Benson H, Greenwood MM, Klemchuk H (1975). The relaxation response: psychophysiologic aspects and clinical application. Int J Psychiatry Med 6:87–98.

Braith JA, McCullough JP, Bush JP (1988). Relaxation-induced anxiety in a subclinical sample of chronically anxious subjects. J Behav Ther Exp Psychiatry 19:193–198.

Critchley HD, Corfield DR, Chandler MP, et al. (2000). Cerebral correlates of autonomic cardiovascular arousal: a functional neuroimaging investigation in humans. J Physiol 523:259–270.

Devinsky O, Morrell MJ, Vogt BA, et al. (1995). Contributions of anterior cingulate cortex to behaviour. Brain 118:279–306.

Dimond SJ, Beaumont JG (1973). Differences in the vigilance performance of the right and left hemispheres. Cortex 9:259–265.

Faglioni P, Scotti G, Spinnler H (1971). The performance of brain-damaged patients in spatial localization of visual and tactile stimuli. Brain 94:443–454.

Farah MJ (1989). The neural basis of mental imagery. Trends Neurosci 12:395–399.

Frankl VE (1960). Paradoxical intention: a logotherapeutic technique. Am J Psychother 14:520–535.

Frumkin LR, Ripley HS, Cox GB (1978). Changes in cerebral hemispheric lateralization with hypnosis. Biol Psychiatry 13:741–750.

Gray CM, Konig P, Engel AK, et al. (1989). Oscillatory responses in cat visual cortex exhibit inter-columnar synchronisation which reflects global stimulus properties. Nature 338:334–337.

Gruzelier J, Brow T, Perry A, et al. (1984). Hypnotic susceptibility: a lateral predisposition and altered cerebral asymmetry under hypnosis. Int J Psychophysiol 2:131–139.

Heide FJ, Borkovec TD (1983). Relaxation-induced anxiety: paradoxical anxiety enhancement due to relaxation training. J Consult Clin Psychol 51:171–182.

Hellige JB (1993). Hemipheric Asymmetry: What's Right and What's Left. Cambridge, MA: Harvard University Press.

Hilgard ER (1965). Hypnotic Susceptibility. New York: Harcourt Brace Jovanovich.

Kabat-Zinn J (1990). Full Catastrophe Living: Using the Wisdom of Your Body and Mind to Face Stress, Pain and Illness. New York: Delacorte Press.

Kosslyn SM (1996). Image and Brain: The Resolution of the Imagery Debate. Cambridge, MA: MIT Press.

Lacy JI (1967). Somatic response patterning and stress: some revisions of activation theory. In: Appley MH, Trumball R, eds. Psychological Stress: Issues in Research. New York: Appleton-Century-Crofts.

Lane RD, Fink GR, Chau PML, et al. (1997). Neural activation during selective attention to subjective emotional responses. NeuroReport 8:3969–3972.

Lazar SW, Bush G, Gollub RL, et al. (2000). Functional brain mapping of the relaxation response and meditation. NeuroReport 11:1581–1585.

Marks IM (1987). Fears, Phobias and Rituals: Panic, Anxiety and Their Disorders. New York: Oxford University Press, pp 457–494.

McGuire PK, Silbersweig DA, Murray RM, et al. (1996). Functional anatomy of inner speech and auditory verbal imagery. Psychol Med 26:29–38.

Moran J, Desimone R (1985). Selective attention gates visual processing in the extrastriate cortex. Science 229:782–784.

Moriguchi A, Otsuka A, Kohara K, et al. (1992). Spectral change in heart rate variability in response to mental arithmetic before and after the beta-receptor blocker, carteolol. Clin Auton Res 2:267–270.

Mountcastle VB (1978). Brain mechanisms for directed attention. J R Soc Med 71:14–28.

Neely JH (1977). Semantic priming and retrieval from lexical memory: roles of inhibitionless spreading activation and limited-capacity attention. J Exp Psychol 106:226–254.

Obrist PA, Webb RA, Sutterer JR, et al. (1970). The cardiac–somatic relationship: some reformulations. Psychophysiology 6:569–587.

Patel C (1984). Yogic therapy. In: Woolfolk RL, Lehrer PM, eds. Principles and Practice of Stress Management. New York: Guilford Press, pp 70–107.

Posner MI, Presti DE (1987). Selective attention and cognitive control. Trends Neurosci 10:13–17.

Pribram KH, McGuiness D (1975). Arousal, activation, and effort in the control of attention. Psychol Rev 82:116–149.

Rainville P, Hofbauer RK, Paus T, et al. (1999). Cerebral mechanisms of hypnotic induction and suggestion. J Cogn Neurosci 11:110–125.

Richmond BJ, Sato T (1987). Enhancement of inferior temporal neurons during visual discrimination. J Neurophysiol 58:1292–1306.

Schultz JH, Luthe W (1959). Autogenic Training: A Psychophysiologistic Approach in Psychotherapy. New York: Grune and Stratton.

Shapiro DH (1982). Overview: clinical and physiological comparison of meditation with other self-control strategies. Am J Psychiatry 139:267–274.

Singer W (1993). Neuronal representations, assemblies and temporal coherence. Prog Brain Res 95:461–474.

Spitzer H, Desimone R, Moran J (1988). Increased attention enhances both behavioral and neuronal performance. Science 240:338–340.

Stephan KM, Fink GR, Passingham RE, et al. (1995). Functional anatomy of the mental representation of upper extremity movements in healthy subjects. J Neurophysiol 73:373–386.

Tiitinen H, Sinkkonen J, Reinikainen K, et al. (1993). Selective attention enhances the auditory 40 Hz transient response in humans. Nature 364:59–60.

Tucker DM, Williamson PA (1984). Asymmetric neural control systems in human self-regulation. Psychol Rev 91:185–215.

Ursin H, Kaada BR (1960). Functional localization within the amygdaloid complex in the cat. Electroencephalogr Clin Neurophysiol 12:1–20.

Wallace RK, Benson H, Wilson AF (1971). A wakeful hypometabolic physiologic state. Am J Physiol 221(3):795–799.

Werner G (1980). Higher functions of the nervous system. In: Mountcastle VB, ed. Medical Physiology, 14th ed, Vol 1. St. Louis: CV Mosby.

Willemsen G, Ring C, McKeever S, et al. (2000). Secretory immunoglogin A and cardiovascular activity during mental arithmetic: effects of task difficulty and task order. Biol Psychiatry 52:127–141.

Wolpe J (1976). Theme and Variations: A Behavior Therapy Casebook. Elmsford, NY: Pergamon, p 17.

Chapter
20

DEFINING MIND–BODY MEDICINE

> The totality that is a human being has been divided for study into parts and systems; one cannot decry the method but one is not obliged to remain satisfied with its results alone. What brings and keeps our several organs and numerous functions in harmony and federation? And what has medicine to say of the facile separation of "mind" from "body"? What makes an individual what the word implies—not divided? The need for more knowledge here is of an excruciating obviousness. But more than mere need there is a fore-shadowing of changes to come . . . Contributions from other fields are to seek from psychology, cultural anthropology, sociology and philosophy as well as from chemistry and physics and internal medicine to resolve the dichotomy of mind and body left us by Descartes.
>
> (Gregg, "The Future of Medicine," 1936)

I have tried to present here, from the perspective of an internist, the essential content of what has come to be known as mind–body medicine.[1] In the early 1980s, in response to what I perceived to be a real need in general medicine, I set out to discover for myself the knowledge that would enable me to understand

---

[1]In some ways an unfortunate designation in that, while meaning to emphasize the unity of mind and body, it may be construed as emphasizing the division.

in physiological and biological terms the processes mediating the most prevalent psychosomatic and somatopsychic phenomena. My intention was to devise an effective approach to the management of patients with psychosomatic disorders, an approach well-suited to the often too busy schedule of the average primary care physician. There seemed to me to be two central questions:

- By what mechanisms is the mind–body unity integrated? To make the relevant processes understandable but also more real for myself, and for my students and colleagues, it seemed important to provide a plausible explanation of how the mind–body link is mediated and, in so doing, to bring the issues into the conceptual framework of medical education—in other words, to describe the processes in terms of biology and physiology. These pages give some pointers to the impressive diversity of these mechanisms and to the clinical syndromes they produce.
- What are the essential components of the successful management of patients with psychosomatic disorders? To successfully manage such patients, are there as many elements to understanding the distressed patient as there are diverse personality types, or are there a few central issues that are common to most patients? In surprising contrast to the multiple mechanisms mediating psychosomatic processes, I was struck by the remarkably limited number of central issues which, if attended to by the doctor, go a long way in helping patients to deal with suffering and situations of crisis. Furthermore, it became increasingly evident that general physicians need to have some familiarity with the powerful therapeutic potential of cognitive-behavioral therapy in the medical context. The role of the doctor as healer should be greatly enhanced by an awareness of these issues, as it seems that many clinical predicaments may be effectively approached with these principles in mind.

One of the most curious aspects of the story presented in this book, however, is not only that it dates back to the first years of the twentieth century, but also that its essential message has been widely overlooked in favor of the onrushing sophistication in the technical aspects of medical science over the same period—much like a sailboat becalmed on an expanse of ocean as a hydrofoil races by on an inexorable course from one horizon to the other. I have been repeatedly impressed in my readings by the surprising contemporary relevance of observations made 50 to 80 years ago about some of the main issues discussed in this book, and this is reflected in the reference lists. Gregg's representation of the mind–body dichotomy in the preceding quotation is more than 60 years old but remains as relevant now as it was when written. In the role of consumer advocate in 1931, Stefan Zweig decried the "objectification and technicalization of therapy in the nineteenth century" that had come to an "extreme excess" in his time, with the interposition of machines between the patient and the doctor (Chapter 1). On the professional side, Kerr, Dalton, and Glebe (1937) commonly encountered patients whose clinical state and suffering derived from "a world undergoing critical social, moral and economic changes." They ruefully observed that patients "are often shunted from one physician to another, and the sins of commission inflicted upon them fill many black pages in our book of achievement" (Chapter 4). *Plus ça change, plus c'est la même chose!*

The disorders discussed in this book have the quality, when persistent, of interfering with daily function and seriously reducing the quality of life. They may even endanger the life of the individual in some cases. While the more intractable cases invariably have a significant psychosocial basis, they may also be the emotional complications of people who have an unremarkable number of worries, an adequately adjusted social existence (i.e., they are in a satisfactory marital or significant-other relationship), and who mostly hold down a stable job.

THE DIAGNOSTIC WEB OF PSYCHOSOMATIC DISORDERS

Multiple States . . .

Psychosomatic problems in clinical practice fall squarely in the arena of general medicine and its subspecialties. It has been said, with some truth, that the existence of specific somatic syndromes is largely an artifact of medical specialization and that there is considerable overlap between patient groups (Wessely et al., 1999). It may, in fact, be stated as a rule that by using any one of the conditions mentioned in this book as an index case, a literature search will invariably show a significant association and overlap with a large group of other psychosomatic conditions. One recent example of many that illustrate this point is the study by Korszun et al. (1998) of 92 patients who fulfilled the criteria for chronic fatigue syndrome, fibromyalgia, or both. Of this group, 42% reported a diagnosis of temperomandibular disorders, 46% had histories of irritable bowel syndrome, 42% of premenstrual syndrome, and 19% of interstitial cystitis. Of the patients with temperomandibular disorders, the great majority had generalized symptoms before the onset of facial pain, yet despite this, 75% had been treated exclusively for temperomandibular disorders, usually with bite splints. Chronic fatigue syndrome has also been documented to overlap with irritable bowel syndrome (Gamborone et al., 1996), sick building syndrome (Chester and Levine, 1997), fibromyalgia (Aaron et al., 2000; White et al., 2000), and temperomandibular disorder (Aaron et al., 2000)—and this does not represent an exhaustive survey.

Among other troublesome syndromes are non–ulcer dyspepsia (gastroenterology), chest pain with normal coronary arteries, mitral valve prolapse (cardiology), chronic Lyme disease (infectious diseases), chronic and recurrent pain syndromes such as chronic pelvic pain (gynecology), tension headaches and migraine (neurology), lower back pain (orthopedic surgery), and atypical facial pain (dentistry, maxillofacial surgery). To this list must be added a spate of very contemporary disorders such as multiple chemical sensitivities syndrome (Ross et al., 1999), sick building syndrome (Ooi and Goh, 1997), candidiasis hypersensitivity, and the Gulf War syndrome (Ford, 1997; Barsky & Borus, 1999; Sillanpaa et al., 1999.)

And Multiple Layers . . .

A widespread difficulty in clinical thinking emanates from the educational doctrine that demonstrable (measurable) changes in organ or tissue structure or function make the likelihood of a psychosomatic disorder more remote, or tends to exclude it. A few examples:

- The altered antibody profile to the Epstein-Barr virus (EBV) in patients with the chronic fatigue syndrome helped sustain, for a number of years, the widespread belief that the clinical state reflected a resurgence of an EBV infection (Chapter 15).
- Symptomatic mitral valve prolapse for many years was seen to be primarily a cardiac disorder. Until recently, the idea that the milder degrees of mitral valve prolapse may be another indication of a physiological state associated with extreme degrees of anxiety or fatigue was never seriously considered (Chapter 13).
- In some reputable textbooks of medicine and medical journals, chest pain with normal coronary arteries is still graced with the name "microangiopathic angina," despite a consistent absence of biochemical evidence of ischemia and an exellent prognosis—for a supposedly ischemic process affecting the myocardium (Chapter 11).
- Two observations in recent years incriminate emotion as a major determinant of prognosis in patients suffering myocardial infarction (Chapter 7). (1) Sympathetic β-receptor blockers are important in secondary prevention, that is, in preventing further significant ischemia and death. (2) Active depression has serious prognostic significance in patients who have suffered a myocardial infarction. But the idea of including the psychological care of these patients in the intensive care or cardiac rehabilitation protocols, much as is done today in most reputable pain clinics for pain syndromes, has yet to catch on.

THE ESSENTIAL ELEMENTS OF MIND–BODY MEDICINE

In writing this book, I strove to place the principles and practice of mind–body medicine squarely in the context of general medical practice. On the one hand, the mechanisms of production of psychosomatic conditions reflect an interplay of brain activity, especially emotion, with familiar biological and physiological processes of the body. On the other, the management of these conditions requires an educated conversation with the patient, which, in order to be effective, is based on understanding the psychosocial and physiological processes involved as well as their likely frame of mind—the specific things worrying them. I reiterate here that for medical practice to be truly effective, the whole person must be evaluated and treated. The following discussion summarizes some of its key elements.

Excluding Organic Diseases

A cardinal requirement of practice in this field is that the appropriate investigations be conducted at the outset to rule out underlying pathology. In the presence of an anxiety state or depressive mood, assuming that the patient's symptoms derive from an emotional state before properly excluding other potential causes is a dangerous mistake. The physician may sometimes feel that investigations will only intensify the patient's anxiety. Especially where symptoms persist, however, all patients should have the benefit of screening investigations that may be considered to reasonably exclude an organic disease process.

Understanding Indirect Communication

The pervasive tendency of patients to express emotional distress as a somatic problem, typical in medical clinics, presents the physician with a formidable clinical challenge. Some patients seem to have a genuine inability to perceive emotion within themselves and tend to focus exclusively on their physical state or symptoms, a condition called alexithymia (Chapter 2). For others, addressing the emotional implications of the symptoms is just too threatening. This usually leads to an aggressive denial of the possibility that the symptom in question might represent psychological distress, an attitude that often convinces the treating physician. This is the classical predicament in many patients with anorexia nervosa. It is also common in the chronic fatigue syndrome, as well as in fibromyalgia and other chronic pain syndromes.

In panic disorder, the almost universal tendency of patients to speak only about their distressing physical symptoms is nearly always triggered by the intense fear component. These patients usually mistakenly assume that the intensity of their fear reaction is a response to, and commensurate with, the sinister implications of the symptom. It is worth emphasizing, however, that an intense fear reaction to virtually any symptom, even chest pain (especially at the onset of the symptom), should arouse the suspicion of panic disorder. In contrast, patients with chest pain due to angina pectoris are almost invariably focused at the onset of their symptoms, on the physical discomfort, not on their fear about the pain's likely implication. In any event, a truly prolonged symptom history in the face of repeated negative investigations should invite a thorough exploration of the patient's psychosocial history.

Risk Factors for Stressed States and Emotional Morbidity

The notion that there are risk factors in the field of emotional health is as valid as in any other field of medicine. A proper awareness of these factors should prove as useful in uncovering functional somatic syndromes as high serum cholesterol, hypertension, and diabetes mellitus are in predicting significant arterial disease or as chronic cigarette smoking is in predicting premature heart or respiratory disease. Substantial epidemiological evidence points to the association of particular life events and social circumstances with an increased frequency of either physical or emotional morbidity. Such events and circumstances include changes in personal or social status, even seemingly desirable ones, fewer years of education, absence of social support, and unemployment, including normal retirement. The stress of chronic illness may also be a risk factor for emotional problems. The circumstances of any patient in relation to these social factors are normally quite easily determined. On the other hand, obtaining an accurate picture of personal relationships and problems within the family—physical or sexual abuse, for example, and exposure to excessive amounts of alcohol and to drugs—may require more time and patience.

The Importance of Control

Regardless of any other factors, a patient's sense of losing control because of symptoms, which arises out of an inability to influence their occurrence or intensity, is a major determinant of stress (Chapter 4). The consequences may vary from a deteriorating clinical state, unresponsive to standard medical treatment, to a noncompliant, uncooperative patient who is nevertheless in real need of the treatment prescribed. There is also a very tight coupling between feelings of control and self-confidence. In practice, the concepts of self-confidence and feelings of control are completely interchangeable in that loss of one means loss of the other. The issue of control is likely to be relevant in any persistently suffering patient. Talking to the patient about the sense of losing control is likely to strike a responsive chord, in that it conveys the feeling that the physician understands the relevant issues.

In the therapeutic encounter, the emphasis is on restoring feelings of control in order to help diminish the intensity and frequency of the symptoms. This is done by utilizing cognitive and behavioral techniques, bearing in mind that acquiring even a small measure of control (where none existed before) may have a substantial therapeutic impact. The elements of control in this context include

- A proper understanding of the true nature of the disorder obtained through a clearly explanation of the disorder.
- Correcting patients' erroneous beliefs about the significance of the symptoms.
- Fostering a much more sensitive awareness of patients' physical responses to different emotional states.

This is usually facilitated by a behavioral therapy program. In addition, once having learned a meditative or relaxation technique, patients will probably then be able to utilize what they have learned and practiced to achieve a state of relaxation as they feel the anxiety or the symptom developing.

The growing popularity of alternative medicine in the West appears to be another expression of the central importance of control for the individual. Beyond the question of efficacy of the treatment chosen, patients are very often in a position of ultimate control in that they are themselves choosing the particular treatment option.

The Multiplicity of Mechanisms

Many mechanisms may mediate psychosomatic processes, as we have seen in preceding chapters (Chapter 8). The mechanisms may be highly directed and specific or very general. With the advent of sophisticated imaging techniques, the extent of central nervous system plasticity has been more clearly defined, both in response to unusual functional demands and in terms of specific pathophysiological processes in organs or tissues. These nervous system changes, both functionally induced and in response to pathological processes in peripheral tissue, help create a *facilitated pathway* between CNS and periphery, leading to the particular expression of the clinical problem.

Anticipatory anxiety (*symptom anticipation*), as in panic disorder, may be an important component of any clinical state characterized by episodic or recurrent symptoms, particularly when the frequency and intensity of symptoms appear to be increasing. The context-related symptom is always worth looking for because it can often be successfully managed by behavioral interventions. The context may be seasonal attacks, cold wind inducing angina pectoris, attacks of Raynaud's phenomenon on getting out of bed in the morning, nausea before committee meetings, or any number of others. The principle is a symptom linked to a defined situation or experience. Examples of nondirected processes include symptoms resulting from hyperventilation or the autonomic lability and mitral valve prolapse that may result from extreme degrees of physical unfitness.

The much quoted "fight-or-flight" reaction of Cannon, which is traditionally presented as the physiological basis of the stress response, is not considered very relevant here. This is not because it is not real, but because the classical fight-or-flight reaction occurs as part of a stress response of such an acute kind that it does not represent a diagnostic challenge, either to the subject or to an observer. It is not difficult to see that the perspiring, trembling individual with dilated pupils, complaining of palpitations, is "stressed," whatever the reason. But most stress responses encountered in clinical practice are much more subtle, and they are frequently mediated by autonomic responses directed toward a specific organ or tissue. This is very different from the fight-or-flight reaction, which depends on an outpouring of epinephrine and norepinephrine. My belief is, furthermore, that the repeated, uncritical representation of the fight or flight reaction as the sole or even the principal physiological mechanism of the stress response has significantly hindered our proper understanding of the subject.

Chronic or recurrent pain syndromes have a special clinical status, especially when they are associated with a degree of suffering that significantly interferes with the patient's quality of life. In these patients, there is always an affective component to the clinical problem and attention to this element is needed in order to alleviate suffering, even without necessarily eliminating the pain. Regardless of the cause for the pain this is generally true. This is the exact situation in which it may be fruitful to regard the pain as a metaphor for an underlying emotional state, most often anger, grief, or guilt. It is important to explore this possibility with the patient. One only has to consider the sometimes remarkable content of dreams to understand that the metaphorical expression of emotion is an inherent, natural activity of the brain and by no means an artificial device created by psychotherapists.

In addition, there is a large group of pain sufferers in whom chronic anxiety plays a central role, and the main mechanism of pain production appears to be a lowered pain threshold. These patients tend to complain mostly of chest or abdominal pain or of muscular tension and pain. The diagnoses they receive include irritable bowel syndrome, esophageal motility disorders, and fibromyalgia.

Considering an Affective Diagnosis

In addition to the clinical conditions referred to above, a number of major psychiatric syndromes that often present first in the medical clinic may prove extremely debilitating or even life-threatening if they are neglected. These include depression, panic disorder, and posttraumatic stress disorder. Patients with chronic fatigue syndrome and some with chronic pain syndromes, in particular, may suffer from extreme lassitude. The latter two conditions are fairly easy to diagnose, but the first three are often missed in the medical clinic, sometimes for long periods. Consequently, only a high index of diagnostic suspicion will help identify these patients in good time.

Beyond the issue of specific diagnoses, however, the practitioner still must regularly confront the central question: In which patients may the clinical deterioration or persistent symptomatology be attributed to emotional factors? I suggest that the extent to which patients are preoccupied with their health problems correlates well with the degree of emotional distress. Such preoccupation has the quality of intrusive thinking and manifests itself when the patient is not specifically distracted by a particular task, such as work-related activity. Thus, asking patients to roughly assess the percentage of their free time occupied by concerns about their health is a good indicator of who may be in need of intervention. When asked in this simple and direct way, patients tend not to realize the implication of the question (namely, that their reply has a direct bearing on their emotional status) and are less likely to be defensive and evasive.

Diagnostic Labels Are Not a Necessity

Patients are often reluctant to acknowledge a psychiatric diagnosis, mainly because of the potential social stigma but also because of the implied emotional instability. In many cases, however, particularly those requiring the cooperation of family members for effective management, a diagnostic label is desirable or unavoidable (depression, panic disorder, PTSD, for example). Often, however, specific diagnosis is virtually irrelevant. In my opinion, it is sometimes wiser to use general terminology, such as "stressed state," and focus on the pressures that lead to the condition, for which an appropriate management program is then proposed. The main discussion then centers on the treatment program rather than the specifics of the diagnosis. Once the program progresses, a more detailed analysis of the evolution of the problem usually becomes less threatening and will probably help patients gain insights that will make it easier to overcome the present crisis and to deal with stress in the future.

The Management of Stressed States and Psychophysiological Disorders

I like to present the management program as an educational package designed to teach individuals how to regain control over their lives. While never promising to eliminate the specific clinical problem that brought the patient to the doctor's office, because this is not a realistic goal, a successful management program usually results in the problem fading into insignificance with time, or at least being transformed into a much more manageable entity. Knowledge, in the context of the frequent uncertainty associated with symptoms and medical conditions, often brings control. Knowledge about the nature of the clinical problem, correction of mistaken beliefs about its significance, increased self-awareness (self-knowledge) through relaxation, meditation, or biofeedback techniques all play an important part in the process. In addition, suggestions about life-style enhancement in terms of regular and appropriate exercise, sufficient holiday time, and healthy eating habits also help strengthen the individual's sense of control because they emphasize the extent to which we are able to influence our own sense of well-being. Physical fitness, for example, contributes significantly to our ability to withstand emotional and physical stress, partly at least by stabilizing autonomic responses.

All the modalities of therapy discussed here may be applied to any of the conditions described in this text. The mix and emphasis may differ, as will the need for using medication and choice of drug, but for the most part these elements of therapy are common to all.

The Patient Is an Active Participant in Planning Therapy

The success of any therapeutic program depends on the patient's willing cooperation. A stress reduction program involving deep relaxation, mindful meditation, or biofeedback training, with or without drug therapy, is usually mentioned in any discussion of therapeutic options. Patients must feel that they are part of the decision-making process, which means that the treatment program will evolve out of a discussion of the various possibilities.

At the same time, if some form of behavioral therapy is chosen, it should be emphasized that although a patient does not have to believe in the process, she or he must nevertheless be genuinely willing to commit to a trial period. I usually commend any skeptical comment by the patient about the likely outcome of the program as evidence of thoughtfulness, which I regard as a favorable sign. I have always found it easier to work with individuals who fully understand what we are doing and why. What motivates such patients to cooperate, besides their sense of helplessness and suffering, is their feeling that the explanation given them sounds relevant to their problem and does offer some possibility of relief. In most cases, my experience has been that as they start to respond their acceptance grows. The patients most unlikely to respond are those who seek consultation because of family or other external pressures. They visit the physician simply to be able to say that they tried but—predictably—the result was another failed therapy.

Mind–Body Medicine Is Cost-Effective Medicine

With burgeoning health costs becoming a major problem worldwide, the mind–body model of medical practice is exceptional in offering an efficacious, low-cost approach to dealing with patients who are major users of health care services. In general, 15%–20% of patients—disproportionately representing the group we are discussing here—utilize more than 80% of medical resources. It would seem to make good economic sense to invest a little more time and effort in dealing with these patients to improve not only their suffering but also the burden they impose on the health care system. Following an initial consultation and assessment, a follow-up visit may comfortably be handled in about 30–40 minutes, including a patient report and physician's reaction, an exercise of deep relaxation (with or without specific content relevant to the patient's particular problem), which takes between 15 and 20 minutes, and then a few more minutes of conversation to examine issues that came up during the exercise. Utilizing the information laid out here, with a knowledge of the patient's predicament, the doctor's questioning can be highly focused.

While providing treatment for symptomatic and suffering patients, the physician also teaches stressed but basically healthy individuals how to deal with that stress in order to remain healthy. In its most comprehensive form, mind–body medicine works to restore the individual to a level of emotional and physical functioning that represents the best chance of a healthy and creative life. It is a paradox of human nature that we seek such guidance only when we are challenged by ill-health or subnormal function. It seems that we have to lose something important before we acquire the motivation to make the effort to value, regain, and safeguard it. But perhaps the sharpest irony is that humanistic medical practice may ultimately take hold more for economic reasons than because of the intrinsic humanity of the medical profession.

THE ESSENTIAL ROLE OF MIND–BODY MEDICINE

Generally, the greatest difficulty physicians face is dealing with the psychiatric aspects of medical practice. This is a paradox because today the majority of practitioners would probably concede the central importance of the patient's emotional state and mental attitude in dealing with stress of any kind, and particularly the stress of illness.

The unease and dissociation that characterize the attitude of many physicians considering a psychiatric diagnosis often give patients a clear signal that the problem belongs elsewhere. Those physicians who are willing to involve themselves actively in treating patients for anxiety and depression will almost invariably use medication, but they mostly feel unqualified or unmotivated to explore through conversation the likely basis for the patient's emotional state or, for that matter, to suggest with conviction alternative approaches, such as psychotherapy, that may help provide a much more satisfactory long-term solution of the problem.

More problematic still is the attitude of physicians toward somatization and chronic pain syndromes. Consider the fact that up to 30% of first catheterizations in patients complaining of chest pain show normal coronary arteries. Of these patients, at least half have diagnosable panic disorder. Yet, for the most part, these patients remain undiagnosed and untreated for extensive periods, even a few years, with the attendant suffering and poor function despite the availability of effective therapy. The inadequate management of such patients has the quality of a serious and very substantial mental block on the part of the treating physician. The attitude, particularly common in specialist practice, is typified as "doing what I have been well trained to do"—and when all the tests are negative, passing the patient on to the next specialist.

In contrast, consider the ease with which medical practitioners approach medical problems of other kinds. With few exceptions, they are comfortable in their assessment and management of an extensive gamut of common clinical problems, whether they touch the heart, lungs, gut, skin, endocrine system. The accepted norm is to treat that which one feels competent treating, and if a problem presents unusual features or seems too complicated, to turn to the specialist for advice or to transfer the patient to the specialist's care. The ease of interaction and fluid bidirectional professional communication in so many areas of medical practice contrast starkly with the stilted, uneasy, inhibited relationship that characterizes the interaction of psychiatry with the rest of the medical profession. Rather than explore the historical reasons for this development, I simply suggest that the mind–body medicine model offers an excellent answer to the problem.

Any practitioner of medicine who has grasped the limited number of important principles described in these pages and who learns to apply them will be much better equipped to deal with most of the psychosomatic problems encountered in medical practice. As with every area of medicine, hands-on involvement promotes familiarity and increased sensitivity in both diagnosis and therapy. The mind–body field provides the generalist with the basic tools for dealing with the common emotional problems in medical practice. The increased confidence that this familiarity brings allows doctors to develop a more professional and self-confident attitude to this field. These tools will suffice for the management of certain patients, and for others, as with the other specialties, patients will have to be referred for formal psychiatric or psychological evaluation and management. And, as in other specialties, there may be patients whose management is shared by collaborative interaction between the primary care physician and the psychotherapist. Perhaps the greatest challenge is the awareness that familiarity with mind–body medicine helps impart a practical approach to virtually any patient encountered, even those who might be regarded as suffering from the most intractable or hopeless of problems. Mind–body medicine promises to help normalize the attitudes of physicians and medical students toward the psychological aspects of medical practice. Its substance helps make everyday medical practice truly humanistic.

REFERENCES

Aaron LA, Burke MM, Buchwald D (2000). Overlapping conditions among patients with chronic fatigue syndrome, fibromyalgia, and temperomandibular disorder. Arch Intern Med 160:221–227.

Barsky AJ, Borus JF (1999). Functional somatic syndromes. Ann Intern Med 130:910–921.

Chester AC, Levine PH (1997). The natural history of concurrent sick building syndrome and chronic fatigue syndrome. J Psychiatr Res 31:51–57.

Ford CV (1997). Somatization and fashionable diagnoses: illness as a way of life. Scand J Work Environ Health 23 (suppl 3):7–16.

Gambarone JE, Gorard DA, Dewsnap PA, et al. (1996). Prevalence of irritable bowel syndrome in chronic fatigue. J R Coll Physicians Lond 30:512–513.

Gregg A. (1936, October). The future of medicine. Harvard Medical Alumni Bulletin.

Kerr WJ, Dalton JW, Gliebe PA (1937). Some physical phenomena associated with the anxiety states and their relation to hyperventilation. Ann Intern Med 11:961–992.

Korszun A, Papadopoulos E, Demitrack M, et al. (1998). The relationship between temperomandibular disorders and stress-associated syndromes. Oral Surg Oral Med Oral Pathol Oral Radiol Endod 86:416–420.

Ooi PL, Goh KT (1997). Sick building syndrome: an emerging stress-related disorder? Int J Epidemiol 26:1243–1249.

Ross PM, Whysner J, Covello VT, et al. (1999). Olfaction and symptoms of multiple chemical sensitivities syndrome. Prevent Med 28:467–480.

Sillanpaa MC, Agar LM, Axelrod BN (1999). Minnesota Multiphasic Personality Inventory-2 validity patterns: an elucidation of Gulf War syndrome. Mil Med 164:261–263.

Wessely S, Nimnuan C, Sharpe M (1999). Functional somatic syndromes: one or many? Lancet 354:936–939.

White KP, Speechley M, Harth M, et al. (2000). Co-existence of chronic fatigue syndrome with fibromyalgia syndrome in the general population: a controlled study. Scand J Rheumatol 29:44–51.

INDEX

Abortion, accidental 28, 38
Adherence to treatment. *See* Compliance in
    drug taking
Affect, imprinting of. *See* Kindling
Agoraphobia, 209, 212, 233
Alexithymia, 9–10, 391
Allostatic load, 48, 60–61. *See also* Stress
Altered state of consciousness. *See also*
    Hypnosis; Meditation; Relaxation
    therapy; Selective attention
  autogenic training, 362
  control in therapy, feeling of 371–72, 372*f*
  critical faculty, suspension of, 367–68
  definition of, 363
  doctor–patient dynamic in, 371–72, 372*f*
  fear of, 363
  guided imagery, 362
  memories, recollection of, 366
  muscular relaxation and, 369–70
  neurophysiology of, 364–69
  recollection of memories and, 366–67
  suggestibility and, 368
  terminology in therapy, 371
Alternative healing practice, 3–4, 393
Amaurosis fugax, 237
Amygdala. *See also* Limbic system
  emotionally charged memories and, 119
  fear response and, 119, 219–20
  kindling of, 121
  paralimbic area, 120
  respiratory response and, 369
  rostral limbic system and, 366
Analgesia
  endogenous mechanisms of, 140
  narcotic, 140
  patient–controlled, 34
  placebo mediated, 140
  rebound headaches and, 167–68
Anorexia nervosa, 23, 307, 391
Anterior cingulate cortex. *See* Selective
    attention
Anticipation. *See also* Symptom anticipation;
    Conditioning
  anticipatory activation of the nervous
    system, 119–20
  anticipatory anxiety, in angina pectoris,
    117, 118

  in asthma, 118, 119
  in vasomotor rhinitis,118
  context–related symptoms, and, 393
  of death, 121–22
  headache fear and, 117
  Mantoux response and, 135. *See also*
    Hypnosis
  operant conditioning, in 114, 119
  placebo effect, and 129
  of recovery with medication, 133–134
  of unemployment, health effects, 55
Antidepression medication. *See also*
    Depression; Drug treatment
  mechanisms of action, 311–12
  plateau effect of efficacy, 340
Anxiety. *See also* Chest pain; Cognitive
    behavioral therapy; Control, feeling
    of; Drug treatment; Education;
    Hyperventilation
  anticipatory, 116, 136, 218–19. *See also*
    Symptom anticipation
  asthma and, 259–60
  autonomic lability, 233–34
  cardiovascular effects, 230–32
  cognitive aspects of, 352, 353–54
  confronting, in therapy 379–80
  corticotrophin–releasing factor and, 220
  effort intolerance and, 230
  free–floating, 359
  hypoglycemia simulating, 93
  iatrogenic, 25–27
  lactate production and, 232
  meditation and, 345
  metabolic effects, 232–33
  palpitations, 214
  physical activity, 230–234
  placebo response and, 132–33. *See also*
    Placebo response, nonspecific factors
  somatic representation of, 115, 189
  respiratory rate and, 369
Arousal. *See also* Hyperventilation;
    Respiration; Sympathetic activation
  attention and, 369
  catecholamine induced, 258
  drug induced, 333, 334, 340
  emotional and blood pressure response,
    113